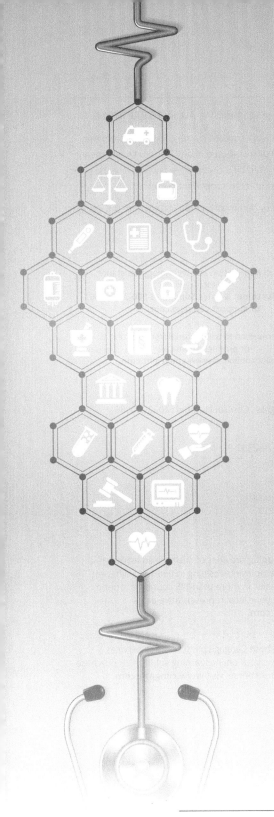

Applied
Law &
Ethics

in Health Care

Wendy Mia Pardew, ESQ.

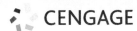

CENGAGE

Australia • Brazil • Canada • Mexico • Singapore • United Kingdom • United States

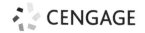

CENGAGE

Applied Law & Ethics in Health Care,
First Edition
Wendy Mia Pardew, Esq.

SVP, Higher Education Product Management:
Erin Joyner

VP, Product Management, Learning
Experiences: Thais L. Alencar

Product Director: Jason Fremder

Senior Product Manager: Stephen Smith

Product Assistant: Dallas Dudley

Learning Designer: Kaitlin Schlicht

Senior Content Manager: Sharon Chambliss

Digital Delivery Quality Partner:
Lisa Christopher

Director, Product Marketing: Neena Bali

Product Marketing Manager:
JoAnn Gillingham

Senior IP Analyst: Ashley Maynard

IP Project Manager: Nick Barrows

Production Service: MPS Limited

Designer: Felicia Bennett

Cover Image Source: Birth Brand/
Shutterstock.com

Interior image Source: Francois Poirier/
Shutterstock.com; Alexander Lysenko/
Shutterstock.com

For product information and technology assistance,
contact us at
**Cengage Customer & Sales Support, 1-800-354-9706
or support.cengage.com.**

For permission to use material from this text
or product, submit all
requests online at **www.copyright.com.**

Library of Congress Control Number: 2022900886

ISBN: 978-0-357-62387-9

Cengage
200 Pier 4 Boulevard
Boston, MA 02210
USA

Cengage is a leading provider of customized learning
solutions with employees residing in nearly 40 different
countries and sales in more than 125 countries around
the world. Find your local representative at
www.cengage.com.

To learn more about Cengage platforms and services,
register or access your online learning solution, or purchase
materials for your course, visit **www.cengage.com.**

Printed at CLDPC, USA, 03-22

Dedication

I dedicate the first edition of *Applied Law & Ethics in Health Care* to you, the health care students who have braved all that comes with chasing your dreams, working late into the night, and making sacrifices so you can serve others. I thank you today for becoming tomorrow's guardians of quality health care.

I also dedicate this book to my three sisters, Debbie Esola, Jill Peace, and Erica Pardew, each of whom provided inspiration, encouragement, humor, and perspectives that made writing this textbook so gratifying.

"Go into the world and do well.
But more importantly, go into the world and do good."
— Minor Myers, Jr.

Wendy Mia Pardew
St. Petersburg, Florida
September 2021

Contents

7 The Health Record   169

8 Introduction to Ethics   193

9 Laws and Ethics of Patient Confidentiality   211

Preface

All health care professionals have a critical need to understand law and ethics as applicable to the health care industry. Maintaining a safe, legal, and ethical health care environment is a shared responsibility of all members of the health care team. To that end, this text is written for a variety of health care professionals, rather than one specific profession. This text can be used in a multidisciplinary health care law and ethics course or by law and ethics courses specific to a health care profession.

The text focuses on legal and ethical topics that apply throughout the health care industry, including the concepts of standard of care, scope of practice, criminal and civil acts, contracts, negligence, health care ethics, and more. This text reflects new health care regulations and technology, and it will prepare future health care professionals for the changing health care environment. The spectrum and depth of topics contained in this text makes it valuable as a resource that would be wise to keep handy long after graduation.

The issues discussed in this text occur in the real world. As a result, actual legal decisions and real-life anecdotes illustrate concepts and enhance understanding. The underlying concept coupled with the cases and anecdotes ensure readers can understand, digest, and apply the material, while also sparking interest and engagement.

Patients' health care needs will continue to expand. And, just as methods of treatment will change, methods of health care delivery and compensation will also change. The law strives to keep pace with the new issues raised due to new maladies, treatments, technology, and regulations. This text serves as an invaluable resource for health care professionals working in the center of this exciting and often challenging time of change.

Organization of the Text

This text is designed to cover the most common legal and ethical issues health care professionals will encounter. Chapters start by exploring the business of health care and the legal system in general (Chapters 1–4) and then move through legal topics students need to know, such as standard of care, employment laws, criminal and tortious acts, contractual issues, negligence, medical malpractice, and more (Chapters 5–7). The conversation then turns to ethics, presenting the basics of health care ethics, and moving on to discussions of the allocation of scarce resources, medical research, reproductive issues, and end-of-life issues (Chapters 8–12). Each chapter is designed in a similar fashion: first providing student focus through Objectives and Key Terms; then presenting concepts coupled with relevant legal cases and news stories; and ending with a summary and activities for students to apply what they have learned.

Features

The key features in this text are designed to support learning and show real-world context of chapter concepts. The following is a brief description of each feature:

- **Quotes:** Relevant and thought-provoking quotes appear at the start of each chapter and throughout the text.
- **Objectives:** Each chapter begins with a list of objectives to focus attention on what students need to learn.
- **Key Terms:** A list of key terms appears at the start of each chapter, and each key term is presented in boldface and defined in the margin of the text where the term first appears in the chapter.
- **News Stories:** Timely examples of legal and ethical health care dilemmas in the news illustrate chapter concepts and promote engaging discussions.
- **Legal Case Studies:** Summaries of actual legal cases highlight the legal issues and actions most prevalent in health care today.
- **Summary:** A bulleted list of key concepts serves as an at-a-glance study tool.
- **Suggested Activities:** Students can complete a list of additional activities to further engage with the chapter material through research, role play, field trips, and other exercises.
- **Study Questions:** These questions quiz students on their ability to understand and apply key chapter concepts.
- **Case for Discussion:** Real and fictional court cases allow students to practice applying what they have learned.

What's New

Applied Law & Ethics in Health Care, first edition, is an evolution of *Law, Liability, and Ethics for the Medical Office Professionals*, sixth edition, and it is intended for a for a variety of health care professionals.

This edition seeks to make health care law and ethics accessible, interesting, and relevant for students in a range of health care disciplines.

As such, chapters have been reorganized to build on content from preceding chapters to deliver a clearer, deeper picture of legal realities in modern health care, and updated content has been added. New content reflects recent legislation, including the Affordable Care Act (ACA), telemedicine, and euthanasia, among other critical topics. In addition, new legal cases and news stories have been added throughout the text to address some of the most recent dilemmas in medical offices and hospitals throughout the United States. Many key term definitions have been revised for greater clarity. To assist with comprehension, summaries at the end of each chapter are tied to the objectives at the start of each chapter to help students further understand core chapter content at-a-glance. Ethics content has also been expanded in Chapter 8 to provide students with more instruction on ethical decision making and ethical theories.

A chapter-by-chapter summary of major content updates is included below:

Chapter 1—The Big Business of Health Care and You

- New content on certification; scope of practice; vicarious liability; health care delivery systems; surprise billing; HSAs; and technology and medicine, including impact of COVID-19 upon telemedicine and health information on personal electronic devices

Chapter 2—Laws and Regulations You Will Encounter

- Additional content on licensing; scope of practice; medical license revocation or suspension; mandatory reporting; chain of custody, workplace sexual harassment; the Americans with Disabilities Act; Medicare and Medicaid; and unions and health care workers
- Expanded "Controlled Substances Acts" section, including information on the Controlled Substances Schedules, Drug Enforcement Agency, and United States Pharmacopeia (USP)

Chapter 3—From the Constitution to the Courtroom

- Additional content on common law and the phases of a lawsuit

Chapter 4—Criminal Acts and Intentional Torts

- Additional content on classifications of murder; fraud, including false billings, and delegation of duties; and defamation of character
- New content on federal and state anti-kickback statutes, including the Stark law
- Expanded and revised "Abuse" section, including content on child abuse, elder abuse, domestic violence, and sexual assault

- Additional content on reporting illegal activities in the health care setting following proper protocol and completing an incident report related to patient care

Chapter 5—What Makes a Contract

- Additional content about collections, bankruptcy, and termination of delinquent patients

Chapter 6—Medical Malpractice and Other Lawsuits

- New content on expert witnesses and health care providers' duty to their patients
- Additional content on statute of limitations; causation; informed consent; the impact of medical malpractice suits; and defensive medicine

Chapter 7—The Health Record

- Additional content on electronic health records
- New content on HITECH; goals and benefits of data interoperability; source of privacy rights and the Tarasoff case; patient and family access to health records; release of patient information; and chain of custody

Chapter 8—Introduction to Ethics

- New content on definition of ethics; morals; development of values; and professional etiquette
- New section entitled "Ethical Theories", including information about deontology, teleology, utilitarianism, and virtue-based ethics
- New section entitled "Ethical Decision Making", explaining common steps in ethical decision making
- New section entitled "Personal Ethics in the Workplace", differentiating personal and professional ethics

Chapter 9—Laws and Ethics of Patient Confidentiality

- Additional content differentiating patient confidentiality, privacy, and privileged communication
- New content on HIPAA, including the Privacy Rule, the Security Rule, HIPAA compliance, the Enforcement Rule, the Breach Notification Rule, violations and penalties, and filing a HIPAA complaint
- New sections entitled "HIPAA-Authorized PHI Uses and Disclosures" and "Patient-Authorized PHI Uses and Disclosures"

Chapter 10—Professional Ethics and the Living

- New content on the allocation of scare resources; the ethics of transplants; and medical tourism

- Additional content on clinical trials and autonomy versus paternalism in health care

Chapter 11—Reproductive Issues and Early Life

- Updated content on artificial insemination and assisted reproductive technology; genetic testing before birth; embryonic stem cells for research; cloning and gene editing; and medicolegal rights of the fetus and the newborn

Chapter 12—Death and Dying

- Updated content on attitudes toward death; dying and the Uniform Determination of Death Act (UDDA); and the right to die

Instructor Resources

Additional instructor resources for this product are available online. Instructor assets include an Instructor's Manual, Solution and Answer Guide, MindTap Educator's Guide, Transition Guide, PowerPoint® slides, and a test bank powered by Cognero. Sign up or sign in at www.cengage.com to search for and access this product and its online resources.

MindTap

MindTap is a fully online, interactive learning experience built upon authoritative Cengage content. By combining readings, multimedia activities, and assessments into a singular learning path, MindTap elevates learning by providing real-world application to better engage students. Instructors customize the learning path by selecting Cengage resources and adding their own content via apps that integrate into the MindTap framework seamlessly with many learning management systems.

    The MindTap includes:

- Polling Activities: Polling questions that engage students in critically thinking about chapter topics
- Concept Checks: Short, low-stakes quizzing designed to assess students' reading comprehension and progression toward mastery of learning objectives
- Case Studies: Scenarios with auto-graded questions
- Writing Assignments: Prompts for students to complete additional research on chapter topics
- Quizzes: Additional multiple-choice questions testing students on learning objective mastery

    To learn more, visit www.cengage.com/training/mindtap.

Acknowledgments

Writing the first edition of *Applied Law & Ethics in Health Care* was a team effort, and I was lucky enough to work with the A-team. Several people deserve acknowledgment, praise, and my most sincere thanks: Stephen Smith, for inviting me to take on another rewarding project and for his boundless professionalism and support; Sharon Chambliss, Senior Content Manager, for expertly and enthusiastically guiding me through the copyediting and other final stages of the textbook's production; and, my family and friends for their support and for enduring the many times I had to say, "I can't, I am writing."

Also, I would like to highlight my thanks to Cengage's Learning Designer Kaitlin Schlicht and her exceptional collaboration. This is the second textbook I have worked on with her. Kaitlin has once again patiently, precisely, and perfectly guided me through the substantive writing process. At every stage and with every draft chapter submission, Kaitlin was focused, meticulous, challenging, and engaged in her feedback. Thank you, Kaitlin.

I am indebted to the first edition reviewers listed below whose experience and willingness to contribute helped make this edition one we can all be proud of.

Wendy Mia Pardew

REVIEWERS

Dawood Guirguis, MD
Dean of Academics and Director of Health Sciences
Eastwick College, Hackensack Campus
Hackensack, NJ

Jason Knight
Assistant Professor
Winona State University
Winona, MN

Mindi Short, CCMA, CPT, CPC, CPB, CPPM, CASCC
Medical Assisting Program Director/Instructor
Dixie Technical College
St. George, UT

Kristin Spencer, PhD, MBA, CMA(AAMA), RMA(AMT), AHI(AMT)
Medical Assistant Program Director/Professor
Jackson College
Jackson, MI

Gladdi Tomlinson, RN, MSN
Professor of Nursing
Harrisburg Area Community College
Harrisburg, PA

Chapter 1

The Big Business of Health Care and You

 Wherever the art of medicine is loved, there is also a love of humanity.

Hippocrates

Objectives

After reading this chapter, you should be able to:

1. Recognize the importance of your role on the front lines of the health care industry.
2. Differentiate among registration, certification, and licensure for health care professionals.
3. Identify proper protocol when a health care professional is asked to perform a task outside of the scope of practice.
4. Summarize what is meant by personal protection and provider protection.
5. Compare standard of care for medical assistants and for different health care professionals.
6. Summarize laws and standards that protect patients.
7. Identify the different types of legal entities.
8. List the main types of managed care organizations.
9. Explain the risks and rewards of telemedicine.

Building Your Legal Vocabulary

Agent
Bylaws
Capitation
Certification
Conglomerate
Directors

Dividends
Fee-for-service
Investment
Joint venture
Legal entity
Licensure

Negligence

Negotiated fee schedules

Notice

Officers

Per capita payment

Reasonable person

Registration

Respondeat superior

Scope of practice

Shares

Standard of care

Stockholders

Utilization review

Vicariously liable

Introduction to the Business of Health Care

Technological advances, mergers of insurance and health care companies, pharmaceutical companies increasingly driven by profit, continued medical malpractice lawsuits, and changes to health care delivery and compensation systems, among others, have all contributed to the health care industry becoming big business. Nationally, the annual health care expenditure grew from $3.0 trillion in 2015 to $3.8 trillion in 2019. From 2019 to 2028, the United States expects to see annual health spending grow at an average rate of 5.4 percent, which would amount to $6.2 trillion by 2028. Centers for Medicaid & Medicare Services. (16 December 2020). Historical. Retrieved from www.cms.gov /Research-Statistics-Data-and-Systems/Statistics-Trends-and-Reports /NationalHealthExpendData/NationalHealthAccountsHistorical.

The business of health care continues to grow increasingly complex. As a health care professional, you will be on the front line of this multi-trillion-dollar industry and how you perform on the front line matters. You will be entrusted with tasks and information that, in the most extreme situation, could mean the difference between life and death. In addition to being familiar with information that will allow you to perform your duties competently and professionally, frontline health care professionals also need to be familiar with the liability and risks that can result in a lawsuit or other undesirable consequences.

The health care industry has many competing interests as providers, nurses, medical office professionals, hospital employees, and others employed in the health care field work to achieve their objectives. Those objectives are most often related to balancing maximum personal financial gain through the health care services provided while delivering quality health care and complying with laws, regulations, and health insurance company protocols. The health insurance companies seek to reduce costs and maximize profits. Employers want to reduce the cost of the health insurance they provide to their employees. The government wants to protect its citizens and manage health care costs. And, patients want the best possible care at the lowest possible price. These competing interests form the framework of the big business of the health care industry.

The industry relies upon competition and regulation to control health care costs. Competition in business has led employers, governments, and health insurance companies to seek control of escalating costs through regulation. Health insurance companies, eager to gain market share, develop new products intended to help manage ever-increasing health care costs. This competitive approach has given rise to managed care organizations (MCOs), which are health care delivery and compensation systems that are different than the traditional pay-for-fee service.

The health care business' framework also includes the legal entities health care businesses use and how health care is delivered and compensated. A solid and well-rounded understanding of these aspects of the health care business will ensure you are the best professional possible while on the front lines.

The Front Line Is You

A patient's first interaction when undergoing care is usually with a frontline health care professional, and this may very well be you. It is the frontline health care professionals who communicate most frequently with patients. What you know and how you conduct yourself can influence patients' experiences and outcomes. The health care industry is a complex maze of laws, regulations, protocols, and interactions that you will want to understand.

To be the best professional you can be, a well-rounded understanding of the health care industry is essential. For your patients, "the best professional" means providing the most professional, efficient, and effective service for them that you can. For your employer, it means representing yourself and your employer in a professional manner, as well as ensuring you do all that you can to prevent complaints, lawsuits, regulatory violations, mistakes, and any other act that creates risk for you, your patient, or your employer.

The Importance of Legal Knowledge

Medical malpractice, licensing and regulations, employment law, federal health care laws, and corporate mergers are just some of the legal issues that arise in the health care industry today. When you understand the nature and scope of these issues, how they arise, and how they affect a business, you can recognize situations that may lead to an unwanted legal action and know what to do when you see such situations brewing.

Today, health care professionals participate in many aspects of the delivery of health care. They are held to a higher **standard of care** than laypersons who do not have your special knowledge and training. Some health care professionals, such as physicians and nurses, are held to the standard of care established by **licensure** and **registration** boards at the national or state level. Professionals who have earned a

standard of care The amount of care that a reasonable person in similar circumstances would exercise.

licensure Completion of basic minimum qualifications required by the state for that profession.

registration Recordation and maintenance of professionals' license-related administrative information.

Table 1-1 Licensure, Registration, and Certification

	Licensure	**Registration**	**Certification**
Definition	completion of basic minimum qualifications required by the state for that profession	recordation and maintenance of professionals' license-related administrative information	endorsement by an accredited professional organization that the holder has specific expertise as evidenced by passing an examination
Objective	indicates the license holder has met the requirements needed to work in a specific profession	verifies and records administrative information about licensed professionals	identifies certain areas of specialty or expertise earned by the licensed professional

certification Endorsement by an accredited professional organization that the holder has specific expertise as evidenced by passing an examination.

scope of practice The tasks and services that a qualified health care professional is considered competent and allowed to perform pursuant to their license, or, if no license, their education, and experience.

certification often have a higher level of skill in a specialized area, and have proven their expertise through testing or other processes. Table 1-1 shows the differences between licensure, registration, and certification.

Part of being a health care professional includes fully understanding what **scope of practice** means with regard to what you do. Many categories of health care professionals are not licensed to practice medicine and must carry out their responsibilities without making medical decisions or acting outside of their area of expertise. If you are ever unsure if a task requested of you is within your scope of practice, ask your employer and ensure you get an answer that you fully understand. This is true even if it is a little uncomfortable to do so. You should be provided with the training, support, and supervision to do your job. You should also have the opportunity to voice concerns about what you are asked to do if you are unsure whether it is within your scope of practice.

Personal and Provider Protection

By understanding basic principles of the law as they pertain to health care, you can better protect yourself from litigation, damage to your professional reputation, and loss of personal assets. You will also be in a better position to protect your employer's interests.

Florida's Medicaid Fraud Control Unit and the Miami-Dade Police Department arrested dental hygienist Julio Suarez, who was accused of Medicaid fraud by delivering care outside his scope of practice. Suarez is alleged to have performed procedures on patients that should have been performed by a licensed dentist and then billing Medicaid for the services. In total, Suarez fraudulently caused the Medicaid program to pay more than $8,000. Suarez was charged with one count of Medicaid fraud, a second-degree felony, and one count of grand theft, a third-degree felony. Should he be convicted, Suarez faces up to 15 years in prison and $10,000 in fines.

"It is utterly despicable that a health care professional would knowingly deceive trusting patients about their licenses and credentials in order to practice unlawful dental procedures," said Florida's Attorney General Ashley Moody. "To further use that deception to scam the Medicaid program out of thousands of taxpayer dollars is inexcusable and criminal."

ADANews. (2021, March 24). Inspector General Reports Two Medicaid Fraud-Related Enforcement Actions. *ADANews*. Retrieved from www.ada.org/publications/ada-news/2021/march/inspector-general -reports-two-enforcement-actions-in-march-related-to-medicaid-fraud.

Providers and corporate employers are liable for their own conduct, as well as being **vicariously liable** for their employees' conduct while the employees are working within the scope of their employment. In the employment setting, this theory of liability is known as **respondeat superior**, which is Latin for "let the master answer." It is sometimes difficult to determine whether an employee is acting within the scope of employment. The test is whether the employee's conduct served the interest of the employer or furthered the employer's business.

Across the health care industry, there are a myriad of relationships that can give rise to a vicarious liability claim. For example, dentists have the right to control the professional activities of dental hygienists working for them and the duty to supervise them. As a result, dentists are vicariously liable for the wrongful acts of dental hygienists that work for them. In this hypothetical case, a dental hygienist loses grip of a pointed instrument, which then lands on the patient's eye. The dropped instrument caused permanent visual damage to the patient. The patient could sue the dentist based upon vicarious liability under the doctrine of respondeat superior for the **negligence** of the hygienist.

vicariously liable Legally obligated for the acts of others who are acting as their agent.

respondeat superior Legal theory that holds employer responsible for the behavior of an employee working within the scope of employment.

negligence Failure to act with reasonable and prudent care given the circumstances.

A patient sustained an injury during an Xray of his shoulder at a New Jersey medical center. The plaintiff alleged that the medical center's radiology technician had plaintiff hold weights during the Xray, which was contrary to the directions provided by the plaintiff's physician. Plaintiff's complaint did not name the technician, and, therefore, the lawsuit was focused only on the medical center's vicarious liability.

To assert a medical malpractice claim in New Jersey under the theory of vicarious liability (respondeat superior) against a health care entity and based

(Continues)

(Continued)

on the negligence of a "licensed professional," the applicable statute requires a sworn statement from an expert with the same type of professional license as the alleged negligent employee.

On appeal, the court ultimately focused on whether the plaintiff met the statute's applicable criteria, which included the submission of a sworn statement from an expert. The appellate court reversed the trial's court's decision and found that no sworn statement was required because the only theory of liability sought was vicarious liability for the technician's wrongful acts, and a radiology technician is not a "licensed professional" for purposes of the statute.

JDSupra. (2021, March 22). Affidavit of Merit May No Longer Be Required for Claims of Vicarious Liability in New Jersey. JDSupra. Retrieved from www.jdsupra.com/legalnews/affidavit-of-merit-may-no-longer-be-7077502/.

As a health care professional, you will want to be aware of your specific scope of practice and the full responsibilities of your employment. Keep in mind that you work in a highly regulated industry. Ignorance of a law or a regulation does not excuse a violation. You are a professional and expected to know the laws and regulations that govern your profession and your job.

As members of society, we are all expected to conduct ourselves in a responsible manner that will not cause harm. This is known legally as holding an individual to a **reasonable person** standard of care. Physicians, nurses, and other health care professionals are all held to a higher standard of care than what is demanded under the reasonable person standard of care because of their specialized training and expertise.

reasonable person A prudent person whose behavior would be considered appropriate under the circumstances.

Locum tenens is used to describe physicians, nurses, and physician assistants who are temporarily performing the duties of another. Providers who are practicing "locum tenens," which is Latin for "to hold the place of," are held to the same standard of care as other providers with the same expertise and certification.

The standard of care takes into consideration the surrounding circumstances, including what a similarly qualified provider would do under the same set of circumstances. An analysis of what a "similarly qualified provider" would do includes factors such as geographic location or physical location. Violations of the standard of care are the basis of medical malpractice lawsuits, certificate or license revocations, and, in some cases, criminal charges.

Besides the agreement never to harm or exploit clients, and to treat them with respect, there is little accord among practitioners in the field about what constitutes proper care. A New York City psychoanalyst's treatment of anxiety is likely to be very different from that of an existentialist's treatment of the same condition in rural Idaho or the local counselor's treatment on an Indian reservation in Arizona. Similarly, a military psychologist or prison social worker are likely to have different sets of loyalties which effect their interventions, disclosures, and other clinical variables. This is why the definition of standard of care is context based. Along these lines the controversial issue of multiple relationships manifests itself or is applied differently in different settings.

Zur, O, Ph.D. (nd). The Standard of Care in Psychotherapy and Counseling. Zur Institute. Retrieved from www.zurinstitute.com/standard-of-care-therapy/.

For many health care professionals, the required standard of care is not well defined. For physicians and nurses, professional guidelines for accepted practices are more clearly defined. When a provider directs a lab technician, for example, to perform certain tasks associated with patient care, (i.e., to act as the provider's **agent**) the delegation of responsibility is based on the premise that the health care professional can perform as well as the person who assigned the task. It also follows that, in those situations, the health care professional may be held to the same standard of care as the provider or nurse for the task performed.

agent One who has authority to act on behalf of another.

Health care professionals are the link between the patient and the provider when arranging office visits, laboratory tests, therapeutic appointments, and hospital admissions. They are crucial in the development of good relations between the patient and the provider. It is important that health care professionals understand the legal issues involved with providing health care and the importance of good patient relations. Positive patient interactions minimize the nonmedical and nonlegal variables involved in malpractice and may prevent a legitimate complaint from developing into a lawsuit.

Patient Protection

Patients trust that they are being treated by qualified health care professionals. State licensure laws protect patients by defining the education and experience required to perform certain procedures before the licensed provider can treat patients. A license indicates that the holder has the basic minimum qualifications required by the state for that occupation.

License requirements also control employers by setting standards for hiring that ultimately protect patients. Licenses are granted by state-run licensing boards, which also have the power to revoke licenses. Although the grounds for revocation may vary slightly from state to state, they always include unprofessional conduct, substance abuse, fraud in connection with examination or application for a license, alcoholism, conviction of a felony, and mental incapacity.

Often health care professionals are closer to the patients and more sensitive to their needs than are providers. The requirements of privacy and respect for the confidential relationship between patient and provider must be met: privacy and confidentiality have ethical and legal bases. Permission to touch and the right to perform certain procedures are interwoven with state medical practice acts.

The Health Insurance Portability and Accountability Act (HIPAA), which is further discussed in Chapters 2 and 9, is a federal law requiring every health plan and provider to maintain "reasonable and appropriate" safeguards to ensure the confidentiality of patient health information.

The Arizona Supreme Court held that the Health Insurance Portability and Accountability Act (HIPAA) can provide guidance as to the standard of care in a negligence claim for wrongful disclosure of medical information. Plaintiff brought suit after his estranged wife picked up a prescription for him and was also given a prescription for erectile dysfunction (ED). The plaintiff's doctor gave him a sample medication for ED, which the plaintiff's pharmacist filled in addition to his usual prescription. The plaintiff decided he did not want to fill the ED prescription and twice asked the pharmacist to cancel it. At the time, the plaintiff sought to reconcile with his estranged wife, and had picked up plaintiff's usual prescription for him. The pharmacy employee also gave her the ED medication. After picking up the prescriptions, plaintiff's now ex-wife ceased all reconciliation efforts and told friends and family members about the prescription.

Initially, the plaintiff complained to the pharmacy, who then apologized and acknowledged that the company had violated HIPAA and its own privacy policy when it disclosed the ED prescription to his ex-wife. Plaintiff then sued, and as part of the case, the court indicated a plaintiff can use HIPAA as evidence of the standard of care for the safeguarding of protected health information in a negligence claim.

This case confirmed that HIPAA standards and rules may be used to establish the standard of care for the use and disclosure of protected health information.

Shepherd v. Costco Wholesale Corp., No. CV-19-0014 (Ariz. Mar. 8, 2021).

In addition to protecting the patient, laws exist that protect the public as a whole. Certain health matters, for example, must be reported by providers in every state, including births and deaths, venereal and other communicable diseases, injuries resulting from violence such as stab and gunshot wounds, child and elder abuse, blindness, immunological proceedings, requests for plastic surgery to change a person's fingerprints, and cases of industrial poisoning, among others.

Patient Bill of Rights   Health care facilities and providers have creeds entitled a "Patient Bill of Rights" that establish standards, including ethical standards, for patient care. A Patient Bill of Rights is not always required by law, so the content will change depending on the provider and facility. A Patient Bill of Rights conveys patients' legal and ethical rights and includes acknowledgment of a patient's right to choose treatment, to consent to treatment, and to refuse treatment, among others (Figure 1-1).

The following is a list of rights that may be included in the Patient Bill of Rights:

- To be treated with courtesy and respect in an environment free from discrimination.
- To be treated confidentially, with access to your records limited to those involved in your care or otherwise authorized by you.
- To be informed by your health care provider about your diagnosis, scheduled course of treatment, alternative treatment, risks, and prognosis.
- To use your own financial resources to pay for the care of your choice.
- To refuse medical treatment, even if your provider recommends it.
- To create Advance Directives and have your provider(s) or hospital staff provide care that is consistent with these directives.
- To be informed about the outcomes of care, treatment, and services that have been provided, including unanticipated outcomes.
- To be provided an estimate of charges for medical care, a reasonably clear itemized bill, and, if needed, an explanation of the charges.
- To receive prompt and reasonable responses to questions and requests.
- To know what patient services are available, including whether an interpreter is available.
- To be informed if medical treatment is for experimental research and to give your consent or refusal to participate.

Figure 1-1 Sample Patient Bill of Rights

The Business Structure: Legal Entities

A health care facility can be a solo practitioner operating from a single office, or it may be a group of providers who have agreed to share the costs and sometimes the liability of a group practice with several office locations. It may be a corporation, or a **conglomerate** controlling hospitals or other health care facilities. Each medical practice has an underlying **legal entity** that governs matters such as ownership, profit distribution, liability, taxes, and control, among others. State, county, or city law governs the structure and requirements. Legal entities include sole proprietorships, partnerships, limited liability companies, professional associations, limited liability partnerships (LLPs), and corporations.

Any legal entity can choose to operate and hold itself out to the public under a name that is different than its registered name. The alternate name is referred to as a DBA, short for "doing business as." Companies that operate as a DBA (sometimes referred to as a trade name, a fictitious name, or an assumed name) usually have to file state or local registrations that identify the people or legal entity that is responsible for the DBA. The main purpose for these filings is to prevent fraud and let the public know with whom they are doing business.

conglomerate A corporation diversifying operations by acquiring varied businesses.

legal entity An individual or organization that has legal capacity to contract, incur and pay debts, and sue and be sued.

Sole Proprietorship

A sole proprietorship is a legal entity that requires no state filing to create it. A sole proprietorship is simply one person operating a business for profit. That person has unlimited personal liability for the business. A sole proprietor can have employees, including other providers. The person who chooses this business structure does so for two main reasons. First, individual ownership is the simplest and most basic business structure and appeals to a person who wants to be independent and free from the laws that govern other legal entities. Second, any financial rewards from the practice are for the owner and do not have to be shared with anyone else. However, any losses are also the owner's.

A sole proprietorship should not be confused with a solo practice, which is a type of health care business where the practice includes just one provider. A solo practice can be one of the many legal entities discussed in this chapter. Most solo practitioners choose legal entities other than a sole proprietorship for liability and tax reasons. In fact, all medical practice types such as solo practices, group practices, and employed provider practices may choose their legal entity type.

Partnership

A partnership, sometimes called a "general partnership" (GP), is two or more people who combine their work, money, and talents to achieve a common goal. It is a more complicated form of legal entity than a sole proprietorship. A partnership is formed when two or more parties agree—in compliance with state and local law—to certain business aspects such as ownership, profit distribution, liability, taxes, and control. Many states require a document or registration that serves as **notice** to the public that the partnership members are doing business together. Unless the terms of the partnership provide otherwise, each partner has a right to participate in managing the business and making decisions.

notice An announcement of pertinent information to those who have a right or obligation to know.

A high degree of mutual trust and confidence must exist between partners. For example, if one partner's personal debts become so large they cannot be satisfied by his or her private assets, creditors may go after that partner's share of the business property, thereby threatening the partnership.

In conducting the affairs of a partnership, all partners are bound by the acts of the others. This affects them as individuals. If, for example, one partner places an order for equipment beyond the financial means of the partnership, the other partners are required to share payment of the bill, possibly by using their personal funds. A notable exception is an LLP. In such cases, personal assets can be protected.

Limited Liability Companies

A limited liability company (LLC) is a legal entity, created by one or more individuals or other legal entities, to further a common goal and to create ground rules for matters such as ownership, profit distribution, liability, taxes, and control. Individuals who have an interest in an LLC are usually referred to as "members." State law, as opposed to federal law, governs LLCs.

Business owners have increasingly used LLCs because they provide protection from being held personally liable and can be advantageous from a tax perspective. LLCs do not always provide the protection from personal liability for the wrongful acts of members or employees, which explains the use of the word "limited." LLCs also require less legal and accounting work to get started. In addition, members can decide among themselves who has authority to perform acts such as hiring or firing employees, contributing capital, and earning profits, among others.

Some states allow for certain professionals, such as providers, lawyers, architects, and accountants, to form professional limited liability companies (PLLCs). A PLLC is very similar to an LLC, but the governing statutes dictate that the limits of liability may only be applied to certain aspects of the business, such as creditors. A PLLC limits the liability protection that certain professionals can expect. In a health care scenario, PLLCs do not allow providers to limit their liability for patient wrongs, such as malpractice.

Corporations

A corporation is a legal entity created by one or more individuals to further a common goal and to make use of corporate tax and legal advantages.

A corporation is formed in accordance with the state laws in which it is registered. State laws usually require that a corporation's name includes a corporate designation such as "Corporation," "Co.," "Corp.," or "Inc."

Much thought is often given to the corporate name. The corporation may use any name, provided it has not been taken by some other legal entity in the state or does not too closely resemble the name of an existing legal entity. Health care providers usually try to choose a name that will instantly indicate to the public the services they provide.

officers Persons holding formal positions of trust in an organization, especially those involved in high levels of management.

directors Those elected and terminated by stockholders to manage a corporation.

stockholders Those who hold an interest in a corporation.

shares Units of stock giving the possessor part ownership in a corporation.

investment Expenditure of resources (money, effort, etc.) intended to secure income or profit.

bylaws Regulations adopted by a corporation or association to govern its internal affairs.

dividends Distributed profits of a corporation.

The life of a corporation does not end upon the death of its **officers**, **directors**, or **stockholders**. Even if all died in a common disaster, **shares** of the corporation would generally be passed on to the officers', directors', or stockholders' heirs. The corporation will not cease to exist until it is dissolved by the requisite legal process. This is true even in a corporation where only one individual holds all of the stock.

One of the most desirable features of a corporation is the protection given to investors. For example, if the corporation loses money and the debts become greater than the assets, the creditors may not collect from the individual owners, known as stockholders. Only the capital of the corporation is available for the payment of debts. It is important to remember that judgments resulting from lawsuits are indeed debts. The most an individual investor may lose is the amount of the original **investment**.

Management responsibility is in the hands of the corporation's board of directors. The number of directors is usually set in the **bylaws** of the corporation, which are adopted at the first stockholders' meeting. Directors answer to the stockholders, who elect and can terminate them. A member of the board of directors is expected to be loyal to the corporation and its shareholders. It is improper for a director to have an interest in any business that competes with the corporation. Officers of a corporation include the president, vice president, treasurer, secretary, and any other officers the board of directors appoints. They are employees of the company and need not be stockholders. Profits of a corporation are distributed to stockholders as **dividends**.

Not-for-profit organizations may also be corporations; there are no shareholders and no dividends. Revenue in excess of expenses is reinvested in the organization.

Similar to a PLLC, a professional corporation (PC) or a professional association (PA) are legal entities that are designed for business endeavors of professionals such as providers, attorneys, architects, and accountants.

Health Care Delivery and Compensation Systems

As cost management in health care rose to crisis levels, alternative delivery and compensation systems have largely replaced traditional health care business practices. In the past, a patient who felt unwell would decide when and whom to visit for health care. The patient would then pay a fee for the provider's service either directly or through an insurance company.

The traditional **fee-for-service** payment system has shown that it encourages increased costs and reduces the quality of care patients receive as compared to other health care delivery systems. Consequently, those with a stake in the matter (health insurance companies, government, employers, patients, and providers) have developed alternative delivery systems that reward cost management, quality care, and efficiency.

fee-for-service Basis of professional billing, either so much per hour or per identified procedure.

Managed care organizations seeking to manage health care costs and improve health care contract with providers and health care facilities to provide health care services for the MCOs insured in accordance with certain requirements. The two longstanding forms of alternative delivery systems are health maintenance organizations (HMOs) and preferred provider organizations (PPOs). Other alternative delivery systems are emerging that bear no resemblance to traditional office-based delivery systems.

Amazon (Nasdaq: AMZN) unveiled major plans to expand its budding home-based care offering, "Amazon Care," across the U.S.....

Since then, home-based care stakeholders have been trying to make sense of the news and figure out what it means for them—and the in-home care patients they serve. Their early evaluations are thus far divided, with some excited by Amazon's ability to bring additional attention to home-based care and others concerned about technology overshadowing the human touch.

Amazon launched Amazon Care—an initiative that uses an app to coordinate in-person care and virtual health care services—about 18 months ago. The company initially began testing the platform as part of an exclusive pilot program for employees and their family members in the Seattle area, but eventually expanded it across all of Washington....

While not much is known about Amazon Care as far as health impacts or utilization, Amazon officials have publicly touted the offering's accessibility, convenience and timeliness.

"I would only caution that people who are integral to the building, running and supervising of this platform are those who know health care, preferably with clinicians and patients on the board," Jinjiao Wang, a nurse scientist in New York, shared via social media. "Algorithms should only serve, not dictate, humans." "We're rebuilding the whole delivery system around the human at the center," Nicole Bell, a business development executive with Amazon Care, said in a promotional video posted to the platform's website. "You just open the app and from there, you can do a text chat with a nurse or a virtual care visit with a provider. If we can't meet your needs in that virtual environment, we bring the health care system to you."

Holly, R. 'We're Rebuilding the Whole Delivery System':
Why Amazon Is Betting Big on Home-Based Care. (2021, March 22).
Home Health Care News. Retrieved from www.homehealthcarenews.com/2021/03
/were-rebuilding-the-whole-delivery-system-why-amazon-is-betting-big-on-home-based-care/.

The Affordable Care Act of 2010 resulted in the promotion of another primary MCO, the accountable care organization (ACO), as well as variations of all three. In addition, Medicare and Medicaid have experienced similar changes as the government seeks to contain costs and improve the quality of health care.

The Affordable Care Act

The Patient Protection and Affordable Care Act (PPACA), more commonly referred to as the Affordable Care Act (ACA), was signed into law on March 23, 2010, but many of its provisions did not take effect immediately. As a result, the government, employers, health care industry, and patients had time to prepare for the changes that the ACA required. The ACA is expansive, and it touches on many subjects including:

- use of electronic medical records,
- prohibition of coverage denials based upon preexisting conditions,
- requirement that insurance companies offer all applicants of the same age and locality the same premium without consideration of most preexisting conditions or age,
- imposition of minimum standards for health insurance companies,
- requirement that, with very narrow exceptions, all Americans have some form of health insurance,
- provision of government subsidies for insurance premiums based upon financial considerations,
- introduction of state run health insurance exchanges that allow comparison shopping for health insurance policies,
- revisions to Medicaid eligibility,
- requirement that dependents can remain on their parents' health insurance until their 26th birthday,
- prohibition on canceling policies when policyholders become ill, and
- requirement that new health insurance plans must fully cover certain preventive treatment and medical tests, without charging co-payments or deductibles.

The ultimate goal of the ACA is to encourage health care that increases the quality and affordability of health insurance, lowers the uninsured rate by expanding public and private insurance coverage, and reduces the costs of health care. The ACA seeks to ensure that all have health care, and since its passage, the number of uninsured Americans has decreased significantly.

Managed Care Organizations

Managed care is a term used to describe a method of delivering and compensating health care with a pointed focus on lowering costs and improving quality. An MCO is simply an organization that provides managed health care. Managed care typically includes a wide spectrum of health care services, including preventative care, diagnosis and treatment of illness, prescriptions, and mental health care. Managed care contracts with physicians, hospitals, clinics, and other health care providers to create provider networks. An in-network provider or health care facility is part of an MCO's network if there is a preexisting agreement between the MCO and the health care provider. The agreement dictates the protocols for patient care and the compensation system. An out-of-network provider is a provider or health care facility that does not have an agreement with the MCO. To discourage the use of out-of-network providers, a patient's reimbursement for services provided by an out-of-network provider is not compensated at the same level as an in-network provider. Managed care focuses on various aspects of health care and can include characteristics such as:

- networks of health care providers or facilities, who have agreed to predetermined protocols and compensation,
- primary care providers (PCPs), who coordinate all of a patient's health care,
- preauthorization for specific treatments,
- limited reimbursement for out-of-network providers,
- claim filing assigned to the provider rather than the patient, and
- tiered coverage of prescription drugs.

There are many different ways that MCO's members contribute to the cost of their health care. A member will typically pay a monthly premium, some or all of which may be paid by a third party, such as an employer or the government. In addition, members may be responsible for satisfying an annual deductible before certain coverages are effective. With a few exceptions, each office or emergency room visit or prescription requires that members contribute in the form of a co-payment. MCOs manage prescription-drug costs by charging members a lower co-payment for drugs that cost the MCO less. See Table 1-2 for an MCO matrix that includes the characteristics of HMOs, POSs, EPOs, and PPOs.

MCOs use PCPs as gatekeepers to control the cost-effectiveness of services offered to members. Gatekeepers control access to specialists. In addition, many MCOs have adopted authorization requirements, meaning that the MCO must approve some procedures before the PCP orders them. The payers are controlling access to health care by denying approval for certain procedures and allowing payment for others. They make decisions that reduce the number of hospital admissions, shorten the time until discharge, control the number of expensive diagnostic procedures, and, in the mental health field, substitute medication for therapeutic counseling treatment. When gatekeepers have an incentive to deny referrals to specialists, limit diagnostic treatments, and shorten hospital stays, the integrity of the patient–provider

Table 1-2 MCO Characteristics Matrix

	Requires PCP	Requires referrals	Requires preauthorization	Pays for out-of-network care	Cost-sharing	Do you have to file claim paperwork?
HMO	Yes	Yes	Not usually required. If required, PCP does it.	No	Low	No
POS	Yes	Yes	Not usually required. If required, PCP likely does it. Out-of-network care may have different rules.	Yes, but requires PCP referral.	Low in-network, high for out-of-network.	Only for out-of-network claims.
EPO	No	No	Yes	No	Low	No
PPO	No	No	Yes	Yes	High, especially for out-of-network care.	Only for out-of-network claims

Source: Verywell

relationship is called into question. When insurance companies make the decision to allow or deny diagnostic testing and hospital admissions, the patient–provider relationship is further eroded, and the well-being of the patient becomes an issue.

MCO's continued search for ways to provide quality care while keeping costs low has also affected the financial well-being of patients. For example, the rise of "surprise billing" resulted in the No Surprises Act, which creates federal rules for out-of-network billing in certain scenarios.

> The No Surprises Act contains key protections to hold consumers harmless from the cost of unanticipated out-of-network medical bills.
> Surprise bills arise in emergencies—when patients typically have little or no say in where they receive care. They also arise in non-emergencies when patients at in-network hospitals or other facilities receive care from ancillary providers (such as anesthesiologists) who are not in-network and whom the patient did not choose.
> Surprise bills lead the list of affordability concerns for many families; 2 in 3 adults say they worry about unexpected medical bills, more than the number worried about affording other health care or household expenses. Surprise bills can number in the millions each year. Among privately insured patients, an estimated 1 in 5 emergency claims and 1 in 6 in-network hospitalizations include at least one out-of-network bill. A health plan that generally doesn't cover out-of-network care, such as an HMO, might deny a surprise bill entirely.

Or plans might pay a portion of the bill, but leave the patient liable for balance billing—the difference between the undiscounted fee charged by the out-of-network provider and the amount reimbursed by the private health plan. Balance billing on surprise medical bills can reach hundreds or even thousands of dollars. Surprise medical bills are not a problem today under public programs—Medicare and Medicaid—that prohibit balance billing.

KFF. (2021, February 4). Surprise Medical Bills: New Protections for Consumers Take Effect in 2022. KFF. Retrieved from www.kff.org/private-insurance/fact-sheet/surprise-medical-bills-new-protections-for-consumers-take-effect-in-2022/.

An MCO's in-network health care providers are typically compensated by a capitated rate, sometimes also known as "per member per month" (PMPM). The MCO, on behalf of all its members, contracts with various health care providers who make themselves available to provide care in exchange for a set fee per month. The fee represents the number of members in the provider's care. In some cases, providers are employees of the MCO, and they work for a salary. In most cases, providers are part of a larger network maintained by the MCO for the members' benefit.

Health Maintenance Organizations   HMOs are comprehensive health care delivery and compensation systems that provide provider and hospital services from participating providers. With the exception of emergencies, HMOs will not cover care provided by out-of-network providers. HMOs require that each member have a PCP who monitors the overall health of the member and provides referrals to specialist in accordance with the HMO's protocols. HMOs typically do not pay for specialist visits that have not been referred by the PCP. HMOs operate on the presumption that maintaining health and preventing illness is less expensive than the cost of treatment for the illness that would otherwise develop.

There are two main HMO provider payment structures: the prepaid group practice (PGP) and the individual practice association (IPA). Prepaid group practices are groups of providers who agree to provide comprehensive health care services for a fixed prospective **per capita payment** to a definite population. The staff model and the group model are two forms of PGPs. Under the staff model, the providers are employees of the HMO, are salaried, and may at the end of the fiscal year receive a portion of any profit. In the group model, the providers are organized as a partnership or corporation in a group practice. The group contracts with the HMO to provide care for HMO members, sometimes called subscribers. The group receives **capitation** payment and a share of the HMO's net income as a group and pays participating providers on a fee-for-service or salary basis.

per capita payment Pay equally according to the number of individuals.

capitation Payment in a lump sum to providers, HMOs, and health care facilities to deliver health care to a segment of the population.

In contrast, IPAs are groups of providers who join together and enter into agreement with other organizations to provide medical services to a defined population. In this structure, the providers practice in their own office on a fee-for-service or capitation basis. Comprehensive health benefits are provided to the designated population for a fixed periodic payment.

HMOs are regulated under the HMO Act of 1973 (42 *United States Code* section 300c-300e-17 [1976 and Supp. III 1979]). Under this Act, member providers must agree to give at least one-third of their time to HMO subscribers. Employers with more than 25 employees must offer an HMO as an alternative choice to conventional health care coverage, if such a choice is available in the area.

In a continued effort to find the best combination of cost savings and quality care, MCO hybrids are routinely introduced. A point-of-service (POS) is a combination of a traditional fee-for-service plan and an HMO. Members are rewarded with lower costs when they choose to use their PCP as a gatekeeper but are not prohibited from choosing out-of-network providers. Members incur higher costs when they receive care from an out-of-network provider.

joint venture A group of persons together performing some specific business undertaking that is limited in duration or scope.

negotiated fee schedules The amount an insurance company or other third-party payer will reimburse for a specific medical procedure.

utilization review A process by which hospitals review patient progress to efficiently allocate scarce medical resources.

Preferred Provider Organizations

PPOs are groups of providers and hospitals that contract with employers, health insurance companies, or third-party administrators to provide comprehensive medical services on a fee-for-service basis to subscribers. A PPO may be sponsored by a hospital, a provider, an employer, or an insurer, or it may be a **joint venture** between a hospital and a medical practice. The mechanisms used to control health care costs include **negotiated fee schedules** and **utilization reviews**. A PPO covers the cost of a preferred provider's care, as well as a reduced portion of a nonpreferred provider's care.

The evolution of PPOs with high deductibles prompted the creation of health savings accounts (HSA), which provide tax breaks for money set aside in an HSA for health care–related expenses.

A health savings account, or H.S.A., can help pay for some medical expenses, if you qualify to have one. And they offer three valuable tax breaks: Money is deposited pretax, can grow tax-free and is not taxed when you spend it, as long as the expenses are eligible. . . . There's a catch, though: The accounts are available only to people with health insurance plans that meet specific criteria, such as a high deductible, which is the amount a person pays for nonpreventive medical care before insurance. For 2020 and 2021, the amount is at least $1,400 for an individual or $2,800 for family coverage. . . . The accounts can pay for a variety of medical and health expenses, including doctor visits, hospital stays, surgery, and vision or dental care. The money can also go toward long-term-care insurance premiums and services. . . . The federal government's pandemic relief program expanded what H.S.A.s can pay for, including nonprescription medicine like pain relief and allergy pills, and menstrual products like tampons and pads. (The I.R.S. has a full list of eligible items.) . . . People often confuse H.S.A.s with other types of health accounts, such as flexible health spending accounts. But unlike F.S.A.s, health savings accounts are portable: If you change jobs or leave the work force, you keep the account. Contribution limits are higher for H.S.A.s, and there is no deadline to spend the cash. Unspent money can be invested for health needs in retirement. . . .

Carrns, A. (2021, March 19). The New York Times. The Triple Tax Break
You May Be Missing: A Health Savings Account. Retrieved from www.nytimes.com
/2021/03/19/business/health-savings-accounts-tax-break.html.

The PPO has emerged as the most commonly used form of health insurance coverage. Consumers like the freedom to choose their own providers, which is frequently cited as one of HMO's drawbacks. As you might expect, the member costs for a PPO is greater than for an HMO.

An exclusive provider organization (EPO) is a hybrid of a PPO and an HMO, where members can choose from a group of preferred providers. An EPO, however, will not pay any percentage of costs associated with a nonpreferred provider.

Accountable Care Organizations   The Affordable Care Act includes guidelines for ACOs and sets the stage for the increased popularity of ACOs. An ACO is a type of MCO that seeks to improve health care and reduce costs by using groups of providers, hospitals, and other health care professionals to coordinate cost-effective, quality health care and to reward positive patient outcomes by sharing cost-savings with providers. It functions similarly to an HMO but without the gatekeeper requirement, and out-of-network providers are covered at a reduced percentage.

Health care providers and health insurance companies are forming ACOs for Medicare patients as well as for patients with private insurance. The ACOs created for Medicare patients include the Medicare Shared Saving Program (MSSP), the Advanced Payment system, the Investment system, the Pioneer system, and the Next Generation system. The variations in the ACO systems differ based upon characteristics such as the way patient outcomes are rewarded, how the providers are compensated, the subset of Medicare patients they serve, or the ACO's level of experience.

Technology and Medicine

Seemingly overnight, technology has worked its way into our health care and some of the risks and rewards are yet to be fully understood. The COVID-19 pandemic sped up the use and acceptance of certain health care technologies. Telemedicine, which was just starting to gain more widespread popularity in 2020, has become a common method of interacting with a provider.

. . . as Covid snaked its way into the fabric of the world, hospital finances suffered, patients avoided care (in some instances, urgently needed care), and clinician capacity far outweighed demand.

If ever there existed a silver lining to a global pandemic, care technology (like remote patient care) catapulting to the stage was, for the good or the bad, warts and all, a glimmer of hope.

Contemplating the remote care "condition" during the heat of Covid I classified health system and clinical readiness in three rather obtuse categories:

1. Those who are comfortable with, and deeply embedded in, telehealth care,
2. Those who were nibbling around the edges of telehealth with varying levels of implementation (discussions, examination, curiosity), and
3. The unprepared (forced to embrace telehealth as the only [short term] means of offering patient visits).

As a refresher, due to Covid, use of telehealth applications increased under the umbrella of a federal Emergency Order which relaxed many regulatory aspects of telehealth and associated remote delivery services. However, once the EO expires, Congress will need to revisit codifying telehealth. That said, it seems the genie is out of the bottle. At this point in Covid's yearlong-plus history, physicians and health systems have learned to either adapt (see #3 above) or thrive (see #1 above) with telehealth.

Gorke, J. (2021, March 19). Deploying Healthcare Technology: How Vulnerable Are You? *Forbes.* Retrieved from www.forbes.com/sites/jeffgorke/2021/03/29 /deploying-healthcare-technology-how-vulnerable-are-you/?sh=4be7ca4fd050.

Our personal electronics tell us to eat less or more, to sleep and when, to take our prescriptions, to relax, and to exercise more, among countless other metrics.

Smartphones have endless apps that monitor these health metrics such as heart rate, meditation and mindfulness, medication, general wellness, weight loss, menstrual cycles, sleep, diabetes, blood oxygen levels, and so much more. Drones are being tested as a method of health care delivery. Thermal cameras are being used to detect elevated temperatures, a common indicator of the COVID-19 virus.

The ever-growing use of electronic records and patient portals to store, report, track, schedule, communicate, and monitor patient health care suggests this practice is here to stay. It also suggests that, as technology in health care grows, so too will the demand for cyber security.

Personal health information has become a lucrative target for illegal actions on the Internet. Health care companies have more liability than just HIPAA violations, and they now need to be stalwart defenders of their technologies' security.

Telemedicine

Telemedicine is a health care delivery system used when the patient is in one location and the treating provider is in another, possibly thousands of miles away.

The COVID-19 pandemic lit a fire under the use of telemedicine, which includes the use of video, as well as the transmission of electronically collected health metrics from the patient to the remote provider. While telemedicine is not new, the recent pandemic brought it front and center stage globally. Medical schools and accrediting organizations are providing classes, best practices, and competencies for those health care provider who will practice virtually. Telemedicine is being used in a wide array of applications and settings, including:

- Psychiatrists, psychologists, licensed social workers, and other mental health care providers often use video and telephone to conduct virtual sessions (driven in large part by the COVID-19 pandemic, which spawned a significant need for mental health care).

- Children's Health Care of Atlanta uses telemedicine for rural pediatric patients, including those who were the victims of sexual assault and who might not otherwise be able to get the specialized health care needed.

- An Arizona neurosurgical practice uses telemedicine so its patients can remember what was said during office visits. Patients have their consultation and follow-up visits videotaped, so the details are available.

In health care's cost-sensitive environment, telemedicine has become prominent, and its applications are many. It offers a way to provide quality care to patients in rural areas or to patients in need of specialized diagnostic evaluation. See Figure 1-2 for a sample timeline of a physician-on-demand videoconference consultation.

There are, however, unanswered legal questions. For example, in which state or county or city is medicine being practiced—where the

9:22 p.m.	Recurrent sinus infection rises to the level where the patient can no longer tolerate the symptoms. She has been too busy all week to schedule an appointment with her primary care provider. It is now late in the evening on a Friday, and she does not want to be sick all weekend. She downloads a smartphone application for a national physician-on-demand service and creates an account. Insurance doesn't currently cover the cost of the visit, which is $40 for each 15 minutes. Her co-pay at her PCP is $25.
9:27 p.m.	Videoconferencing begins. The physician asks about patient's symptoms, history of sinus infections, and current medications. Physician concurs that the signs of a sinus infection are present and that an antibiotic is in order.
9:35 p.m.	Videoconference concludes and the physician electronically sends an antibiotic prescription to the patient's local pharmacy.
9:44 p.m.	Pharmacy calls the patient to report that the prescription is ready for pickup.
10:02 p.m.	Prescription is in the patient's hands, and she takes the first dose that night.
Three days later	Patient receives an email from the physician-on-demand company reminding the patient to follow up with her primary care provider if symptoms have not improved and that her treatment history is available in the smartphone application.

Figure 1-2 Timeline of Physician-on-Demand Videoconference Consultation

patient is or where the provider is located? Does the provider need a license to practice medicine in each state where he or she consults with a patient? Some issues affect the provider engaged in practicing. Others affect the medical profession as a whole.

i   Nathan Jones (not his real name) is 57 and had recently been hospitalized with the rare autoimmune condition dermatomyositis, which can cause a strange rash, muscle pains, and facial swelling. He'd also experienced difficulty swallowing.

Since going home, Mr. Jones had been diligently taking his medications, but when our telemedicine visit began, I noticed severe swelling around his lips. He also reported a strange phenomenon of his voice changing when lying flat.

Quickly, I instructed him to open his mouth, and I saw that his tongue was swollen. Concerned that his airway was closing, I immediately arranged for an ambulance to transfer him to the hospital. In less than an hour, Mr. Jones was in the care of our medical intensive care unit at Stony Brook University Hospital on Long Island, New York.

Without telemedicine, I might not have known about my patient's critical condition. Not one "to make fanfare," Mr. Jones says he would never have sought an in-person medical appointment to address these pressing health issues—and his follow-up appointment was not for several weeks, which, in retrospect, would have been too late.

Noel, K. (2021, March 24). What Every Doctor Needs to Know About Telemedicine. AAMC. Retrieved from www.aamc.org/news-insights/what-every-doctor-needs-know-about-telemedicine.

The use of teleradiology is increasing and is in sync with the way businesses now operate globally. Hospitals contract with provider groups in India, for example, to read x-ray, computerized tomography, and magnetic resonance images. Likewise, some radiology groups have established branch locations in places like Hawaii to provide more round-the-clock service to health care providers in other time zones.

Another increasing use of telemedicine is in the field of home health care. More patients are being monitored at home to ensure their well-being. This may require the patient "reporting in" by computer, or it may be a device that sends signals to the medical provider without requiring the patient to do anything.

Companies that deliver provider-on-demand services are popping up to address the needs of patients in rural areas, patients who lack the ability to leave their homes, busy parents or professionals, and patients on vacation. Some of the provider-on-demand services come in the form of a house call by a provider and some provide care by videoconferencing. Employers are adding telemedicine options to its employee benefits.

As experience with telemedicine supports it as a cost-effective health care delivery system, you can expect to see it as a common health care insurance offering. A handful of states already have laws that relate to telemedicine and health insurance coverage.

☑ SUMMARY

- The health care industry is a big business.
- What you do on the front line matters.
- Understanding the laws that apply to health care is important for employees to protect themselves, their employer, and the patient.

- Because medicine is closely regulated by state and federal law, it is necessary for employees to be aware of statutes and regulations that define the procedures they are permitted to perform.
- Health care professionals work in the delivery of health care and are held to a higher standard of care than laypersons without special knowledge and training.
- There are several types of legal entities, all of which are governed by state law.
- The Affordable Care Act made expansive changes to the way the health care industry does business.
- Managed care organizations include HMOs, PPOs, and ACOs, and they all seek to reduce costs and deliver quality health care.
- Technology in health care is booming, and telemedicine has fast become a widely accepted health care delivery system.

SUGGESTED ACTIVITIES

1. Does the area of health care you plan to work in require licensing or registration in the state where you will practice? Does it have certifications that identify those who have expertise in specific areas? Who issues those certifications?

2. Find the website for your state's department of corporations. This is the department that registers businesses. Find a local business' registration material on the department of corporation's website. Can you tell what kind of legal entity it is? Can you tell what year it was created? What else does the business' online registration tell you?

3. If given the choice, what type of health insurance would you prefer: an HMO, PPO, ACO, or something else? Why? What details should you know about your health insurance?

4. Have you or someone you know ever been a telemedicine patient? How was the experience? What do you think would have been different about the visit had it been in person?

STUDY QUESTIONS

1. How can frontline health care professionals help prevent a medical malpractice lawsuit?

2. Identify the major disadvantage of a sole proprietorship or a partnership.

3. How does a corporation differ from a partnership?

4. Summarize the conflicts that exist when an MCO provides bonuses to providers for providing fewer tests.

5. What are the risks associated with technology in health care?

CASES FOR DISCUSSION

1. Brackenridge Hospital admitted Plaintiff to its intensive care unit following a serious car accident. Medical resident Dr. Villafani and attending physician Dr. Harshaw performed a tracheostomy and inserted a breathing tube. Several days later, plaintiff experienced bleeding from the surgical wound. Dr. Villafani examined plaintiff but did not immediately share plaintiff's condition with Dr. Harshaw. Plaintiff went into cardiac and respiratory arrest resulting in permanent and severe brain damage. At the time of plaintiff's treatment, Dr. Villafani was enrolled in a general surgery residency program operated by St. Joseph's Hospital. Central Texas Medical Foundation, an institution participating with St. Joseph's placed Dr. Villafani at Brackenridge Hospital, and had a contractual agreement with St. Joseph's to do so. The Foundation and Brackenridge dictated the details of how and when Dr. Villafani performed his residency responsibilities while at Brackenridge. The contract between St. Joseph's and the Foundation prevented St. Joseph's from having any direct control over Dr. Villafani's work while at Brackenridge. Plaintiff sued several defendants, including St. Joseph's, who was found vicariously liable for plaintiff's injuries under the theory of respondeat superior. On appeal, the court reversed. Who, if anyone, should be held vicariously liable for Dr. Villafani's treatment of plaintiff?

2. Ms. SoderVick was a patient at Parkview Health System's OB/GYN practice and arrived at Parkview's offices for an appointment. A certain Parkview employee was charged that day with updating patient information in the electronic health record system. Parkview had provided the employee with patient privacy issues and HIPAA compliance training. The employee had signed a "Confidentiality Agreement and Acknowledgement Regarding Access to Patient Information," which made clear that the release of patient information could be a violation of HIPAA and Parkview's policies and that an employee could be immediately terminated if the employee released such information. When Ms. SoderVick arrived, she submitted a completed patient information sheet to the employee who recognized Ms. SoderVick's name as someone who had commented on a photo of the employee's husband on his personal social media account. The employee suspected that Ms. SoderVick might be engaged in an extramarital affair with her husband, and she texted

her husband that Ms. SoderVick was a patient. The employee's texts included information, such as the patient's name, her job title, and the reasons for the appointment. The employee falsely texted her husband that Ms. SoderVick was HIV-positive and was promiscuous. Parkview ultimately learned of the employee's texts to her husband about the patient and launched an investigation that included notifying the patient of the disclosure of her protected health information. Ms. SoderVick then sued and asserted the legal theory of respondeat superior. Should Parkview be held liable? Was the employee's conduct incidental to her job duties? Should Parkview be held liable for the employee's acts?

Chapter 2

Laws and Regulations You Will Encounter

 Law is an ordinance of reason for the common good, promulgated by him who has care of the community.

Thomas Aquinas

Objectives

After reading this chapter, you should be able to:

1. Describe the government's influence on the practice and licensing of medicine.
2. Identify circumstances that require mandatory reporting.
3. Describe controlled substances acts.
4. Summarize basic workplace discrimination and harassment laws.
5. Summarize basic laws impacting employee wages and benefits.
6. Summarize Occupational Safety and Health Act (OSHA) regulations for the health care industry.
7. Describe the purpose and components of job descriptions, procedures manuals, and employee handbooks.
8. Explain the purpose of unions.

Building Your Legal Vocabulary

Bargaining unit
Censure
Collective bargaining
Disparate impact
Disparate treatment
Facially neutral
Inference

Interstate commerce
Mitigating
Negligent per se
Probable cause
Quality assurance
Risk management

Introduction to Health Care Laws, Regulations, and Business Protocols

In addition to the health care business framework details discussed in Chapter 1, the laws and regulations that touch health care and those who work in the industry are also an important part of that framework. As a health care professional, you will want to be aware of various medical practice laws and regulations, the nature of your employment, discrimination, sexual harassment, health care laws and regulations, and, in some situations, union membership and collective bargaining. In addition, it is helpful to remember that you work in a field that is highly regulated by federal and state legislation. Ignorance of a law or a regulation does not excuse a health care professional's violation. You are a professional and expected to know the laws and regulations that govern your profession.

Medical Practice Laws

Medical practice laws control the practice of medicine. State legislatures establish state medical boards with the authority to control health care provider licensing. In all states, individuals who are not physicians are prohibited from practicing medicine, yet not every state defines what "practicing medicine" means. Medical practice acts may include nursing practice acts, or the two may exist independently. State law, if any, governs the licensure of other health care professionals.

Licensure statutes were originally established to prevent unqualified people from practicing medicine. In *Hawker v. New York* (170 U.S. 189 [1898]), the U.S. Supreme Court extended physician licensure decisions to include standards of behavior and ethics, holding that in a physician, "character is as important a qualification as knowledge."

censure A formal statement of disapproval.

Licensing boards not only grant licenses but also renew and revoke licenses. They may fine, reprimand, and **censure.** In so doing, the board must follow due process. Due process requires that a provider be put on notice that there is a pending suspension or revocation, be given an opportunity for a prompt hearing, and be given the rights to confront the accuser, prepare an effective defense, retain counsel, and cross-examine any witnesses.

One ground for the revocation or suspension of a medical license is permitting unlicensed physician to perform procedures or tasks that are outside of the scope of their practice. Physicians should be aware of the risks of assigning medical procedures to nonphysicians, including license suspension or revocation or a medical malpractice lawsuit. As a health care professional, understanding your scope of practice is your responsibility, as is the need to question the assigning provider about tasks assigned to you that you believe may be outside the scope of your practice.

State Board of Registration

State medical licensing laws regulate a state's board of registration. These boards, which are known by many different names depending on the state, are typically overseen by people who have the expertise to understand and enforce the applicable laws. A board learns about provider complaints through anonymous communications, newspaper articles, patients, hospitals, other health care providers, insurance companies, and the provider's employees. The board has the power to perform investigations and make formal conclusions according to its rules. During an investigation, a board may have access to records involving the health care provider's practice—prescriptions, hospital records, reimbursement claims—as long as information that can be used to identify the patient in the record is withheld.

> Washington state health officials have restricted the license of a Spokane County osteopathic physician and surgeon after reviewing charges and evidence accusing him of malpractice.
>
> Jason Adam Dreyer is accused by the Washington State Department of Health of performing extensive spine surgeries on patients for financial gain. He currently works for MultiCare in Spokane. . . .
>
> In the statement of charges, the Board of Osteopathic Medicine and Surgery Department says Dr. Dreyer "overstated the Patient's diagnosis of 'dynamic instability' to justify spinal fusion surgeries, overstated treatments performed during spine surgeries, and inadequately charted in Patient's records" at Providence St. Mary's.
>
> Until the charges are resolved, Dr. Dreyer cannot perform spine surgeries.
>
> Nelson, M. (2021, March 16). Spokane Physician Stripped of License After Reports of Excessive Surgeries. KREM2. Retrieved from www.krem.com /article/news/health/spokane-physician-stripped-license-reports-excessive-surgeries /293-14893f1d-7c72-4ddd-b362-61f7672e73bc.

Mandatory Reporting

Under certain circumstances, providers are required to submit reports to governmental agencies. Some of these reports are required by all practicing health care providers, and these include births, deaths, and communicable diseases. Generally, health care providers are required to report injuries and suspicious or "unnatural" deaths to the local coroner or medical examiner. To whom and when the reports are submitted are factors that vary from state to state. In many states, failure to report specific injuries or deaths can result in misdemeanor charges.

Abuse

Providers, nurses, and other health care professionals are required in most states to report the abuse of children, elderly, and patients. The Child Abuse Prevention and Treatment Act requires that states meet certain uniform standards to be eligible for federal assistance in setting up programs to identify, prevent, and treat problems caused by child abuse and neglect. It also protects the reporter of abuse against liability and includes a penalty clause that permits the prosecution of professionals who have knowledge of but do not report abuse.

Being on the front lines of healthcare, nurses have unfortunately needed to report cases of abuse and neglect. As mandated, they are trained to identify signs and symptoms of abuse or neglect and are required by law to report their findings. Failure to do so may result in discipline by the board of nursing, discipline by their employer, and possible legal action taken against them.

If a nurse suspects abuse or neglect, they should first report it to a physician, nurse practitioner, or physician assistant. Notifying a supervisor may also be required, depending on the workplace. If the victim is with a suspected abuser, the exam should take place without that person in the room. Nurses should provide a calm, comforting environment and approach the patient with care and concern. A complete head-to-toe examination should take place, looking for physical signs of abuse. A chaperone or witness should be present if possible as well. Thorough documentation and description of exam findings, as well as patient statements, non-verbal behavior, and behavior/statements of the suspected abuser should also be included.

The nurse should notify law enforcement as soon as possible, while the victim is still in the care area. However, this depends on the victim and type of abuse. Adults who are alert and oriented and capable of their decision-making can choose not to report on their own and opt to leave. Depending on the state, nurses may be required to report suspicious injuries to law enforcement whether or not the patient consents or wishes to press charges.

Depending on the type of abuse, the nurse is required to call Adult Protective Services or Child Protective Services and follow it up with a written report. Contacting additional resources, such as social services, may also be a requirement (depending on the organization). . . .

Nurses should be familiar with their state's mandated reporter laws. Employers are typically clear with outlining requirements for their workers, but nurses have a responsibility to know what to do in case they care for a victim of abuse.

Bucceri Androus, A., RN, BSN. (2021, November 23). What Should a Nurse Do If They Suspect a Patient Is a Victim of Abuse? RegisteredNursing.org. Retrieved from www.registerednursing.org/articles/what-should-nurse-do-suspect-patient-victim-abuse/.

Even if you are not considered a mandatory reporter, remember that you are still an agent of your supervising provider. A suspected case of child or elder abuse should be carefully documented and office policy should be closely followed.

Elder abuse is handled at the state and national level, and virtually every state has some form of elder abuse law. Exactly who is protected and from what the legal protection is provided varies from state to state. Federal acts that seek to protect various forms of elder abuse include The Elder Justice Act of 2009, The Older American Acts, and Elder Abuse Victims Act of 2009. See Chapter 4 for a more detailed discussion of elder abuse.

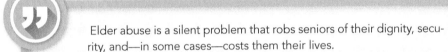

Elder abuse is a silent problem that robs seniors of their dignity, security, and—in some cases—costs them their lives.

Up to five million older Americans are abused every year, and the annual loss by victims of financial abuse is estimated to be at least $36.5 billion. . . .

How many older Americans are abused?

Approximately one in 10 Americans aged 60+ have experienced some form of elder abuse. Some estimates range as high as five million elders who are abused each year. One study estimated that only one in 24 cases of abuse are reported to authorities.

Who are the abusers of older adults?

Abusers are both women and men. In almost 60% of elder abuse and neglect incidents, the perpetrator is a family member. Two thirds of perpetrators are adult children or spouses.

National Council on Aging. (2021, February 23). Get the Facts on Elder Abuse. National Council on Aging. Retrieved from www.ncoa.org/article /get-the-facts-on-elder-abuse.

Controlled Substances Acts

A controlled substance is a drug or a chemical whose manufacture, storage, distribution, and use are controlled by the government because of its potential for misuse or abuse. Notably, not every drug that is controlled is considered to have the potential to be abused. Controlled substances acts restrict the distribution, classification, sale, handling, storage, prescription, and use of controlled substances. These acts cover everyone from criminals who are not involved in health care delivery to health care providers, who hold licenses to write prescriptions, to manufacturers of drugs. Because different states have varying prescription and over-the-counter drug regulations, a federal Controlled Substances Act of 1970 (CSA) was implemented. Most states have enacted the Uniform Controlled Substances Act, which is similar to the CSA.

Despite laws and regulations enacted to ensure the legal and proper dispensing and use of controlled substances, the acts are not foolproof. Controlled substances are not always used for their intended purpose, which has given rise to a black market for prescription drugs.

Methods of Obtaining Prescription Drugs

A review of multiple studies demonstrates a variety of ways individuals obtain prescription drugs. The following summarizes the studies' findings.

- 55% free from a friend or relative
- 20% from a prescriber
- 10% purchased from a friend or relative
- 5% stolen from a friend or relative
- 5% purchased from a drug dealer
- 2% from multiple doctors
- 1% from theft from medical practice or pharmacy
- Less 1% from internet

Preuss, C., Kalava, A., King, K. (2021, February 17). Prescription of Controlled Substances: Benefits and Risks. National Center for Biotechnology Information. Retrieved from www.ncbi.nlm.nih.gov/books/NBK537318/.

Opioids are one example of a controlled substance that has acquired a significant black market. Due to its highly addictive properties, opioid addiction has been a significant concern in the United States. According to The United States Department of Health and Human Service - Substance Abuse and Mental Health Services Administration, "[a]mong people aged 12 or older in 2019, 3.7 percent (or 10.1 million people) misused opioids in the past year."

Substance Abuse and Mental Health Services Administration. (2020, September). Key Substance Use and Mental Health Indicators in the United States: Results from the 2019 National Survey on Drug Use and Health.

Seven years ago, as the opioid epidemic tightened its hold on Erie, Taylor Miller launched an effort to help recovering addicts like herself.

Miller, then 20, said she wanted to do all she could to get her hometown through the heroin-fueled crisis.

Her advocacy, including a candor that made her message so heartfelt and genuine, has been cut short.

Miller, 27, died Sunday at her family's residence in Fairview. She "lost her battle with mental illness and addiction," her family said in her obituary, published in the Erie Times-News on Thursday.

. . . Miller started a Facebook group, H.O.P.E., for Heroin Overdose Prevention in Erie, that raises the awareness of deaths resulting from heroin overdoses. . . .

Palattella, E. (2021, 15 April). Taylor Miller, Advocate in Erie's Opioid Fight, Dies at 27: 'She Fought So Hard'. GoErie. Retrieved from www.goerie.com/story/news/crime/2021/04/16/taylor-miller-opioid-crisis-heroin-advocate-eries-fight-dies-27-losing-battle/7234867002/.

Controlled Substances' Schedules

Controlled substances are further classified into five schedules, which reflect the drug's accepted medical use and its potential for abuse.

Drug Scheduling

Drugs, substances, and certain chemicals used to make drugs are classified into five (5) distinct categories or schedules depending upon the drug's acceptable medical use and the drug's abuse or dependency potential. The abuse rate is a determinate factor in the scheduling of the drug; for example, Schedule I drugs have a high potential for abuse and the potential to create severe psychological and/or physical dependence. As the drug schedule changes—Schedule II, Schedule III, etc., so does the abuse potential—Schedule V drugs represents the least potential for abuse. A Listing of drugs and their schedule are located at Controlled Substance Act (CSA) Scheduling or CSA Scheduling by Alphabetical Order. These lists describe the basic or parent chemical and do not necessarily describe the salts, isomers and salts of isomers, esters, ethers and derivatives which may also be classified as controlled substances. These lists are intended as general references and are not comprehensive listings of all controlled substances.

Please note that a substance need not be listed as a controlled substance to be treated as a Schedule I substance for criminal prosecution. A controlled substance analogue is a substance which is intended for human consumption

(Continues)

(Continued)

and is structurally or pharmacologically substantially similar to or is represented as being similar to a Schedule I or Schedule II substance and is not an approved medication in the United States. (See 21 U.S.C. §802(32)(A) for the definition of a controlled substance analogue and 21 U.S.C. §813 for the schedule.)

Schedule I

Schedule I drugs, substances, or chemicals are defined as drugs with no currently accepted medical use and a high potential for abuse. Some examples of Schedule I drugs are:

heroin, lysergic acid diethylamide (LSD), marijuana (cannabis), 3,4-methylenedioxymethamphetamine (ecstasy), methaqualone, and peyote

Schedule II

Schedule II drugs, substances, or chemicals are defined as drugs with a high potential for abuse, with use potentially leading to severe psychological or physical dependence. These drugs are also considered dangerous. Some examples of Schedule II drugs are:

Combination products with less than 15 milligrams of hydrocodone per dosage unit (Vicodin), cocaine, methamphetamine, methadone, hydromorphone (Dilaudid), meperidine (Demerol), oxycodone (OxyContin), fentanyl, Dexedrine, Adderall, and Ritalin

Schedule III

Schedule III drugs, substances, or chemicals are defined as drugs with a moderate to low potential for physical and psychological dependence. Schedule III drugs abuse potential is less than Schedule I and Schedule II drugs but more than Schedule IV. Some examples of Schedule III drugs are:

Products containing less than 90 milligrams of codeine per dosage unit (Tylenol with codeine), ketamine, anabolic steroids, testosterone

Schedule IV

Schedule IV drugs, substances, or chemicals are defined as drugs with a low potential for abuse and low risk of dependence. Some examples of Schedule IV drugs are:

Xanax, Soma, Darvon, Darvocet, Valium, Ativan, Talwin, Ambien, Tramadol

Schedule V

Schedule V drugs, substances, or chemicals are defined as drugs with lower potential for abuse than Schedule IV and consist of preparations containing limited quantities of certain narcotics. Schedule V drugs are generally used for antidiarrheal, antitussive, and analgesic purposes. Some examples of Schedule V drugs are:

cough preparations with less than 200 milligrams of codeine or per 100 milliliters (Robitussin AC), Lomotil, Motofen, Lyrica, Parepectolin.

United Stated Drug Enforcement Administration. (n.d.). Drug Scheduling. United Stated Drug Enforcement Administration. Retrieved from www.dea.gov/drug-information/drug-scheduling.

Prescribing controlled substances is highly regulated. According to the Shands Jacksonville Drug Report, "Federal law states that a prescription for a controlled substance may be issued only by individual practitioners who are authorized to prescribe controlled substances by the DEA in the jurisdiction where they are licensed to practice their profession. The term 'individual practitioner' includes physicians (MD and DO), dentists (DDS), veterinarians (DVM), and podiatrists (DPM). In the state of Florida, mid-level practitioners such as nurse practitioners, nurse midwives, nurse anesthetists, clinical nurse specialists, and physician assistants are not authorized to prescribe controlled substances."

On June 1, 2010, the Electronic Prescribing for Controlled Substances (EPCS) rules took effect to streamline and improve tracking by eliminating paper prescriptions. According to the DEA, "The rule revises DEA regulations to provide practitioners with the option of writing prescriptions for controlled substances electronically. The regulations also permit pharmacies to receive, dispense, and archive these electronic prescriptions. These regulations are an addition to, not a replacement of, the existing rules. The regulations provide pharmacies, hospitals, and practitioners with the ability to use modern technology for controlled substance prescriptions while maintaining the closed system of controls on controlled substances."

Drug Enforcement Agency

In the health care industry, the DEA is primarily charged with enforcing the Controlled Substances Act, including the distribution, classification, sale, handling, storage, prescription, and use of controlled substances.

> The mission of the Drug Enforcement Administration (DEA) is to enforce the controlled substances laws and regulations of the United States and bring to the criminal and civil justice system of the United States, or any other competent jurisdiction, those organizations and principal members of organizations, involved in the growing, manufacture, or distribution of controlled substances appearing in or destined for illicit traffic in the United States; and to recommend and support non-enforcement programs aimed at reducing the availability of illicit controlled substances on the domestic and international markets.
>
> DEA. (n.d.). Who We Are /About. DEA. Retrieved from www.dea.gov/divisions/about.

United States Pharmacopeia (USP)

The United States Pharmacopeia (USP) is a collection of drug information and standards published by the United States Pharmacopeial Convention. The USP defines standards for prescription drugs, over-the-counter drugs, drugs intended for humans as well as animals, dietary supplements, and some food ingredients. If a specific drug or drug ingredient has a USP quality standard, it is noted via a "USP-NF" marking. And, if that marking is present, the drug or drug ingredient must match the USP standards.

The USP standards are a reference guide for regulating entities, who use them as a benchmark to ensure the products meet the standards. Drug manufacturers also use the USP to ensure its products meet regulatory requirements. Both prescription and over-the-counter drugs must meet the applicable USP standards.

Employment Law

The federal law described in this Employment Law section seeks to ensure employees can work in an environment that is free from discrimination and harassment.

Equal Opportunity Employment

While everyone cannot reach the highest rung on the corporate ladder, the Civil Rights Act of 1964 tells us that the opportunity to do so cannot be denied employees on the basis of race, color, religion, sex, or national origin.

interstate commerce The movement of goods and services, or services that rely on the movement of goods, which cross state borders within the United States.

Title VII of the act prohibits employment discrimination and applies to all employers of 15 or more employees whose business involves **interstate commerce**, to labor unions of 15 or more members, to employment agencies, as well as to state, local, and federal employees. The Equal Employment Opportunity Commission (EEOC) administers and enforces Title VII. Illegal discrimination may be shown by either **disparate treatment** or **disparate impact**.

disparate treatment A marked difference between the way two things are handled.

Disparate Treatment   The most obvious form of discrimination occurs when an employer treats similarly situated employees differently because of their race, sex, religion, or national origin. Because of the difficulty in proving a disparate treatment situation, courts allow plaintiffs to prove disparate treatment indirectly. **Inferences** may be drawn from the acts of the employers. If an employer has been shown to discriminate in the past, the inference will be stronger that the present act involves discrimination.

disparate impact Disproportionate result that seemingly fair practices or policies have upon a protected group.

inference A process of reasoning by which a fact is deduced as a logical consequence of other facts.

Plaintiffs prove their disparate treatment cases by proving the required elements: (1) the plaintiff must be a member of one of the groups protected by Title VII, (2) the plaintiff must be capable of doing the job, and (3) he or she must have been discriminated against.

Disparate Impact   Some employment policies are **facially neutral**, in that they appear to treat all employees equally, but have a "disparate" or "adverse" impact on a particular protected group. For example, a minimum height requirement may discriminate against women, or a maximum weight requirement may discriminate against men.

facially neutral On the surface the matter appears to be impartial.

An employer, faced with the charge of disparate impact, may counter that the policy is justified by business necessity and is related to job performance. In the following case, an employer's business necessity defense was upheld by the court.

Gregory Backus, RN, requested placement as a full-time registered nurse in the labor and delivery section. The hospital refused the request on the basis that it did not employ male RNs on the obstetrics and gynecology units and gave as a reason their concern for female patients' privacy and personal dignity. Backus filed a sex discrimination complaint with the EEOC, alleging that the hospital's refusal to transfer him to the labor and delivery section was discriminatory based on sex.

Testimony in the hospital's defense relied on its policy of recognizing and respecting the privacy rights of its patients. Hospital policy required that catheterizations be performed by individuals of the same sex as the patient. The hospital's policy of restricting nursing positions in labor and delivery came from the fact that obstetrical patients continually have genitals exposed and that there are few duties that a nurse performs that are not sensitive or intimate in nature.

The court decided against Backus and found merit in the hospital's argument that the majority of women patients would object to intimate contact with a member of the opposite sex in the labor and delivery room. The court commented that "in addition to offending patients, a male nurse would necessitate the presence of a female nurse to protect the hospital from charges of molestation. . . . The court refused to consider a male nurse analogous to a male doctor because the doctor, and not the nurse, had been chosen by the patient."

Backus v. Baptist Medical Center, 510 F. Supp. 1191 (1980)

Filing with the EEOC   Most EEOC actions begin with the filing of a Charge of Discrimination by an individual who believes they have been discriminated against. A Charge of Discrimination must be filed within 180 days following the incident, unless the facts warrant an exception that extends the period to 300 days. After a Charge of Discrimination is filed, the EEOC will conduct an investigation.

probable cause Having more evidence for than against.

If the EEOC finds **probable cause** and that Title VII may have been violated, attempts are made to mediate the matter. If the parties are not able to reach agreement, the EEOC issues a Right to Sue Letter to the complaining party, who is free to pursue the matter in a court of law.

Interviewing

Discrimination law has made many changes in the employment interview situation necessary. Employers are not allowed to ask interview questions involving race, religion, age, or whether the interviewee is pregnant. Interview questions must have a legally permissible and non-discriminatory purpose. Sometimes, the mere phrasing of a question can render the question discriminatory. See Table 2-1 for "Interview Questions to Avoid and What to Ask Instead."

Table 2-1 Interview Questions to Avoid and What to Ask Instead

Instead of This	Ask This
How many children do you have?	What days and hours are you able to work?
How old are your children? Or: What arrangements do you have for child care?	Do you have nonwork–related responsibilities what will interfere with specific requirements for the job?
What is your religion? Or: Will you need personal time for particular religious holidays?	Are there specific times that you cannot work?
Do you own a car?	Do you have a reliable method of transportation to get to work?
What is your national origin? Or: Where did you live while growing up?	Are you legally eligible to be employed in the United States?
What is your maiden name?	Have you ever been employed under a different name?
Do you have any disabilities?	Can you perform the duties of the job for which you are applying?
Are or have your wages ever been garnished?	Credit references can be used if in compliance with the Fair Credit Reporting Act of 1970 and the Consumer Credit Reporting Reform Act of 1996.
Do you own your own home?	How long have you resided at your current address? What was your previous address? How long did you live there?
When did you graduate from high school or college?	Do you have a university or college degree, a high school diploma, or equivalent? (Ask only if relevant to job performance.)

Source: Jeanine D'Alusio, J. (2020, February 5). Hiring in Healthcare: Interview Questions to Avoid and What to Ask Instead. Relias. Retrieved from www.relias.com/blog/hiring-in-healthcare-interview-questions-to-avoid-what-to-ask.

It is surprising that a simple interview question can leave your organization vulnerable to risk, but it is true. In fact, an Associated Press and CNBC poll conducted by The Associated Press-NORC Center for Public Affairs Research found that:

- 35% of job seekers have been asked whether they were married (which is against federal law)
- 21% of job seekers have been asked about their medical history or a disability (which can open employers to discrimination lawsuits)
- Overall, 51% of job seekers said they were asked at least one inappropriate or personal question.

Jeanine D'Alusio, J. (2020, February 5). Hiring in Healthcare: Interview Questions to Avoid and What to Ask Instead. Relias. Retrieved from www.relias.com/blog /hiring-in-healthcare-interview-questions-to-avoid-what-to-ask.

Preemployment Testing

Employers are allowed to test potential employees as part of the hiring process, but such tests must be carefully constructed, usually by experts, to ensure that they only measure the skills and abilities necessary to do the job. In *Griggs v. Duke Power Company*, a landmark case in discrimination law, the U.S. Supreme Court established a strict standard, called the business necessity test, for business practices that have an adverse impact on various minority groups. Some forms of testing were determined to be a subtle means of discrimination:

Duke Power Company, a large power-generating corporation in the Carolinas, for years limited blacks to the labor department, the lowest-paying area of the company, and refused to approve requests for transfers to other departments. When Title VII was passed, the company instituted a policy which stated that employees who wanted transfers from the labor department had to present a high school diploma or pass a high school aptitude test. Black employees sued, contending that the company was trying to lock them into their jobs as laborers by imposing unnecessary transfer requirements that they would be unable to meet because of unequal educational opportunities.

(Continues)

(Continued)

The U.S. Supreme Court found that the transfer policies were unlawful because neither the high school completion requirement nor the aptitude test was shown to bear a demonstrable relationship to successful performance of the jobs for which it was used. Under Title VII, the Court declared, "practices, procedures, or tests, neutral on their face, and even neutral in terms of intent, cannot be maintained if they have a discriminatory impact on minorities and are unrelated to measuring job capability." Selection practices that are fair in form but discriminatory in operation can be used only if they are justified by a "business necessity."

Griggs v. Duke Power, 401 U.S. 424 (1971)

Drug Testing

Another area of preemployment testing in which the Supreme Court has made decisions relates to drug testing. Because many hospital employees have responsibilities that directly affect patient care, an argument could be made that drug testing is needed to ensure the public's safety. On the issue of safety, *National Treasure Employees Union v. Von Raab*, 489 U.S. 656 (1989) could be analogous to the situation of health care workers. The Court determined in this decision that mandatory drug tests for applicants and employees seeking promotions to sensitive positions in the U.S. Customs Service were constitutional and permissible. The Supreme Court had previously ruled that drug testing of employees is a "search and seizure" within the realm of the Fourth Amendment, and that each case must be resolved on a case-by-case basis using a balancing test between individual rights and public safety. The *Von Raab* decision considered public policy with public safety outweighing concerns about employees' rights to privacy. Preemployment drug testing is now considered routine in many health care settings, particularly hospitals. The law specifically requires tests that provide "qualitative data" on the presence of drugs or alcohol. The intent of the law is to determine whether the employee is fit for duty.

Chain of Custody   An important aspect of preemployment drug testing is ensuring the specimen is reliable and that it is protected from tampering. A chain of custody form documents information related to the specimen and contains the information shown on Figure 2-1, including:

- Information to identify the person who gave the specimen
- The reason for the tests and the tests being requested
- The type of specimen
- The date, time, and place of the specimen collection and any related comments

- The name of the person who collected the specimen
- Information as to where the specimen was analyzed and how it got there
- The names of other people who had custody of the specimen

Accuracy and completeness are crucial when completing a chain of custody form. The consequences of an incomplete or inaccurate chain of custody form include test result reporting delays, the need to re-run tests, and inaccurate or incomplete results.

USA LABS
ID#
Referred by

Health Care Provider
Address
Phone

DO NOT WRITE IN THIS AREA

CHAIN OF CUSTODY

STEP 1 — TO BE COMPLETED BY EMPLOYER/COLLECTOR.
DONOR IDENTIFICATION—PLEASE PRINT

LAST NAME
FIRST NAME M.I.
SOC. SEC. NO. — —
EMPLOYEE NO.
DONOR I.D. VERIFIED ☐ PHOTO I.D. ☐ EMPLOYER REPRESENTATIVE

SIGNATURE OF EMPLOYER REP.

REASON FOR TEST (CHECK ONE)
☐ (1) PRE-EMPLOYMENT ☐ (2) POST ACCIDENT ☐ (3) RANDOM
☐ (4) PERIODIC ☐ (5) REASONABLE SUSPICION/CAUSE
☐ (6) RETURN TO DUTY
☐ (99) OTHER (SPECIFY)

TESTS REQUESTED: TOTAL TESTS ORDERED ☐

SPECIMEN ☐ Urine ☐ Blood (SUBMIT ONLY ONE SPECIMEN WITH EACH REQUISITION)

STEP 2—COLLECTOR, FOR URINE SPECIMENS, READ TEMPERATURE WITHIN FOUR MINUTES OF COLLECTION.
CHECK THE BOX IF TEMPERATURE IS WITHIN THE SPECIFIED RANGE ☐ 90°–100°F / 32°–38°C
OR RECORD ACTUAL TEMPERATURE HERE: ______

STEP 3—TO BE COMPLETED BY COLLECTOR. COLLECTION SITE

COLLECTION DATE ______ TIME ______ ☐AM PM
ADDRESS
REMARKS ______
CITY STATE ZIP
( )
PHONE

I certify that the specimen identified on this form is the specimen presented to me by the employee identified in Step 1 above, and was collected, labeled and sealed in the donor's presence.

COLLECTOR'S NAME PRINT (FIRST, M.I. LAST) SIGNATURE OF COLLECTOR

STEP 4—TO BE INITIATED BY THE DONOR AND COMPLETED AS NECESSARY THEREAFTER.

PURPOSE OF CHANGE	RELEASED BY SIGNATURE	RECEIVED BY SIGNATURE	DATE
A. PROVIDE SPECIMEN FOR TESTING			
B. SHIPMENT TO LABORATORY			
C.			

COMMENTS:

Self-stick Identification
Labels for sealing specimen:
(123) (123) (123) (123)

SPECIMEN PACKAGE INTEGRITY WAS ☐ACCEPTABLE ☐UNACCEPTABLE WHEN RECEIVED IN LAB.
RECEIVER'S INITIALS

FOR OFFICE USE

Figure 2-1 Sample Chain of Custody Form

Genetic Information Nondiscrimination Act of 2008

Health care insurers and group health care plans may not deny coverage or charge higher premiums based solely on an individual's likelihood of developing a disease in the future. The Genetic Information Nondiscrimination Act of 2008 (GINA) also prohibits employers from using genetic information when hiring, firing, training, or promoting employees. Recent amendments to GINA include requirements that employee wellness programs be voluntary and that the wellness programs cover spousal participation.

Sexual Harassment

Sexual harassment is unwelcome sexual attention at an employee's workplace that establishes a hostile work environment, negatively affects the employee's ability to do their job, or which results in a detrimental change in their job responsibilities. It is one form of discrimination. The harasser can include peers, subordinates, supervisors, customers, vendors, and clients. The prohibited range of behavior includes verbal comments, subtle or overt pressure for sexual activity, leering, pinching, patting, and other forms of unwanted touching as well as rape and attempted rape.

Sexual harassment has been a long-time problem in the workplace, and the health care industry is no exception.

As a leading health care institution, Mayo Clinic has committed to a culture of fairness, equity and safety. To demonstrate its commitment and transparency, Mayo Clinic reviewed all sexual harassment complaints and investigations from September 2017 to September 2019 and published the results in an article, "Addressing Sexual Harassment in the #MeToo Era: An Institutional Approach," in Mayo Clinic Proceedings, a monthly peer-reviewed journal....

Charanjit Rihal, M.D., a Mayo Clinic cardiologist and chair of the Personnel Committee, which oversees physician and scientist employment issues, said Mayo Clinic, as did many other institutions, experienced an increase in sexual harassment allegations in late 2017 and early 2018.

The hospital has "developed a rigorous approach to effectively and consistently address all allegations of harassment." The article reviews how these complaints were handled and whether the process aligned with institutional policies.

Mayo Clinic's Sexual and Other Harassment Policy was updated in 2017, just before the #MeToo movement gained prominence nationally. The policy defines all types of harassment and how complaints are investigated and addressed....

"Clinical care, scientific research and health care education require highly functional teams," says Gianrico Farrugia, M.D., Mayo Clinic's president and CEO, and a study co-author. "When harassment occurs, victims experience serious and potentially lasting damage, team dynamics break down, and patient care may be affected. Clear policies and processes must be in place for addressing harassment of all kinds, but they're only effective if the organization's leaders are committed, set zero-tolerance expectations and follow through."

Insurance Journal. (2020, September 3). How One Hospital Addresses Sexual Harassment Claims and Culture. *Insurance Journal*. Retrieved from www.insurancejournal.com/news/national/2020/09/03/581423.htm.

There are federal and state laws that prohibit sexual harassment in the workplace and require that allegations of sexual harassment be filed with the EEOC before filing a lawsuit. Among other actions it may take, the EEOC may file a federal lawsuit seeking damages on the behalf of the employee, as it did in the following case.

An RN at a pediatric medical practice was allegedly approached by one of the group's physicians, who pressed his groin against her while she was seated at her desk. Approximately two months later, the RN stepped aside to allow the same physician to pass her in the hallway. The physician is alleged to have grabbed and squeezed the RN's hip as he passed.

The RN then reported the incidents to her direct supervisor, the office manager, who directed her to report the physician's conduct to the group's human resources department. Human resources interviewed the RN, and shortly thereafter, informed the RN that it was unable to verify her allegations. The next day, the RN was transferred to another of the group's offices.

The RN shared with the human resource director that the transfer would cause her personal hardship and that a transfer was not needed because the office manager had arranged for the RN and the physician to work on opposite sides of the office. Human resources indicated that there was nothing they could do to change the physician's behavior and working in the new office would allow her to be more at ease.

The RN's role at the new office was to sit at the front desk, answer phones and schedule patient appointments instead of working with patients as she had done at the prior office. The RN's hours were reduced, and she was prohibited from working overtime.

Brent, N., MS, JD, RN. (2020, August 10). EEOC Files Sexual Harassment Lawsuit on a Nurse's Behalf. Nurse.Com. Retrieved from www.nurse.com/blog/2020/08/10/eeoc-files-sexual-harassment-lawsuit-on-a-nurses-behalf/.

The conduct of the medical practice was unlawful under Title VII when it retaliated against the RN for reporting the health care provider's sexual harassment to its human resource personnel. Her sharing of the harassment resulted in a retaliatory change of employment.

The change of employment caused the RN unwarranted difficulty, took away her ability to practice nursing care, reduced her pay, and made working conditions at the new site so difficult she was forced to resign.

Federal Age Discrimination Act

The Federal Age Discrimination in Employment Act of 1967 (FADA) covers age discrimination and protects the rights of older workers. It provides that workers over the age of 40 years cannot arbitrarily be discriminated against in any employment decisions because of age. This includes hiring, discharge, layoff, promotion, wages and other terms and conditions of employment, referrals by employment agencies, and membership in and activities of unions.

The FADA applies to employers with more than 20 employees, and to public and private employers, including state and local governments and their agencies. States individually may have separate laws further protecting workers. The act is administered by the EEOC.

Americans with Disabilities Act

The ADA covers people who have physical as well as mental disabilities in employment, public services, public accommodations, and telecommunications. A *disability* is defined as a physical or mental impairment that substantially limits one or more of the major life activities of an individual, or a record of such impairment, or being regarded as having such an impairment. Specifically, the ADA covers people who have conditions ranging from AIDS to cancer to intellectual disabilities but excludes certain antisocial conditions such as kleptomania, pedophilia, and active illegal drug addiction.

Title I of the act prohibits employment discrimination and places the burden on an employer to prove that the requirements of a specific job could not be changed to accommodate a disabled applicant.

Titles II and III of the act, in part, guarantee the disabled access to the workplace. Professional offices of health care providers are in the public sector and, as such, require an employer to make "reasonable modifications" for disabled people to gain access.

Under the ADA, an employer has a duty to provide reasonable accommodation to the known mental or physical limitations of a qualified individual with a disability. The following case, *Jones v. McDonough*, was brought under The Rehabilitation Act, which provides the exclusive remedy for discrimination claims asserted by federal employees and mirrors the ADA's standard for determining disability. Case law interpreting the ADA has helped to define further what is meant by "disability."

The plaintiff worked as a Financial Accounts Technician with the Department of Veterans Affairs Mid-South Consolidated Patient Account Center ("CPAC") in Smyrna, Tennessee from April 1998 until she retired on December 31, 2014. For several years before she retired, her productivity was at unacceptable levels. During this time, the plaintiff was repeatedly coached on her productivity and advised of the various resources available to help her. In January 2014, the plaintiff was placed on a performance improvement plan (PIP), which if not complied with could result in termination. Plaintiff's performance continued below acceptable productivity levels. The plaintiff's parents both passed away in September 2014, and prior to their death, plaintiff had been the primary caregiver for them. While discussing her performance with her supervisor, she shared that caring for her parents before their deaths, stress, anxiety, lack of sleep, and a possible surgery had put her in crisis. With a continued PIP in place and additional conversations about her productivity, the plaintiff provided a doctor's note indicating that she has had difficulty concentrating. CPAC chose to proceed with a last chance agreement that gave the plaintiff a "last chance" to perform at acceptable productivity levels. Plaintiff declined the last chance agreement, chose to retire, and subsequently filed a discrimination complaint. Defendants filed a motion for summary judgment. The court's Order addressed, among other things, plaintiff's claim that CPAC failed or refused to provide "reasonable accommodation" to allow her to continue working while she addressed an alleged disability.

"Courts are required to make a case by case determination of whether an individual qualifies as 'disabled.'" Doe v. Salvation Army in U.S., 531 F.3d 355, 357 (6th Cir. 2008) (citing Albertson's, Inc. v. Kirkingburg, 527 U.S. 555, 566 (1999)).

Consistent with the statutory definition, courts typically break the disability inquiry into three parts. See, e.g., Bragdon v. Abbott, 524 U.S. 624, 631 (1998). In assessing whether a person has a "disability," a court must determine: "(1) whether the plaintiff has a physical or mental impairment; (2) whether that impairment impacts 'one or more major life activities'; and (3) whether the claimed disability imposes a 'substantial limit[ation]' on that identified major life activity." Hentze v. CSX Transp., Inc., 477 F. Supp. 3d 644, 660 (S.D. Ohio 2020) (citing Bragdon, *Bragdon*, 524 U.S. at 631).

The defendant here focuses on the question of whether the plaintiff has established, as a threshold matter, that she has a "physical or mental impairment." In particular, he points out that the plaintiff has not provided any medical documentation to support the existence of a recognized impairment.

(Continues)

(Continued)

Although the defendant does not provide case support for his suggestion that medical documentation is required to prove disability—and that is a debatable proposition under prevailing law—the court finds that, under the circumstances presented here, some documentation is required. The court, therefore, agrees that the plaintiff has failed to establish that she suffers from a mental (or other) impairment.

The only "medical" evidence of a "mental impairment" that the plaintiff has offered—and, indeed, the only medical evidence in the court's record—is Dr. Ahmad's note dated October 6, 2014. As quoted above, Dr. Ahmad's note identified only the functional limitations the plaintiff herself had described to him: Jones told him that she was having "difficulty concentrating and her productivity has been going down." (Doc. No. 34-7.)

. . .

In sum, the court finds, as a matter of law, that depression and anxiety, in order to qualify as an impairment under the ADA, must actually have been diagnosed by a medical professional, even if the condition does not actually meet all of the criteria for a disorder as defined by the DSM.

Susan H. Jones v. Denis R. McDonough, Case 3:19-cv-00310 M.D. Tenn (2021, March 15).

In *Griece Mills v. Derwinski*, 967 F.2d 794 (2d Cir. 1992), a hospital was not required to accommodate the request of a head nurse suffering from depression to report to work at 10:00 a.m., as such accommodation would have imposed "undue hardship" on the hospital. In defining *undue hardship*, the ADA requires consideration of the following factors:

- the nature and cost of the accommodation needed,
- the overall finances of the facility,
- the overall resources of the covered entity, and
- the type of operation or operations of the covered entity.

Notably, an employer is obligated only to accommodate "known" physical or mental limitations of a disabled worker.

Employee Wages and Benefits

Equal Pay Act

Violations of the Equal Pay Act are a form of gender discrimination actionable under Title VII. The Act was passed in 1963 to end the practice of paying women less than men for the same job. Equal work is defined as work requiring substantially similar "skill, effort, and responsibility." It does not mean equal pay for comparable work. The comparable worth theory is based on the premise that particular jobs have been traditionally underpaid because they have been held primarily by women. The 2009 Lilly Ledbetter Fair Pay Act ensured that victims of unequal pay would have enough time to commence a lawsuit. The Act made clear that the 180-day statute of limitations for filing an equal-pay lawsuit begins with each paycheck issued.

Fair Labor Standards Act

State and federal laws regulate employees' wages, hours, and working conditions. The Fair Labor Standards Act (FLSA) establishes a federal minimum wage, mandates extra pay for overtime work, regulates the employment of children, and is administered by the Department of Labor.

Under the FLSA, Congress periodically adjusts the minimum wage rate. The minimum wage applies to all employers who are involved in interstate commerce but exempts executives, administrators, professional employees, outside salespersons, state employees, and agricultural workers. Overtime is considered to be any hours worked in excess of 40 hours per week and must be compensated at one and one-half times the employee's regular rate of pay.

Health care professionals are often confronted with issues involving overtime pay. Note, however, that employees who are paid an annual salary are not paid overtime. Overtime must be paid to hourly employees for work permitted but not necessarily required. For example, an employee may voluntarily work overtime without being required by the employer to put in extra hours, or it may be necessary for an employee to work through lunch or after hours to complete the job. In either case, the employee is entitled to overtime pay.

Family and Medical Leave Act

The Family and Medical Leave Act of 1993 (FMLA) requires employers of 50 or more people to provide up to 12 weeks of unpaid leave each year for the "serious health condition" of an employee or member of the employee's immediate family or for the birth or adoption of a child. The FMLA covers:

- all public employers,
- private employers who have 50 or more employees on the payroll during each of 20 or more calendar workweeks in either the current or preceding calendar year, and
- employees who have been employed for at least 12 months and who have worked at least 1,250 hours in the 12 months preceding commencement of the FMLA leave.

In 2010, the Department of Labor clarified the FMLA definition of "son and daughter" to "ensure that an employee who assumes the role of caring for a child receives parental rights to family leave regardless of the legal or biological relationship." In 2015, the Department of Labor issued a final rule that amended the regulatory definition of "spouse" under the FMLA. The amended definition makes clear that "eligible employees in legal, same-sex marriages will be able to take FMLA leave to care for their spouse or family member, regardless of where they live. This will ensure that the FMLA will give spouses in same-sex marriages the same ability as all spouses to fully exercise their FMLA rights."

Workers' Compensation

Workers' compensation laws are administered by state governments and create a mandatory insurance system that reimburses employees for losses sustained because of work-related injury or disease, regardless of fault. Losses include the cost of medical care, lost income, and rehabilitation expenses. It also provides continuing payments to the spouses and/or children of workers who die of occupational disease or injury. The law applies to all industrial, service, private, state, and local government employees and is paid for by the employer.

Social Security

Social security includes several related programs: retirement, disability, and dependent's/survivor's benefits. Each part has its own set of rules regarding who is qualified to receive benefits and has its own schedule of payment of benefits. Benefits are paid to the retired or disabled worker and/or the worker's dependent or surviving family. The amount paid is based on the worker's average wages while working in employment covered by social security during his or her working life.

To receive social security benefits, an individual must accumulate a predetermined number of work credits in qualified employment. Work credits are measured in quarters of a year (three months) during which time the individual was employed earning the required minimum wage or more.

Retirement Benefits   Retirement benefits require a total of 40 quarters or 10 years of work credit from covered employment. An individual becomes eligible for retirement benefits at age 62 years. If the person chooses to retire at 62 years of age, the monthly benefit payment will be considerably less than if retirement takes place at 65 years of age. Under new regulations, retirement benefits will not be available until 67 years of age.

Disability Benefits   Disability benefits are paid to individuals who are disabled. Any medical condition that prevents an individual from being gainfully employed may be considered a disability, particularly if it is included on the list of disabling conditions found on the Social Security Administration's list. There are special provisions for people who are blind.

Dependent's Benefits   Certain dependents of a retired or disabled worker are eligible for monthly dependent's benefits if the worker is eligible for retirement or disability benefits.

Survivor's Benefits   Surviving family members of a deceased worker may be entitled to survivor's benefits. To ensure fair and equitable distribution of survivor's benefits, the Social Security Administration lists survivors who are eligible.

Medicare and Medicaid

Medicare is a federal insurance program for people who are entitled to Medicare from their social security contributions and payment of premiums. Everyone 65 years of age or older, regardless of income, is entitled to Medicare coverage, as are some people on social security disability and everyone with permanent kidney failure.

Medicare Hospital Insurance, known as Part A, provides basic coverage for inpatient hospitalization and posthospital nursing and home health care. In addition, it provides limited coverage for rehabilitation in nonacute care hospital facilities. There is a yearly deductible.

Medicare Medical Insurance, known as Part B, pays 80 percent of "reasonable" charges for health care providers' fees, outpatient hospital and laboratory work, medical equipment and supplies, home health care, therapy, and so on. A monthly premium is charged for Part B.

In 2005, in response to rapidly increasing costs of prescription drugs, Congress passed a significant expansion to Medicare, creating Part D, coverage for many medications that was effective January 1, 2006. Enrollment is voluntary; there is a deductible, and a co-payment, and a "donut hole."

> The Medicare Part D donut hole or coverage gap is the phase of Part D coverage after your initial coverage period. You enter the donut hole when your total drug costs—including what you and your plan have paid for your drugs—reaches a certain limit. In 2021, that limit is $4,130. While in the coverage gap, you are responsible for a percentage of the cost of your drugs.

(Continues)

(Continued)

How does the donut hole work?

The donut hole closed for all drugs in 2021, meaning that when you enter the coverage gap you will be responsible for 25% of the cost of your drugs. In the past, you were responsible for a higher percentage of the cost of your drugs.

Although the donut hole has closed, you may still see a difference in cost between the initial coverage period and the donut hole. For example, if a drug's total cost is $100 and you pay your plan's $20 copay during the initial coverage period, you will be responsible for paying $25 (25% of $100) during the coverage gap.

How do I get out of the donut hole?

In all Part D plans, you enter catastrophic coverage after you reach $6,550 in out-of-pocket costs for covered drugs. This amount is made up of what you pay for covered drugs and some costs that others pay. During this period, you pay significantly lower copays or coinsurance for your covered drugs for the remainder of the year. The out-of-pocket costs that help you reach catastrophic coverage include:

- Your deductible
- What you paid during the initial coverage period
- Almost the full cost of brand-name drugs (including the manufacturer's discount) purchased during the coverage gap
- Amounts paid by others, including family members, most charities, and other persons on your behalf
- Amounts paid by State Pharmaceutical Assistance Programs (SPAPs).

Medicare Rights Center. (n.d.). The Part D Donut Hole. Medicare Rights Center. Retrieved from www.medicareinteractive.org /get-answers/medicare-prescription-drug-coverage-part-d /medicare-part-d-costs/the-part-d-donut-hole.

Medicaid is a program jointly administered by the federal government and state government. For that reason, rules vary from state to state. Medicaid is provided for low-income individuals and is obtainable through local social services or welfare departments. States can, and do, change both the eligibility requirements and the reimbursement rates in response to changing budget realities. In addition, many providers will not accept Medicaid patients because the reimbursement is so low.

Employee Retirement Income Security Act

The Employee Retirement Income Security Act (ERISA) protects and regulates pensions. A pension is an agreement between an employee and an employer under which each contributes a certain amount of money while the employee works for the employer. These contributions create a fund from which the employee is paid a certain amount of money upon retirement, usually at the age of 65 years.

In the past, many employers and employees contributed to pension plans, but employees often did not collect or benefit at retirement for the following reasons: People changed jobs and had to leave their pension rights behind; workers were terminated just before they reached retirement age; and pension plans, or whole companies, went out of business.

Since the passage of ERISA in 1974, some of the abuses of pensions have been controlled. The act sets minimum standards for pension plans guaranteeing that a worker's pension rights cannot be unfairly denied.

Health Insurance Portability and Accountability Act of 1996   The Health Insurance Portability and Accountability Act of 1996 (HIPAA) is an expansion of ERISA and an outgrowth of managed care. HIPAA amends ERISA by guaranteeing renewal and transferability of health insurance coverage to those who already have coverage and to their dependents. One of the HIPAA's mandates has been to prohibit discrimination in issuing health insurance coverage. The HIPAA nondiscrimination provision generally prohibits group health plans and group health insurance issuers from discriminating against participants or beneficiaries based on any "health factor."

In forming its patterns for analyzing discrimination, HIPAA used the term "similarly situated" to identify different groups: full-time versus part-time, northerners versus southerners, male versus female, those with diabetes versus those without, different occupations, and so forth. An example of illegal discrimination is a group health insurance plan that excludes individuals who participate in certain recreational activities, such as motorcycling.

HIPAA has many rules, and compliance is required for Medicare reimbursement. Compliance is mandatory for all health care organizations that send or receive standard electronic transactions for health claims or other health plan information. Emphasis is placed on patient privacy regulations (covered more completely in Chapter 10) and staff training. Regulations regarding health care are increasing at the state and federal level, with the most significant being the Health Information Portability and Accountability Act of 1996 (HIPAA).

Occupational Safety and Health Act

Congress enacted the Occupational Safety and Health Act (OSHA) in 1970. This act now is in effect in hospitals and other health care facilities. The OSHA rules and regulations are intended to prevent injuries and promote job safety, and OSHA is authorized to enforce its standards through complaint, inspection, and investigation.

The OSHA places employers under the general duty to provide a workplace free from "recognized hazards"—for example, undue exposure to toxic substances, inoperable safety equipment, poor air quality, and excessive noise levels. In addition, OSHA requires detailed records of job-related injuries and may conduct unannounced workplace inspections to assess an employer's compliance.

OSHA can assess penalties of as high as \$136,532 for repeated or willful violations. Although OSHA protects employees' rights, it also imposes responsibilities on employees. Employees may not be discharged or discriminated against for filing a complaint or testifying against an employer due to violations of OSHA regulations.

Employee Right to Know

Right-to-know regulations, originated by OSHA for the protection of industrial workers, now extend to cover health care workers. The right-to-know legislation grew directly out of concerns about hazardous substances and their health effects. The underlying purpose of the law is to make certain that all employees have an opportunity to know what chemicals they are handling, the potential health effects of those chemicals, and ways to prevent or reduce health risks.

These regulations give each employee the right to (1) a complete list of all hazardous chemicals used in the workplace, (2) the contents of every product and the hazards involved in its use, (3) education about hazardous chemicals with which an employee may come in contact, and (4) protective equipment to use when handling dangerous chemicals.

The law addresses toxic and poisonous chemicals, corrosive irritants, flammable materials, and carcinogens. It requires that each product be labeled. There are three types of labels: written labels with extensive information about the chemical; an encoded label with fire, reactivity, and health hazards categories coded 1–4 for severity; and symbolic labels.

Material Safety Data Sheets (MSDSs) on every product must be made available to each employee upon request. These sheets list every ingredient in the product. Every health care should have an MSDS notebook, which is updated regularly.

Special regulations regarding chemical spills prevent workers from cleaning up a spill until the MSDS has been checked to determine whether there are any hazards or necessary precautions. Each spill requires an incident report listing the name of the chemical and the details of the spill—where it took place, the time, the date, who was involved, and what was done to clean it up.

Regulations for Blood-Borne Pathogens

Providers must comply with OSHA's Bloodborne Pathogens regulation (29 CFR 1910.1030), which establishes standards for exposure incidents involving blood-borne pathogens. OSHA defines an exposure incident as "a specific eye, mouth, other mucous membrane, non-intact skin, or parenteral contact with blood or other potentially infectious materials (OPIM), as defined in the standard that results from the performance of a worker's duties." OSHA. (2011, January). Bloodborne Pathogens—Bloodborne

Pathogen Exposure Incidents. See Figure 2-2. The regulations cover both administrative and clinical aspects of practice.

Potentially infectious materials, in addition to products made from human blood, include semen, vaginal secretions, cerebrospinal fluid, synovial fluid, pleural fluid, pericardial fluid, saliva in dental procedures, any body fluid that is visibly contaminated with blood, and all body fluids in situations where it is difficult or impossible to differentiate between body fluids.

Regulations require universal precautions: a written exposure control plan; a list of all job classifications in which employees have occupational exposure; engineering and work practice controls; procedures for disposal of waste and sharps; availability of protective equipment, including gloves; a written schedule and method for housecleaning and decontamination, including laundry; postexposure evaluation processes; and employee training. Orange-red or fluorescent orange warning labels with the biohazard legend must be affixed to containers of regulated waste, to refrigerators and freezers containing infectious materials, and to containers used to transport them.

The regulations order employers to offer hepatitis B vaccines free of charge to every employee who can be reasonably anticipated to have skin, eye, mucous membrane, or parenteral contact with blood or other potentially infectious materials. The employee has no obligation to accept the employer's offer of a free vaccine. Figure 2-2 identifies what to do in the case of an exposure incident.

Evaluating and Controlling Exposure

Studies show that as many as one-third of all sharps injuries occur during disposal. Nurses are particularly at risk, as they sustain the most needlestick injuries. The Centers for Disease Control and Prevention (CDC) estimates that 62 to 88 percent of sharps injuries can be prevented simply by using safer medical devices.

. . .

Post-exposure Evaluation

According to the NIOSH Alert Preventing Needlestick Injuries in Health Care Settings, it is estimated that 600,000 to 800,000 needlestick injuries (NSIs) and other percutaneous injuries (PIs) occur annually among health care workers. PIs are caused by sharp objects such as hypodermic needles, scalpels, suture needles, wires, trochanters, surgical pins, and saws. Additional exposure incidents include splashes and other contact with mucous membranes or non-intact skin. Post-exposure management is an integral part of a complete program for preventing infection following exposure incidents.

United States Department of Labor. (n.d.). Bloodborne Pathogens and Needlestick Prevention. United States Department of Labor. Retrieved from www.osha.gov /bloodborne-pathogens/evaluating-controlling-exposure.

OSHA® FactSheet

Bloodborne Pathogen Exposure Incidents

OSHA's Bloodborne Pathogens standard (29 CFR 1910.1030) requires employers to make immediate confidential medical evaluation and follow-up available for workers who have an exposure incident, such as a needlestick. An exposure incident is a specific eye, mouth, other mucous membrane, non-intact skin, or parenteral contact with blood or other potentially infectious materials (OPIM), as defined in the standard that results from the performance of a worker's duties.

Reporting an Exposure Incident

Exposure incidents should be reported immediately to the employer since they can lead to infection with hepatitis B virus (HBV), hepatitis C virus (HCV), human immunodeficiency virus (HIV), or other bloodborne pathogens. When a worker reports an exposure incident right away, the report permits the employer to arrange for immediate medical evaluation of the worker. Early reporting is crucial for beginning immediate intervention to address possible infection of the worker and can also help the worker avoid spreading bloodborne infections to others. Furthermore, the employer is required to perform a timely evaluation of the circumstances surrounding the exposure incident to find ways of preventing such a situation from occurring again.

Reporting is also important because part of the follow-up includes identifying the source individual, unless the employer can establish that identification is infeasible or prohibited by state or local law, and determining the source's HBV and HIV infectivity status. If the status of the source individual is not already known, the employer is required to test the source's blood as soon as feasible, provided the source individual consents. If the individual does not consent, the employer must establish that legally required consent cannot be obtained. If state or local law allows testing without the source individual's consent, the employer must test the individual's blood, if it is available. The results of these tests must be made available to the exposed worker and the worker must be informed of the laws and regulations about disclosing the source's identity and infectious status.

Medical Evaluation and Follow-up

When a worker experiences an exposure incident, the employer must make immediate confidential medical evaluation and follow-up available to the worker. This evaluation and follow-up must be: made available at no cost to the worker and at a reasonable time and place; performed by or under the supervision of a licensed physician or other licensed healthcare professional; and provided according to the recommendations of the U.S. Public Health Service (USPHS) current at the time the procedures take place. In addition, laboratory tests must be conducted by an accredited laboratory and also must be at no cost to the worker. A worker who participates in post-exposure evaluation and follow-up may consent to have his or her blood drawn for determination of a baseline infection status, but has the option to withhold consent for HIV testing at that time. In this instance, the employer must ensure that the worker's blood sample is preserved for at least 90 days in case the worker changes his or her mind about HIV testing.

Post-exposure prophylaxis for HIV, HBV, and HCV, when medically indicated, must be offered to the exposed worker according to the current recommendations of the U.S. Public Health Service. The post-exposure follow-up must include counseling the worker about the possible implications of the exposure and his or her infection status, including the results and interpretation of all tests and how to protect personal contacts. The follow-up must also include evaluation of reported illnesses that may be related to the exposure.

Figure 2-2 OSHA Fact Sheet: Bloodborne Pathogen Exposure Incidents

Written Opinion

The employer must obtain and provide the worker with a copy of the evaluating healthcare professional's written opinion within 15 days of completion of the evaluation. According to OSHA's standard, the **written opinion** should only include: whether hepatitis B vaccination was recommended for the exposed worker; whether or not the worker received the vaccination, and that the healthcare provider informed the worker of the results of the evaluation and any medical conditions resulting from exposure to blood or OPIM which require further evaluation or treatment. Any findings other than these are not to be included in the written report.

Additional Information

For more information, go to OSHA's Bloodborne Pathogens and Needlestick Prevention Safety and Health Topics web page at: https://www.osha.gov/SLTC/bloodbornepathogens/index.html.

To file a complaint by phone, report an emergency, or get OSHA advice, assistance, or products, contact your nearest OSHA office under the "U.S. Department of Labor" listing in your phone book, or call us toll-free at **(800) 321-OSHA (6742)**.

This is one in a series of informational fact sheets highlighting OSHA programs, policies or standards. It does not impose any new compliance requirements. For a comprehensive list of compliance requirements of OSHA standards or regulations, refer to Title 29 of the Code of Federal Regulations. This information will be made available to sensory-impaired individuals upon request. The voice phone is (202) 693-1999; teletypewriter (TTY) number: (877) 889-5627.

For assistance, contact us. We can help. It's confidential.

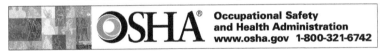

**OSHA® Occupational Safety
and Health Administration
www.osha.gov 1-800-321-6742**

DSG 1/2011

Figure 2-2 (Continued)

Working Conditions

The working conditions in a health care office should be defined in individual job descriptions, office handbooks, and procedure manuals.

Job Description

Each position in an office should have a job description. There are as many formats for job descriptions as there are jobs. At a minimum, job descriptions include the responsibilities and skills required for that position. Figure 2-3 shows excerpts from actual job descriptions found online.

Example: Dental Assistant Job Description Excerpt of Responsibilities and Skills

Responsibilities include:

- Work as a team and utilizes expertise as a dental assistant in assisting the dentist in all clinical procedures. Effectively prepare operatory with materials and instruments for dental procedure.
- Maintains material knowledge up to date as provided by manufacturers.
- Properly prepare dental restorative materials in a timely and effective manner.
- Properly prepare necessary solutions on a daily/weekly basis required for dental use.
- Appropriately maintain state equipment and instruments through lubrication, sterilization and daily cleaning.
- Accurately expose and file digital x-rays.
- Accurately document records as instructed by dentist and the CHD Standard Operating Procedures.
- Handles Behavior Management cases as dictated by the American Association of Pediatric Dentistry
- Accurately enters patient information into approved electronic health record
- Schedules clinic appointments in Eaglesoft, registers clients in HMS, controls flow of dental clinic patients and clinic schedules.
- Maintain patient records
- In a courteous and accurate manner, inform public of clinic procedures, CHD services and refer to other agencies as needed.
- Travel to all clinics as requested.
- Complies with security procedure guidelines.
- Adheres to uniformity of dental procedures countywide as approved by Dental Service Manager
- Instruct patient/parents (guardian) in oral hygiene utilizing appropriate aids

Knowledge, Skills and Abilities necessary for this position:

- Knowledge of dental procedures, expanded functions, dental materials, dental terminology, and behavior management.
- Knowledge of Electronic Records and digital radiographs.
- Skills on preparation of dental materials, skills on sterilization and infection control, skills on equipment maintenance.
- Skills on delivery of expanded functions, skills on record keeping, computer skills, skills on efficient patient flow.
- Ability to communicate with children, parents, co-workers, in general.
- Ability to learn insurance procedures
- Ability to work well with others.
- Ability to avoid and resolve conflict in a professional manner.
- Ability to drive to satellite clinics.

Figure 2-3 Excerpts of Responsibilities and Skills from Online Dental Assistant Job Descriptions

---

Example: Medical Assistant Job Description Excerpt of Job Responsibilities

- Should be able to schedule and change appointments on the telephone and electronically
- Should show care and compassion to patients, including newborns, young children, adolescents and parents.
- Responsible in taking patients to the room and keeping rooms clean and tidy.
- Responsible for sanitizing rooms following each patient.
- Responsible for checking vital signs, including heights, weights, temps, blood pressures, heart rate, pulse-ox, vision, and hearing evaluations
- Must be efficient in documenting in electronic medical record accurately.
- Must be experienced in safe and accurate vaccination administration and documentation.
- Must be able to call patients with normal lab results or telephone messages from the health care provider.
- Must have excellent time management skills, able to multitask and prioritize work.
- Should help with inventory; access state immunization records; prepare school forms.
- Must be able to work well with others, as well as independently.
- Must have excellent written and verbal communication skills in English.

Figure 2-3 *(Continued)*

Procedures Manual

In addition to the job description, each office should have a procedures manual, which describes in detail how to perform the responsibilities included as part of your job description. It is an invaluable educational tool for new employees, as well as an invaluable resource for substitutes when a regular health care professional is out of the office. Written standard office procedures help maintain high standards of patient care, protect against the omission of important steps, ensure compliance with government and third-party regulations, and—when followed—decrease the possibility of a malpractice action. They help to address the **risk management** goals for the office, as well as maintaining **quality assurance**.

If a patient is injured during a procedure and the guidelines for performing the procedure as written in the procedures manual were not followed, the health care employee could be **negligent per se** without **mitigating** circumstances. If an employee is injured during the performance of a procedure and the guidelines for performing the procedure were not followed, the employee could be found contributorily negligent. In contrast, following the procedures manual could prove the employee and/or the health care provider did nothing negligent.

risk management The practice of considering the risk of actions taken and taking steps to minimize the undesired risks of those actions.

quality assurance Procedures and protocols that maintain a stated level of quality of care received by patients.

negligent per se Conduct that is not aligned with the applicable standard of care and without more can be deemed negligence.

mitigating Make less severe due to considerations of fairness and mercy.

Employee Handbook

The Employee Handbook typically provides personnel policies and related instructions. It includes information about work hours, sick leave, pension benefits, evaluation procedures, dress code, conduct toward colleagues and patients, and so on. If the company is unionized, the handbook cannot be changed without negotiating with the union, whereas if the employees are not protected by a union, handbook changes are usually placed in a prominent place to put employees on notice prior to company policy change. The handbook is an important document that you should review and understand in the early stages of your employment.

Unions and Health Care Workers

The history of the organization of health care workers dates back to 1919, when the first known attempt to organize hospital employees took place in San Francisco. The issues at the time were shorter hours and improved working conditions. In 1936, the American Federation of Labor organized engine room, laundry, and dietary employees; nurse's aides; and orderlies in three San Francisco hospitals. Since 1946, the ANA (American Nurses' Association) has supported **collective bargaining**, and most registered nurses have chosen their state nurses' association as their collective bargaining representative. In August 1974, Public Law 93-360 amended the National Labor Relations Act (NLRA) to include nonprofit hospitals and health care institutions. By bringing hospitals, convalescent homes, HMOs, health clinics, nursing homes, and extended care facilities under the NLRA, Congress set the stage for the collective bargaining relationship between management and employees in these institutions.

collective bargaining
Procedural attempt to achieve collective agreements between an employer and accredited representative of a group of employees, to improve the conditions of employment.

i

In September, after six months of exhausting work battling the pandemic, nurses at Mission Hospital in Asheville, N.C., voted to unionize. The vote passed with 70%, a high margin of victory in a historically anti-union state, according to academic experts who study labor movements.

The nurses had originally filed paperwork to hold this vote in March but were forced to delay it when the pandemic began heating up. And the issues that had driven them toward unionizing were only heightened by the crisis. It raised new, urgent problems too, including struggles to get enough PPE, and inconsistent testing and notification of exposures to COVID-positive patients.

They're far from alone in their complaints. For months now, front-line health workers across the country have faced a perpetual lack of personal protective equipment, or PPE, and inconsistent safety measures. Studies show they're more likely to be infected by the coronavirus than the general population, and hundreds have died, according to reporting by KHN and The Guardian.

Many workers say employers and government systems that are meant to protect them have failed. . . .

"The urgency and desperation we've heard from workers is at a pitch I haven't experienced before in 20 years of this work," said Cass Gualvez, organizing director for Service Employees International Union-United Healthcare Workers West in California. "We've talked to workers who said, 'I was dead set against a union five years ago, but COVID has changed that.'"

Labor experts say it's too soon to know if the outrage over working conditions will translate into an increase in union membership, but early indications suggest a small uptick. Of the approximately 1,500 petitions for union representation posted on the National Labor Relations Board website in 2020, 16% appear related to the health care field, up from 14% the previous year.

A nurse for 30 years, Amy Waters had always been aware of a mostly unspoken but widespread sentiment that talking about unions could endanger her job. But after HCA Healthcare took over Mission Health in 2019, she saw nurses and support staff members being cut and she worried about the effect on patient care. Joining National Nurses United could help, she thought. During the pandemic, her fears only worsened. At times, nurses cared for seven patients at once, despite research indicating four is a reasonable number.

Pattani, A. (2021, January 11). For Health Care Workers, The Pandemic
Is Fueling Renewed Interest in Unions. Kaiser Health News.
Retrieved from www.npr.org/sections/health-shots/2021/01/11/955128562
/for-health-care-workers-the-pandemic-is-fueling-renewed-interest-in-unions.

People join unions for many reasons, primarily because of dissatisfaction with wages, benefits, or working conditions. The job you hold determines the **bargaining unit** you may join. When a union is organized, the employer and the union are obligated to bargain in good faith with one another.

Among nurses, collective bargaining is relatively well established but still is a controversial and emotional subject. Unions have had mixed results in organizing hospital clerical personnel. Health maintenance organizations and other alternative health delivery systems offer a fertile field for union organizers. Whether to join a union is a personal decision that depends on an individual's philosophy. It requires considerable self-examination and a weighing of the positive and negative aspects of union membership.

bargaining unit The labor union, or group of employees with similar interests, authorized to conduct negotiations on behalf of the employees who are members of the union or group.

☑ SUMMARY

- Because medicine is heavily regulated by state and federal law, health care professionals need to be aware of laws and regulations that define the areas they work in, procedures they are permitted to perform, and the licensing of providers, nurses, health care professionals, etc.
- There are some circumstances that require mandatory reporting of injury, deaths, or child or elder abuse.
- The Controlled Substances Act regulates the prescription and use of controlled substances.
- Discrimination, including sexual discrimination, is an issue in the hiring and promotion of employees, and there are laws to prevent and punish it.
- The Equal Pay Act prevents the practice of paying women less than men for the same job. The FLSA establishes a federal minimum wage, mandates extra pay for overtime work, and regulates the employment of children. The ERISA involves pensions.
- The OSHA affects health care workers, particularly with regulations involving right-to-know laws and blood-borne pathogens.
- Workers' compensation and Social Security affect every employer and employee.
- Medicare and Medicaid are government-sponsored health care delivery and compensation systems.
- Procedures manuals, job descriptions, and employee handbooks are all part of the business side of a medical practice.
- People join unions for many reasons, primarily because of dissatisfaction with wages, benefits, or working conditions.

SUGGESTED ACTIVITIES

1. It has become more common for the news to report on incidents of workplace sexual harassment. The "#MeToo" movement that encouraged those who had experienced workplace harassment to stand up also provided a platform to discuss the specifics of their stories. Have you learned of specific instances of harassment that you did not realize were considered harassment? What were they? Did learning about them change your behavior in any way?

2. Find the website for a cleaning product you like. Does it have an MSDS posted anywhere on the website? Do they have a number

to call if you want the product's MSDS or can you download a pdf from the manufacturer's website? Are there any ingredients on that product that you are allergic to or try to avoid? Will you still use the product now that you know what it is made of?

3. Have you or someone you know ever been asked an inappropriate interview question? What was it? Was there a way the question could have been phrased so it was not discriminatory?

STUDY QUESTIONS

1. Draft two interview questions that should be asked during an interview for your expected area of expertise and two interview questions that should not be asked.

2. Explain whether it is discriminatory to ask an interview question that seeks to find out if the candidate has had a COVID-19 vaccine? Does your answer change if the interview is for a job as a nurse in an emergency room? What if the candidate in this scenario was interviewing for a remote medical bill coder position?

3. What Act would you reference if a coworker asked you if she would be able to take time away from work for several weeks to care for her sick child?

4. You experience an accidental needle stick with a needle that had been used for a patient. What should you do? What must your employer do?

CASES FOR DISCUSSION

1. Joan Leikvold was hired by Valley View Community Hospital as an operating room supervisor in 1972. She did not have a contract for a specific duration, nor was she told that the hospital would not discharge her except for cause. She was provided with a policy manual and told that the policies were to be followed in her employment relationship with the hospital. In 1978, she became the director of nursing. In October 1979, she requested a transfer back to her former position in the operating room. The chief executive officer (CEO) felt that it was inadvisable for someone who had been in a managerial position to take a subordinate position. Leikvold withdrew the transfer request but was subsequently fired. Her personnel record indicated "insubordination" as the reason for discharge.

Leikvold was an at-will employee. *At-will* means that there is a contract made for an indefinite duration and either party, employer or employee, may terminate the contract at any time for any reason, or without reason, provided the reason is not discriminatory. Can the CEO fire Leikvold?

2. Lavette Midstread was a single, mid-level executive in a close-knit hospitality company that socialized together after hours. Angelo Markus, a married, out-of-town senior executive joined the rest of the staff for drinks when he was in town. During the first outing that Midstread attended with Markus, he made a very direct sexual proposal, to which Midstread diplomatically declined. Thereafter, the executive would stop in Midstread's office and make small talk that made her feel uncomfortable. He would ask about Midstread about her personal life and who she was dating. And, in most instances, he would request that Midstread be the one who drove him back to his hotel after the staff was out socializing. At no time did Midstread tell Markus his conduct was unwelcome for fear of reprisal. One night while other executives were in town and staying at the same hotel, Midstread suggested Markus ride back to the hotel with the other executives. After making a bit of a fuss, Markus rode home with the other visiting executives. The following week, the president called Midstread into his office to say that he and Markus had lost confidence in Midstread's ability to do the job, and he created some unrealistic objectives for her to complete to prove otherwise. She left the company shortly thereafter. Was Markus' conduct harassment? If so, at what point was it considered harassment? When he made the first sexual proposal or at some point later on? If not, why was it not harassment?

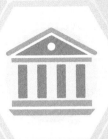

Chapter 3

From the Constitution to the Courtroom

 The powers not delegated to the United States by the Constitution, nor prohibited by it to the States, are reserved to the States respectively, or to the people. **"**

Tenth Amendment to the Constitution of the United States (1791)

Objectives

After reading this chapter, you should be able to:

1. Explain how the Constitution's Supremacy Clause supports a federalist government.
2. Describe the three branches of government.
3. Identify the three levels of the judiciary.
4. Differentiate between federal and state law.
5. Differentiate between origins of statutory, administrative, and common law.
6. Differentiate between criminal and civil law.
7. Describe the four phases of a lawsuit.
8. Explain how a medical record can be used in a lawsuit.
9. Describe techniques that aid in being a good witness.

Building Your Legal Vocabulary

Adjudicate
Arbitration
Assault
Battery
Beyond a reasonable doubt
Civil
Common law
Concurrent
Contingency

Criminal
Cross-examination
Defendant
Deposition
Deterrence
Direct examination
Enumerate
Interrogatory
Judgment

Mediation

Motion

Negligent act

Negotiation

Perjury

Plaintiff

Preponderance of the evidence

Pretrial conference

Reformation

Restraint

Retribution

Standard of proof

Strict liability

Tort

It All Starts with the Constitution

The American system of government and its legal system flow from the Constitution. The Constitution determines whether federal or state law is applicable and enforceable. Federal, state, administrative, and common law all recognize the Supremacy Clause of the U.S. Constitution.

The legal system dictates how disputes are resolved in courts. Once a plaintiff files a lawsuit, the sequence of events is generally the same regardless of whether it is filed in federal or state court. Testifying as a witness in a lawsuit is a serious matter, and preparation is imperative.

When the U.S. Constitution was enacted in 1787, it included a Preamble and seven statements, called Articles, which broadly described how the new nation would function. Since then, 27 Amendments to the Constitution have been added. The Preamble, the Articles, and the Amendments make up the Constitution that provides the structure for federal and state government in the United States.

The Constitution's first three Articles address the separation of powers, which expressly separates the federal government into three distinct branches: the executive (president), the legislative (Congress), and the judicial (federal courts). It is this separation of powers that allows for a system of "checks and balances," where no one branch of government is more powerful than another. The system of checks and balances prevents abuse of power by ensuring that the powers of each branch of government can be reviewed by another branch of government.

concurrent Two or more events happening at the same time.

The concept of "federalism" arises in the Constitution's next three Articles. Federalism is a system of government that, in the United States, recognizes two **concurrent** government structures: the federal and state governments, where each has specific powers. Some of these powers are overlapping. The states govern a majority of everyday legislation and services pursuant to the Constitution. The Supremacy Clause, discussed later, ensures that the federal government can legislate certain matters that fall under one of its enumerated powers, including interstate commerce and foreign relations.

Article I, Section 8 of the Constitution and subsequent Amendments **enumerate** the federal government's powers and responsibilities. These powers and responsibilities are referred to as enumerated powers. The Tenth Amendment clarifies that "[t]he powers not delegated to the United States by the Constitution, nor prohibited by it to the states, are reserved to the states respectively, or to the people."

The first 10 Constitutional Amendments (also referred to as the "The Bill of Rights") define issues of social liberty and justice afforded to U.S. citizens. The remaining 17 Amendments further define issues of social liberty and justice, government structure and protocol, and powers of the federal government. You can find a copy of the Constitution and the Bill of Rights at www.archives.gov.

enumerate To list a number of things.

The Supremacy Clause

A fundamental part of the U.S. government's federalist structure is Article VI, Clause 2 (also referred to as "the Supremacy Clause"), which reads, "[t]his Constitution, and the laws of the United States which shall be made in pursuance thereof; and all treaties made, or which shall be made, under the authority of the United States, shall be the supreme law of the land; and the judges in every state shall be bound thereby, anything in the Constitution or laws of any State to the contrary notwithstanding." Consequently, when there is a conflict between federal and state law, the Supremacy Clause tells us that federal law will govern. There are, however, exceptions to this rule.

Enumerated Powers

The Constitution enumerates the federal government's powers, as well as concurrent powers shared with the states. States may legislate issues that have been constitutionally reserved for the federal government provided the state laws do not conflict with the federal laws.

The Constitution could not expressly define every enumerated power the federal government needs to govern effectively. As a result, disputes arise that challenge the federal government's authority to enact or implement a law. In these instances, courts use legal analysis to decide whether the disputed action by the federal government falls within its enumerated powers.

The Interstate Commerce Clause The Commerce Clause (Article I, Section 8, Clause 3) describes enumerated powers found in the U.S. Constitution. The clause states that the U.S. Congress shall have the power "[t]o regulate commerce with foreign nations, and among the several states, and with the Indian tribes." The Interstate Commerce Clause specifically refers to the federal government's power to legislate "among the several states."

When an act of commerce involves more than one state, the Interstate Commerce Clause is often used as legal authority for Congress to exercise legislative power over state activities. Over many years and many different lawsuits, courts have expanded the definition of "commerce" as it pertains to whether Congress may legislate. A narrow definition of "commerce" is a business transaction. The broad definition includes many types of interaction, both of a business and a social nature.

The Necessary and Proper Clause (Article 1, Section 8, Clause 18) is frequently used together with the Interstate Commerce Clause to further justify Congress' authority to make certain laws. The Necessary and Proper Clause states that Congress is authorized to "make all laws which shall be necessary and proper for carrying into execution the foregoing powers, and all other powers vested by this Constitution in the government of the United States, or in any department or officer thereof." As a result, the Necessary and Proper Clause gives Congress the power to pass laws that are "necessary and proper" to carry out its express powers, which can be interpreted in many ways.

Three Branches of Government

The federal government is divided into three branches: the executive (the president), the legislative (Congress), and the judiciary (federal courts).

Executive Branch

The president and the president's cabinet make up the executive branch. The president appoints the cabinet members, who are then confirmed by the Senate. The cabinet is an advisory committee comprised of the vice president and the heads of 15 federal agencies (each head, with a few exceptions, holds the title of "Secretary"). The federal agencies represented in the cabinet are Department of State, Department of the Treasury, Department of Defense, Attorney General, Department of the Interior, Department of Agriculture, Department of Commerce, Department of Labor, Department of Health and Human Services, Department of Housing and Urban Development, Department of Transportation, Department of Energy, Department of Education, Department of Veterans Affairs, and Department of Homeland Security. The executive branch is responsible for carrying out and executing laws made by Congress.

Congress

Congress is made up of the House of Representatives and the Senate, who together pass legislation. See Figure 3-1, *How an idea becomes a law*. Legislation is also referred to as "statutory law" or "statutes" or "law." Article I, Section 8 of the Constitution enumerates all of Congress'

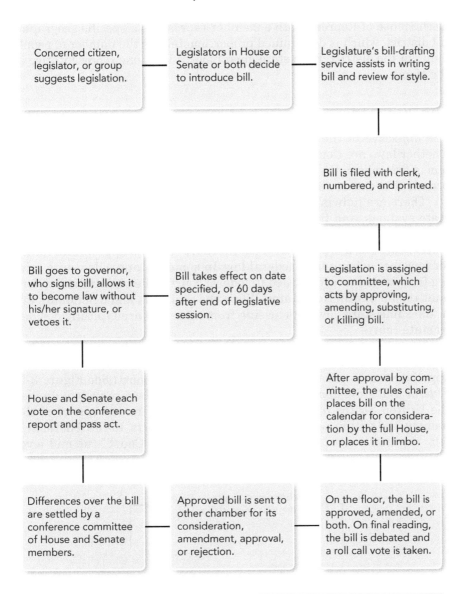

Figure 3-1 How an Idea Becomes a Law

express powers, including the power to tax and to spend those taxes for the citizens' welfare, to borrow money, to create money, to declare war, to regulate immigration, among many others.

Congress has 535 voting members, including 435 Representatives and 100 Senators. Each state has two senators elected to serve 6-year terms. The members of the House of Representatives are each elected for a 2-year term, and there may be no more than 435 at any one time.

Each House of Representative member represents a specific geographical district, which is determined proportionately by the number of people living in the district. Each state must have at least one representative in the House.

The Judiciary

The objective of the federal judicial branch is, in part, to interpret whether laws are Constitutional. As part of the checks and balances system of federalism, the judiciary reviews laws passed by Congress and the president to ensure the laws are Constitutional.

There are judicial branches of government in both the federal and state systems, and they operate very similarly. There are many rules related to jurisdiction, which determines whether a lawsuit belongs in a federal court or a state court. Federal courts are the appropriate forum for lawsuits arising from federal law. In some instances, lawsuits arising from state law are decided in federal court if the plaintiff and defendant reside in different states. When the plaintiffs and defendants are in the same state, lawsuits arising from state law are typically decided by state courts.

The structures of the federal and state legal systems are comparable. There are usually three levels of courts: the trial court, the mid-level appellate court, and the highest-level appellate court. See Figure 3-2, *Federal and state appellate processes*. The federal court system divides the United States into Circuits representing certain regions of the country, and within each Circuit are several Districts. In the federal system, the trial court is referred to as the "District Court," the mid-level

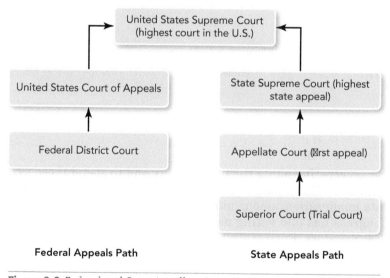

Figure 3-2 Federal and State Appellate Process

appellate court is the "Circuit Court," and the highest court in the land is the "U.S. Supreme Court." There is but one Supreme Court, which is located in Washington, D.C.

Health Care: Federal or State Law?

Health care professionals today regularly face a confusing mix of federal and state law. But this was not always the case. For the most part, in United States' early years, the federal government did not legislate health care. The Constitution does not contain any express federal powers or rights related to health care. The enumerated powers, including the Interstate Commerce Clause, the Supremacy Clause, and the Necessary and Proper Clause have, however, played a part in allowing the federal government to legislate health care.

After the Great Depression in the early 1930s, President Franklin D. Roosevelt instituted The New Deal programs focused, in part, on citizen welfare, including Social Security. The spirit of these programs was continued when President Lyndon B. Johnson created additional federal programs related to health care in the 1960s. Medicare was created then as a federal health insurance program that assists qualifying citizens with disabilities and those who are at least retirement age. Medicaid was, and still is, a joint federal and state effort to provide health care to citizens whose incomes are below the federal poverty threshold, citizens who are disabled, and older people. In addition, President Johnson enacted several programs focused on health through nutrition, including Food Stamps and school lunch programs. Often, health care programs are federally controlled programs that are often run by states in accordance with a mix of state and federal regulations.

The federal government's involvement in health care matters has fluctuated depending on the then-current president's view of federalism. Some presidents believed that the federal government should be less involved with health care matters and that the states should be more involved, while other presidents sought to increase the federal government's involvement and lessen the state's involvement. The tension between the federal and the state governments is a hallmark of federalism. As a result, the federal and state governments have become increasingly intertwined in health care funding, regulation, and administration.

The Health Insurance Portability and Accountability Act of 1996 (HIPAA) is an example health care–related federal law. HIPAA ensures that patients across the United States have the same right of privacy, and that insurance companies and health care providers have the same obligations to protect patient health information regardless of the state in which they conduct business. At the same time, states have enacted laws that mirror HIPAA and are sometimes more stringent. Health care professionals should be aware of the federal HIPAA regulations, as well as the state patient privacy regulations of the state where they work.

Administrative and Common Law

Administrative law governs the activities of administrative agencies of government. Both federal and state governments have administrative law. To enable the federal government to exercise its authority and enforce the law, Congress delegates authority to administrative agencies. Administrative agencies then make rules and regulations pertaining to the agency's specialty. Congress may give certain agencies power to **adjudicate** disputes involving the application of those rules to particular parties under certain circumstances. In carrying out their responsibilities, agencies usually perform one or more of the following functions: (1) rule making, (2) adjudication, (3) prosecution, (4) advising, (5) supervision, and (6) investigation. Examples of federal agencies include the Federal Aviation Administration, Centers for Disease Control and Prevention, Federal Emergency Management Agency, Drug Enforcement Agency, among many hundred others.

Common law is different, but no less valid, from law enacted by Congress (statutory law) and administrative law (regulatory law). Common law is court-made law that arises, in part, from judges' interpretation of statutory or regulatory law. The interpretations are found in judicial decisions, which are written records of the facts at hand, the applicable law, and the conclusion based upon the application of the facts to the law. Judges are bound to adhere to the principle of *stare decisis*, which is Latin for "let the decision stand." Simply put, judicial decisions from the past whose underlying facts or issues are substantially the same as the current one being litigated require that judicial decisions adhere to the prior conclusion unless the court distinguishes the prior decision from the current situation. *Stare decisis* gives stability and predictability to the court system yet allows for flexibility when there are new or different facts.

The Distinction Between Criminal and Civil Law

In both the federal and the state court systems, there are two major divisions of law: **criminal** and **civil**. In a criminal case, the state is the **plaintiff**; the person charged with the crime is the **defendant**; and the defendant may face imprisonment.

A crime is defined as the performance of an act forbidden by law or the omission of an act required by law. In either case, the criminal defendant is punished by society. Crimes are divided into felonies and misdemeanors. A felony is a crime punishable by death or imprisonment. A misdemeanor is a crime punishable by imprisonment in jail for less than 1 year or a fine. State and federal legislatures define conduct that determines whether an act is a crime and whether the act is a felony or misdemeanor. In a criminal case, the defendant is found guilty or not guilty. In a civil case, the defendant is found liable or not liable.

adjudicate To decide a disputed matter.

common law Law created as a result of judicial decisions.

criminal The system of law concerned with offenses prosecuted by and deemed prohibited by state or federal law, or a person who has been proven guilty of such an offense.

civil The system of law concerned with disputes between individuals or, where the case does not relate to the violation of a criminal statute, between an individual and the state.

plaintiff A person or party who brings a civil court action against a person or party with whom they have a dispute.

defendant A person or party against whom a civil plaintiff has initiated a lawsuit to settle a dispute; in a criminal matter, a person or party that has been charged with a crime and who is being prosecuted.

It is also possible to have a civil case arising from a criminal act. A defendant in a civil case, however, does not face the possibility of imprisonment. When a civil defendant is found liable, the court system typically seeks to make the plaintiff whole by requiring that the defendant pays the plaintiff money damages. For example, in an **assault** and **battery** criminal prosecution, the state prosecutes a defendant for the crime of assault and battery. A defendant that is found guilty is then punished by the state. The victim of the assault and battery in such a case is neither a plaintiff nor a defendant in the criminal case. The purposes of punishment are **reformation**, **restraint**, **retribution**, and **deterrence**. In some instances, the victim may then attempt to collect damages from the defendant by bringing a civil lawsuit for assault and battery. In some cases, a defendant who is not guilty of a criminal charge can be found liable for damages in a subsequent civil suit. See Figure 3-3, *The civil case process.*

assault Any intentional act, attempt, or threat to inflict bodily injury on another person with the apparent ability to do so.

battery Intentional touching of another person without permission.

reformation The rehabilitation of a criminal.

restraint Restriction of personal liberty.

retribution Something given or demanded as a punishment for criminal wrongdoing.

deterrence Punishment used to discourage crime.

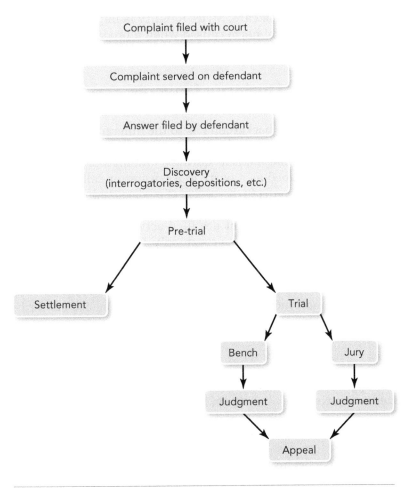

Figure 3-3 The Civil Case Process

The case of O.J. Simpson provides a good example. Simpson was accused and found not guilty of murdering his ex-wife Nicole and her friend Ron Goldman. Even though Simpson was found not guilty, the Goldman family members sued Simpson in civil court for the wrongful death of their son and were awarded damages of $33.5 million. The reason Simpson was found liable in the civil lawsuit and not guilty in the criminal lawsuit is due to the different **standard of proof** required in each type of case. The standard of proof in a civil case is **preponderance of the evidence**. The standard in a criminal case—**beyond a reasonable doubt**—is more difficult to prove than a civil case.

The most common civil lawsuit in the health care industry is an action known as a **tort**. Tort liability is based on one of the following grounds: intentional acts, **negligent acts**, or **strict liability**. Intentional torts may be actions toward property or a person that are done deliberately. Negligence is the result of an act or omission that does not meet the applicable standard of care. Strict liability is imposed on a seller or manufacturer for physical harm caused when a product is defective and unreasonably dangerous.

What Happens During a Lawsuit

Now that you have some background as to the different types of laws and lawsuits, it makes sense to talk about a lawsuit's progression. The next section is a summary of what happens during a lawsuit and what might happen should you be named as a party in a lawsuit or called as a witness. Chapter 6 contains an in-depth discussion of medical malpractice cases.

Medical malpractice attorneys estimate that fewer than 10 percent of the malpractice lawsuits that are filed actually go to trial. It is also estimated that of those that go to court, only 10 percent result in a final **judgment**. The remaining cases are settled out of court either by agreement, **arbitration**, or **mediation**. Settling may take place at any time, including before a case is filed, after judgment, or during or after an appeal. Medical malpractice lawsuits follow the same steps described in the following sections.

Phase I

The first phase is when the alleged negligence occurs and the patient becomes aware that they have been injured.

Phase II

The second phase begins when the patient seeks the advice of an attorney who specializes in medical malpractice about the alleged negligence. The attorney will obtain a copy of the patient's medical records. This may

standard of proof Level of proof required, which is established by considering all evidence and witnesses.

preponderance of the evidence The greater weight of the evidence that is more likely than not.

beyond a reasonable doubt Evidence so strong and credible that it leaves no more than a remote possibility that there is another explanation for what happened.

tort A wrong or injury, other than breach of contract, for which a court will provide a remedy.

negligent act Failure to take reasonable precautions to protect others from the risk of harm.

strict liability Responsibility of a seller or manufacturer for a defective product that causes injury.

judgment A court's decision regarding the rights and obligations of the parties in a lawsuit.

arbitration A hearing held between two or more parties who disagree on an issue but agree in advance to abide by the decision of an impartial third party.

mediation A neutral party meets with parties to a dispute with the intent of persuading them to settle their dispute.

be done by asking the patient to obtain their records or by having the patient sign an authorization to allow the provider to release the records to the attorney. Providers and health care facilities often charge for providing the medical records to authorized parties other than the patient.

Insurance companies require their insured (the provider) to file an incident report at the earliest possible time upon learning of a potential lawsuit. Failure to do so can often allow the insurance company to deny coverage for the claim. Incident reports collect facts but do not admit fault. If the provider was previously unaware of the patient's allegations of negligence, the request from an attorney for a patient's medical records is an indicator that there may be a lawsuit coming.

The original medical records should *never* be released. You should only release a copy of a patient's medical records after verifying that a signed release form is in the patient's chart. Always document who received what records and when, how the records were delivered, and the amount paid for the records, if any. The fees charged for the medical record copies must be reasonable and customary, and only those documents specifically requested should be provided.

The patient's lawyer will have one or more experts review the records and may have an independent health care provider examine the patient. Medical malpractice attorneys often only take malpractice cases on a **contingency** basis, which means that the lawyer will not be paid unless the plaintiff recovers monetary damages. If the plaintiff does not recover any monetary damages, the lawyer is not owed any fees.

When a plaintiff files a medical malpractice lawsuit, the plaintiff puts their medical condition and health at issue. In doing so, the plaintiff's medical records will be given to the defendant, their attorney, and experts. In addition, the plaintiff's medical records will be discussed at trial and will likely be entered into evidence.

At this point, the insurance company, the health care provider, and the attorney for the patient may negotiate a settlement. If these **negotiations** do not result in a settlement, the patient's attorney files a "complaint," which details the facts of the case and the allegations of what went wrong, who is to blame, and how the plaintiff has been hurt. When a complaint is filed, the patient officially becomes the plaintiff and the provider (as well as others who may bear some responsibility for the alleged negligence) becomes the defendant. The defendant then files an "answer" in response to the complaint. Often the parties will meet with the judge assigned to the case, where they will create a schedule for the rest of the case. At this point, the parties will begin "discovery," which is a name for the various ways that the parties collect factual information regarding the case. Discovery includes **depositions**, **interrogatories**, **motions**, and witness identification, among others.

The end of the second phase of the lawsuit comes when discovery is complete, a **pretrial conference** is held, and the judge declares the case is ready for trial.

contingency Something that may occur but is dependent on a different and uncertain future event to happen first.

negotiation Exchange and consideration of offers with the objective of reaching an agreement.

deposition A sworn verbal statement given out of court in response to questions posed by attorneys involved in the case and transcribed by a court reporter.

interrogatory Written questions about a case addressed to one party or witness by another party.

motion The application made to a judge to take a specific action in a case.

pretrial conference A meeting of the parties and the judge to discuss the readiness for and details of trial process.

Phase III

A trial is a means of settling a dispute between two parties before a judge and jury. A jury determines what facts are credible, and the judge determines what specific laws are involved in the matter. The jury then takes the facts apply it to the law, as instructed by the judge, to decide the case. A bench trial is one where the judge takes the place of the jury. The plaintiff presents the facts of the case as he or she sees them, and the defendant has the opportunity to present the facts of the case as he or she sees them. The finder of fact—the jury, or the judge, if it is a bench trial—determines what facts are credible. The judge oversees the trial and makes decisions about the relevant law. Rarely is a trial as dramatic and colorful as those portrayed on television and in the movies.

The attorneys are doing their jobs by presenting their clients' cases. The judge is trying to offer both parties a fair hearing, as well as to keep cases moving through the court. The witnesses are ordinary people who have been subpoenaed, voluntarily or involuntarily, to provide testimony about what they observed or knew. In most medical malpractice cases, one or both sides will present evidence through the use of an expert witness, who has special knowledge of the issues involved that are not known to a layperson. Testimony of a medical expert can go beyond the facts of the case and can include medical issues that affect the condition of the plaintiff or the treatment by the defendant. The members of the jury are trying to listen attentively, so that they can render a fair decision.

At the start of a trial, the attorneys for the parties make opening statements, which tells the fact finder their theory of what happened. The plaintiff then presents evidence through witnesses, documents, and expert opinions. The defense then presents its defense of the case through witnesses, documents, and expert opinions. Once the defense concludes the presentation of the defense case, a plaintiff may be provided with the opportunity to rebut certain aspects of the defense case. Then, both parties have an opportunity to present a closing statement, which summarizes the evidence presented. If there is a jury (rather than a bench trial), the judge will read the jury instructions, which tell the jurors about how they are to deliberate and the applicable law.

Once the jury concludes its deliberation, the verdict, also called the decision or the judgment, is announced in the courtroom. After the verdict is announced and damages, if any, are awarded, the lawsuit moves to Phase IV.

Phase IV

Either side has the right to appeal the decision provided there is a legal basis to do so. Usually, the losing party pursues an appeal. There is a long list of legal basis that will allow an appeal. What does not constitute a legal basis for appeal, however, is that one of the parties did not like the outcome of trial and wants a "do over." The appeal of lawsuits tried in the state court system will be heard in the respective state's court of appeals. In the federal judicial system, appeals go to the federal appellate courts, also called the Circuit Courts. The highest court in the United States is the Supreme Court, who reviews the requests and accepts fewer than 2 percent of cases it receives from lower appellate courts.

You As a Witness

Most lawsuits are won outside of the courtroom. The preparation of the attorney and the witnesses is crucial to winning a lawsuit. When considering your testimony as a witness, look at both sides and see where you fit into the total picture before you get to the deposition, trial, or other hearing. Try to anticipate what defense the other side will offer to your remarks. Try to be objective about your strong points and weak arguments, and follow the instructions given to you by your attorney.

- Pay attention. Trials, depositions, and other legal proceedings can sometimes become very boring and hard to follow. If you are a testifying witness, know that the judge and jury are trying to determine whether you are a credible witness. If you give deposition testimony, everything you say is being recorded. If your trial testimony conflicts with your deposition testimony, it can be used to show the inconsistency in your testimony. In some cases, where the witness has a valid reason for not being able to attend trial to give testimony, the witnesses' deposition may be read into the record at trial. So, deposition testimony is extremely important.

- Behave in a professional manner. The people who are listening to you testify do not know you. The way you look and present yourself is important when the judge and jury are assessing your credibility. Respond clearly and in your own language to the questions. Sit up straight and do not chew gum, tap your fingers, or twirl your thumbs or hair. Dress in a manner consistent with the competent professional that you are. The opposing party's attorney will be evaluating not only your words but also how you present yourself.

- Answer the question asked and only the question asked. Do not offer information if it is not requested. When someone asks you a question, do not give flippant or offhand responses. Do not make a joke or answer quickly in an attempt to conclude the proceeding quickly. Think about what you are saying. If you are given something to read, make certain that you read it thoroughly. In addition, if you do not know an answer or do not understand the question, say so. Do not make up any answer, and always be truthful.

- Cooperate with your attorney. If your attorney objects to a question, do not answer unless and until the court or your attorney instructs you to do so.
- Honesty is the best policy. Remember, you are testifying under oath. Any false statement, no matter how small, may ruin your credibility as a witness. **Perjury** is a crime.

perjury A false statement under oath.

Criminal and civil procedures are covered in volumes of material and take at least two semesters to study in law school and years to perfect in the courtroom. The material covered in this chapter will provide you with a basic idea of how you fit into the picture if you must testify in a lawsuit.

The Art of Examination

The method used to present the facts to the judge and jury is adversarial. This means that both the plaintiff and defendant try to win their case by interviewing their own witnesses and cross-examining witnesses from the opposing side. Asking questions in an attempt to reveal certain information is a skilled endeavor. A witness should be prepared for both **direct examination** and **cross-examination**, which require different questioning techniques by the attorney and responses from the witness. Your attorney or the attorney representing the party for whom you are a witness will ask you questions on direct examination. These questions will be open-ended and narrative. Questions on cross-examination, which will be asked by the other party's attorney, are called leading questions. This is because the lawyer will usually ask questions in the form of a statement that leads the witness to agree or disagree with the statement.

direct examination Attorney's interrogation of a witness by the party for whom the witness has been called.

cross-examination Attorney's interrogation of a witness by the other party's attorney.

A witness on cross-examination should not try to explain his or her responses. Instead, the witness should let his or her lawyer follow up with questions to clarify after the attorney conducting the cross-examination is finished. A witness on cross-examination should simply and precisely answer the questions asked.

☑ SUMMARY

- All law in the United States—both federal and state—flows from the Constitution.
- The federal government concurrently exists with state government, which is the basis for a federalist system of government. Federal and state governments each regulate different aspects of the health care industry. In some instances, both governments regulate.
- The Supremacy Clause tells us that if there is a conflict between federal and state law, that federal law will govern.

- The federal government is divided into three branches: the executive, the legislative, and the judiciary.
- The judicial branch of law, both in the federal and state governments, is responsible for settling legal disputes.
- Administrative law governs the activities of administrative agencies of government. Common law is court-made law that arises, in part, from judges' interpretation of statutory or regulatory law. The interpretations are found in judicial decisions, which are written records of the facts at hand, the applicable law, and the conclusion based upon the application of the facts to the law.
- In a criminal case, the state is the plaintiff; the person charged with the crime is the defendant; the defendant, if found guilty, may face imprisonment. A civil case concerns disputes between individuals and the defendant cannot face imprisonment but may be found liable and have to pay damages to the plaintiff.
- Each lawsuit that goes to trial follows four general phases: injury, pre-trial, trial, appeal.
- A plaintiff's medical records will be part of any medical malpractice trial.
- It is important that a witness in a deposition or trial prepare for testimony. A witness' dress and demeanor should enhance and not detract from the witness testimony.

SUGGESTED ACTIVITIES

1. Watch the short video (available online) "I'm Just a Bill" by Schoolhouse Rock, which summarizes the law-making process in an unforgettable way.
2. Watch the movie *The Verdict* with Paul Newman, an excellent portrayal of a medical malpractice cause of action. It accurately demonstrates legal procedures, the problems of the legal profession, the agony of the plaintiff, the role of the judge, the effect of politics on the court, and an example of a "real-life witness" who is involved in a malpractice action in a position similar to that of a health care professional.
3. While watching *The Verdict*, rate the witnesses as excellent, adequate, or poor on the following items:
   - The attention span of the witness;
   - Whether the manner of the witness matched the part that was being played;

- Whether the witness answered the questions directed to him or her; and
- Whether the witness was cooperative.

4. Find a recent court case, preferably one with medical involvement, and prepare to role-play the parts of witness, plaintiff's attorney, and defendant's attorney. Practice being a credible witness, forming and answering direct examination questions, and forming and answering cross-examination questions. This will give you some idea of how it feels to be a witness and how to answer the different types of questions.

STUDY QUESTIONS

1. What is the purpose of the Constitution's Supremacy clause? How is it tied to the United States' federalist system of government?
2. What are the three branches of government? Why is it necessary to separate the government in this way?
3. What are the three levels of the judiciary? And what is the name of the highest court in the United States?
4. Can federal agencies make their own rules and prosecute those who violate the rules?
5. Explain the major distinction between criminal and civil law.

Chapter 4

Criminal Acts and Intentional Torts

 Crime and punishment grow out of one stem.

Ralph Waldo Emerson

Objectives

After reading this chapter, you should be able to:

1. Summarize types of felonies.
2. Identify and define types of abuse that mandate reporting.
3. Recognize some of the indicators of an abused child or older adult.
4. Explain the steps involved in mandatory reporting, following federal and state guidelines.
5. Determine proper protocol for reporting an illegal activity in the health care setting.
6. Describe types of fraud in the health care industry.
7. Distinguish between criminal and civil causes of action.
8. Summarize types of intentional torts.

Building Your Legal Vocabulary

Conspiracy
Euthanasia
Felony
Larceny
Malice
Manslaughter

Misdemeanor
Murder
Qui tam lawsuit
Robbery
Theft
Wanton

Criminal Acts

Criminal acts are an unfortunate reality in a health care setting. From euthanasia to the theft of prescription drugs to reporting child or elder abuse, a health care professional will encounter issues associated with crimes along the way.

The two main classifications of crimes are misdemeanors and felonies. A **misdemeanor** is an offense classified lower than a felony and generally punishable by a fine or imprisonment other than in a penitentiary. A **felony** is defined as a crime of grave or more serious nature than those designated as misdemeanors. Under federal law and many state statutes, it is any offense punishable by imprisonment for a term exceeding 1 year or death. The crimes discussed in the following sections are all classified as felonies.

misdemeanor A crime that is generally punishable by a fine or imprisonment of less than a year.

felony A crime that is generally punishable by imprisonment for a sentence longer than a year.

robbery The forcible stealing of the personal property of another either from their person or in the immediate presence of the victim.

theft Taking property without the property owner's consent.

Robbery

An individual is guilty of **robbery** if, while carrying out **theft**, the victim is physically injured or has been threatened and put in fear of bodily injury. Robberies in a health care setting are rare, but they do happen. Often the perpetrator is looking for prescription drugs or prescription pads.

The defendant Arrington entered a Maryland drug store wearing a surgical mask and latex gloves and armed with a handgun. Arrington entered the restricted area of the pharmacy while pointing the gun at the pharmacist and demanding oxycodone. After directing the pharmacist to open the cash register, he fired a round into the pharmacy ceiling, and removed cash drawer from the register. Two police officers stopped Arrington in the pharmacy as he was leaving.

Arrington faces a maximum sentence of 20 years in federal prison for robbery; a maximum sentence of 10 years in federal prison for being a felon in possession of a firearm; and a mandatory minimum of 10 years, consecutive to any other sentence, and up to life in prison for using, carrying, brandishing and discharging a firearm in a crime of violence.

United States Department of Justice. (2021, April 8). Temple Hills Felon Convicted After a Three-Day Federal Trial for Robbery, Brandishing and Discharge of a Firearm, and Being a Felon in Possession of a Firearm. United States Department of Justice, U.S. Attorney's Office, District of Maryland. Retrieved from www.justice.gov/usao-md/pr/temple-hills-felon-convicted-after-three-day-federal-trial-robbery-brandishing-and.

Murder

An act done with intent to kill another person constitutes **murder**. In a criminal case, the prosecuting body (i.e., state or federal) must prove the accused's guilt beyond a reasonable doubt. In addition, there are classifications of murder: first-degree murder, second-degree murder, and manslaughter, among others, all of which are defined either by state or federal statute. The classification as to the degree depends upon several factors, including whether there was premeditation, how the murder was committed, and whether the murder occurred during the course of a felony.

murder An act done with intent to kill the victim.

An Ohio doctor was charged with killing 25 patients by prescribing and, in some cases, administering overdoses of fentanyl, a highly potent, effective painkiller intended for seriously ill patients. While the COVID-19 pandemic delayed the trial, the prosecution claims the amount of fentanyl administered to the patients was 5 to 20 times the amount that would be medically appropriate. The doctor's attorney claims the doctor prescribed the medication to increase the comfort of terminally ill patients. The trial will require evidence as to how to treat terminally ill patients.

Healy, J., Farr, I., Feiger, L., Duffy, C. (2019, October 11). One Doctor. 25 Deaths. How Could It Have Happened? *The New York Times*. Retrieved from www.nytimes.com /2019/10/11/us/ohio-doctor-overdose.html.

Attempted Murder

An attempt to commit a crime is itself a crime. To prove that a defendant is guilty of an attempt, three things must be proven beyond a reasonable doubt: that the defendant had a specific intent to commit that particular crime; that the defendant took an overt act toward committing that crime, which was part of carrying out the crime, and came reasonably close to actually carrying out the crime; and that the defendant's act did not result in a complete crime.

For example, if the Ohio doctor who prescribed high doses of fentanyl and was charged with the murder of 25 patients had prescribed a lethal dose of fentanyl to a patient, but the nurse who was to administer the dose did not do so, the doctor could be charged with attempted murder.

Euthanasia

According to *Black's Law Dictionary*, **euthanasia** is the act or practice of painlessly putting to death someone suffering from incurable and distressing disease as an act of mercy. While suicide is not a crime in many states, helping someone die by suicide can have criminal implications. With the exception of a handful of states that allow for physician-assisted suicide or those who have no relevant statute, it is a criminal act to help

euthanasia An intentional action or lack of action causing the merciful death of someone suffering from a terminal illness or incurable condition.

someone end their life. Notably, penalties for acts of euthanasia tend to be more lenient than for murder. Euthanasia is further discussed in Chapter 12, Death and Dying.

Manslaughter

manslaughter The killing of a person without premeditation.

malice An unjust intention to commit an illegal act to injure someone.

wanton An act done with reckless disregard of another's rights or needs.

Manslaughter is the unlawful killing of another without **malice**. A manslaughter conviction requires proof that there was **wanton** or reckless conduct.

Every provider makes errors in judgment at some point in their career, but an error in judgment is not necessarily wanton or reckless conduct. A misdiagnosed condition or error in treatment may result in civil liability (malpractice) but will not be considered criminal conduct, provided the judgment had some recognizable foundation in medicine.

Manslaughter is typically the charge when a provider does not practice in good faith, uses a form of treatment not generally accepted by the medical profession, or practices under the influence of drugs or alcohol, causing death to a patient. In the following case, former provider Conrad Murray was convicted of manslaughter in the death of famed entertainer Michael Jackson.

> Conrad Murray was a physician hired by Michael Jackson to serve as his personal physician for the "This Is It" tour in 2009. Mr. Murray was a cardiologist with a specialty in internal medicine. While in rehearsals for the tour, Mr. Murray would arrive at Mr. Jackson's home every night to, among other things, ensure Mr. Jackson was able to sleep. As part of his care of Mr. Jackson, Mr. Murray used a spectrum of prescription drugs, some of which are not typically used outside of a hospital setting, including: Propofol, Benoquin, Lorazepam, Midazolam, and Lidocaine. At trial, the evidence showed that almost every night for two months before Mr. Jackson's death, Mr. Murray administered Propofol. The prosecution showed that the bedroom did not have the requisite monitoring devices normally used with Propofol, an anesthesia. On the night of Mr. Jackson's death, he returned from rehearsals and was unable to sleep. Throughout the night, Mr. Murray administered several doses of valium, Lorazepam, Midazolam, and at some point Propofol. The subsequent autopsy showed that Mr. Jackson had a number of drugs in his system at the time of his death, including Propofol, Lidocaine, Valium, Ativan, Midazolam, and Ephedrine. The coroner concluded that Mr. Jackson's death was caused by Mr. Murray's administration of Propofol and benzodiazepines; that the treatment administered was not medically indicated; Propofol should not have been used for insomnia; and that the use of an anesthesia in a non-hospital setting was inappropriate.
>
> *People v. Murray*, unpublished decision (Cal App. 2014)

Conspiracy

A **conspiracy** is a scheme between two or more people formed for the purpose of committing some unlawful or criminal act, or some act that is lawful in itself but becomes unlawful when done by the concerted action of the conspirators. A conspiracy is a separate crime. To prove a defendant guilty of conspiracy, three things must be proven beyond a reasonable doubt: that the defendant joined in an agreement or plan with one or more other persons; that the purpose of the agreement was to do something unlawful; and that the defendant joined the conspiracy knowing of the unlawful plan and intending to help carry it out.

conspiracy An agreement among two or more people to undertake an illegal act.

Larceny

Larceny is taking the personal property of another with the intent to permanently deprive that person of their property. To prove a defendant guilty of larceny, three things must be proven beyond a reasonable doubt: that the defendant took and carried away the property; that the property was owned or possessed by someone other than the defendant; and that the defendant took the property with the intent to permanently deprive that person of the property. An example of larceny in a health care setting would be office employees stealing drug samples or medical supplies.

larceny Taking the personal property of another with the intent to permanently deprive that person of their property.

Abuse

The current annual estimates of child abuse (4.4 million incidents reported), elder abuse (5 million victims), or domestic abuse (10 million victims) are staggering. It is likely that you will encounter a situation where your patient's injuries resulted from child abuse, elder abuse, or abuse at the hands of someone in the patient's home. As a result, it is essential to remember that all states require that health care providers report patient injuries that arise from child or elder abuse. Domestic violence is required to be reported in most states where the patient indicates the injuries were inflicted by someone in the patient's home.

Child Abuse

Child abuse is one of the few situations where the law mandates that health care providers report the medical condition of their patients. Statistics support the need for mandatory reporting of child abuse cases. Child's rights advocate group American SPCC reports:

- 1,840 children died from abuse and neglect in 2019.
- 4.4 million child abuse cases reported annually.
- 5 children die per day from cases of child abuse.

- 73% of child fatalities suffered from some form of neglect.
- 92% of cases parents are the abuser.

American SPCC. (n.d.) National Child Maltreatment Statistics. American SPCC. Retrieved from https://americanspcc.org/child-abuse-statistics/.

Key findings in the 2019 report included:

- In 2019, data shows eighty-four and a half percent of victims suffer a single type of maltreatment, sixty-one percent are neglected only, 10.3 percent are physically abused only, and 7.2 percent are sexually abused only.
- In 2019, an estimated 1,840 children died from abuse and neglect at a rate of 2.50 per 100,000 children in the population. The 2019 estimate increased from 2018's estimate of 1,780 children who died from abuse and neglect.

Children's Bureau (Administration on Children, Youth and Families, Administration for Children and Families), U.S. Department of Health and Human Services. (2019). Child Maltreatment 2019. Retrieved from www.acf.hhs.gov/cb /report/child-maltreatment-2019.

Legislative Response   The Federal Child Abuse Prevention and Treatment Act (1974) requires states to mandate that health care providers report instances of physical and mental "injury . . . under circumstances which indicate that the child's health or welfare is harmed or threatened." In response, every state legislature has made child abuse a crime. Any reporter of child abuse is granted full immunity from liability (both criminal and civil) arising from the reported incident.

Mandated Reporters of Abuse   Teachers, nurses, and other licensed health care providers are also identified as mandated reporters under state statutes. At times, mandated reporting may cause personal conflict to the health care provider and other members of the health care team who have been caring for an entire family. But the child, not the parent, is the patient, and it is universally held that confidentiality in the patient–provider relationship does not exist when parents abuse children. At the same time, it is important for reporters to maintain interpersonal relationships with the family in spite of the possibility of being expected to produce evidence against them. In private life, anyone—family, neighbor, or concerned adult—may file a child abuse complaint with a protective agency. When you are working in a health care facility, and unless your job function is listed as a mandatory reporter in the applicable state, health care professionals should file a complaint only when delegated that task by your supervising health care provider.

Professionals Required to Report

Approximately 47 States, the District of Columbia, American Samoa, Guam, the Northern Mariana Islands, Puerto Rico, and the Virgin Islands designate professions whose members are mandated by law to report child maltreatment. Individuals designated as mandatory reporters typically have frequent contact with children. The professionals most commonly mandated to report across the States include the following:

- Social workers
- Teachers, principals, and other school personnel
- Physicians, nurses, and other health-care workers
- Counselors, therapists, and other mental health professionals
- Child care providers
- Medical examiners or coroners
- Law enforcement officers

Additional professionals who are mandated to report suspected or known maltreatment by some States include the following:

- Commercial film or photograph processors (12 States, Guam, and Puerto Rico)
- Computer technicians (in 6 States)
- Substance abuse counselors (14 States)
- Probation or parole officers (17 States)
- Directors, employees, and volunteers at entities that provide organized activities for children, such as camps, day camps, youth centers, and recreation centers (13 States)
- Domestic violence workers (6 States and the District of Columbia)
- Animal control or humane officers (7 States and the District of Columbia)
- Court-appointed special advocates (11 States)
- Members of the clergy (28 States and Guam)
- Faculty, administrators, athletics staff, or other employees and volunteers at institutions of higher learning, including public and private colleges and universities and vocational and technical schools (11 States)

Reporting by Other Persons

In approximately 18 States and Puerto Rico, any person who suspects child abuse or neglect is required to report. Of these 18 States, 15 States and Puerto Rico specify certain professionals who must report but also require all

(Continues)

(Continued)

persons to report suspected abuse or neglect, regardless of profession. The other three States—Indiana, New Jersey, and Wyoming—require all persons to report without specifying any professions. In all other States, territories, and the District of Columbia, any person is permitted to report. These voluntary reporters of maltreatment are often referred to as "permissive reporters.""

Child Welfare Information Gateway. (2019). Mandatory Reporters of Child Abuse and Neglect. Washington, DC: U.S. Department of Health and Human Services, Children's Bureau. Retrieved from www.childwelfare.gov/topics/systemwide /laws-policies/statutes/manda/.

A provider's failure to report child abuse is a matter being addressed by medical societies across the country. It is also being addressed by district attorneys:

Two Child Protective Service workers in West Virginia were fired and charged with misdemeanors relating to the abuse of a 4-year-old boy who died. Breeana Bizub and Tabetha Phillips-Friend were charged with involuntary manslaughter, failing to report suspected abuse and neglect, and violating child abuse reporting procedures. The charges were related to a criminal case involving the boy's mother and her boyfriend.

Associated Press. (2021, April 13). 2 child services workers fired, charged in fatal abuse case. API. Retrieved from https://apnews.com/article /fairmont-west-virginia-child-abuse-56f66caf6c85a672d22ff64bec1ca55d.

Most states specify in statute the types of information that should be included in a report of suspected abuse or neglect. The reporter will be asked to provide as much information about the child's situation as he or she can, including the names and addresses of the child and the child's parents or other persons responsible for the child's care, the child's age, conditions in the child's home environment, the nature and extent of the child's injuries, and information about other children in the same environment.

Child Welfare Information Gateway. (2017). Making and Screening Reports of Child Abuse and Neglect. Child Welfare Information Gateway. Washington, DC: U.S. Department of Health and Human Services, Children's Bureau. Retrieved from www.childwelfare.gov/pubPDFs/repproc.pdf.

Filing a Complaint   Procedures for reporting suspected child abuse begin by telephoning the child protective services agency in your state. Be prepared to give a candid and detailed description of the circumstances that led you to believe the child had been abused.

Child protective agencies screen the complaint after a report has been filed. Agency social workers determine whether the child is "at risk," monitor care for the child at home or in foster placement, escort the complaint through the legal system, and establish criteria to achieve the goal of the child's return home. The substantiation, or confirmation, of abuse is critical to the well-being of the child and family. Nationwide, about 40 percent of all reports are substantiated.

The agency also decides whether to refer the complaint to the district attorney. When the case is referred to the district attorney, the matter becomes criminal, and the penalty for the abuser may be prison.

Legal Process   Cases that reach the courts are often known as petitions for care and protection. Many attorneys are involved in care and protection proceedings. When the petition is presented in court, the child is identified by the attorney representing the protective agency. Additional attorneys are appointed for the child, the parents (often individually), and possibly the grandparents, as well as a court investigator and/or guardian ad litem. The guardian ad litem serves in the best interest of the child, whereas the attorney appointed for the child advocates for the position of the child. The court investigator serves as an extension of the court and investigates the family's history: educational, economic, medical, and psychological. The attorneys for the other members of the family represent and advocate only in their clients' interests.

The Medical Record   In any court procedure, evidence must be offered to the trier of fact in an effort to convict or defend the defendant. In child abuse cases, the medical record often holds critical information that is used in determining whether a child is returned to the parents. Physical examinations document the physical injuries, psychological examinations document the extent of mental abuse and the effect of the family dynamics on the child, and therapists' progress notes are critical in determining whether the family is motivated to change to meet the standards set by society.

Confidentiality   Every attorney wants, but is not necessarily entitled to, every medical report. Access to medical records is protected by patient–provider confidentiality statutes, and the patient holds the privilege to withhold or release the records. Usually, parents hold the right to exercise the patient–provider confidentiality privilege for their children, but when the family is involved in a child abuse investigation, the patient–provider privilege is held by the protective agency, and permission for release of information about the child must be received from the agency. The parents still maintain the right to withhold or release their own medical records.

Sections of the medical record may cover the issue of fault. Usually, the provider will ask a child, "How did this happen?" and the health care provider will document the answer. It is common practice for an emergency room staff to separate caretaker from child on arrival at the hospital to interview each person individually. The staff members then compare notes before determining whether the child is at risk and whether it is necessary to place the child in emergency protective custody. This information becomes part of the medical record but may not be given as much weight as documented injuries because of the lack of experience of the interviewers in ascertaining truth.

Access to Child Abuse Records   The records of a minor in any situation are confidential. In a child abuse case, all medical, school, court, department of social services, and department of youth services records are covered by Health Insurance Portability and Accountability Act of 1996 (HIPAA). These records cannot be released by anyone to anyone without proper authorization. The final course of action available to access a record involves the filing of a complaint seeking a court order compelling the release of the record.

Behavioral Indicators of Child Abuse   Children who are abused physically or emotionally display certain types of behavior. Many of these are common to all children at one time or another, but when they are present in sufficient number and strength to characterize a child's overall manner, they may indicate abuse:

- Overly compliant, passive, undemanding behaviors aimed at maintaining a low profile, avoiding any possible confrontation with a parent that could lead to abuse.

- Extremely aggressive, demanding, and rageful behaviors, sometimes hyperactive, caused by the child's repeated frustrations at not getting basic needs met.

- Role-reversed "parental" behavior, or extremely dependent behavior. Abusive parents have been unable to satisfy certain of their own needs appropriately and so turn to their children for fulfillment, which can produce two opposite sets of behavior in children.

- Lags in development. Children who are forced to siphon off energy, normally channeled toward growth, into protecting themselves from abusive parents may fall behind the norm for their age in toilet training, motor skills, socialization, and language development.

Physical Indicators of Child Abuse

- Bruises and welts
- Burns
- Lacerations and abrasions
- Skeletal injuries
- Head injuries
- Internal injuries caused by blows to midline of abdomen

Elder Abuse

> How many older Americans are abused?
>
> Approximately one in 10 Americans aged 60+ have experienced some form of elder abuse. Some estimates range as high as five million elders who are abused each year. One study estimated that only one in 24 cases of abuse are reported to authorities.
>
> Who are the abusers of older adults?
>
> Abusers are both women and men. In almost 60% of elder abuse and neglect incidents, the perpetrator is a family member. Two thirds of perpetrators are adult children or spouses.
>
> National Council on Aging. (n.d.). (2021, February 23). Get the Facts on Elder Abuse. NCOA. Retrieved from www.ncoa.org/article /get-the-facts-on-elder-abuse.

As the population of the United States grows older and lives longer, opportunities for elder abuse increase.

Elder Abuse Defined   The World Health Organization defines elder abuse as "a single or repeated act or lack of appropriate action, occurring within any relationship where there is an expectation of trust which causes harm or distress to an older person."

Types of Abuse

1. Unintentional Neglect

   Esther, approximately 85 years of age, brings her sister, Martha, into the medical office for a visit with the provider. For the past several weeks, Martha has not been eating well, has been vomiting a bit, and appears generally run down. The medication that the provider prescribed 6 months ago has been depleted, and no one has renewed the prescription. Martha's clothes are rumpled, her hair is stringy, and she appears unkempt, as does Esther. Prior to this time, Esther has been able to adequately take care of Martha but apparently can no longer do so. Martha is an example of a passively neglected elder.

2. Intentional Neglect

A home-based caretaker was charged with the death of her 72-year-old female patient. Physical and mental ailments prevented the patient from caring for herself. The caretaker did not give the patient her medication, did not take her to medical appointments, and did not provide her with her prescribed nutritional supplements. These intentional acts ultimately led to the patient's death.

3. Financial Abuse

Other dimensions of abuse involve money. For example: "You won't believe what happened," reiterated a distraught woman. "My husband's aunt was at home. Sure, she was a bit confused but not ready for a nursing home. Last Friday, Almeida and her daughter, cousins of the aunt, arrived and the next day Auntie was in the hospital. Three days later she was admitted to a nursing home. This morning, the postman stopped and asked if anyone had been to see Auntie lately. He was just there and water was trickling out the front door.

I went to the home, let myself in, and found water everywhere. Someone had left the water faucet on in the second-floor bathtub. Two days later, all of Auntie's bank accounts were depleted and the cousins were off to their home, 1500 miles away."

The above is a classic example of financial abuse: A relative arrives on the scene, usually at the death of the older person, takes every article in sight and leaves before the sun comes up, never to be seen again. In this case, the relatives could not wait for the aunt to die. As part of their plan, they implicated a provider in the hospital and nursing home admission process. The court unknowingly cooperated and issued a temporary guardianship to the cousins. The abusive relatives left a legal entanglement that survived the death of the aunt and enriched the pockets of several attorneys. This type of abuse can be identified as financial on the part of the cousins and passive neglect on the part of the provider.

4. Physical and Psychological Abuse

The following involves physical and psychological abuse and is viewed from the perspective of the employee abuser. "I've been fired," she cried over the telephone, "and it's so unfair. This patient . . . he hit me . . . he kicked me . . . I was only protecting myself. It wasn't my fault his leg got broken. I want to sue . . ."

Joanne had been taking care of an elderly patient in a local nursing home. He was a difficult patient, cantankerous at times, verbally abusive, and, lately, physically abusive. Joanne was getting him ready for bed at night and he "kicked" her. She stated that she grabbed his foot while he was in bed and pushed against it toward his body with her body to protect herself. She heard a "snap," then a "scream" from the patient, and then remembered nothing but confusion. The next day Joanne was called into the supervisor's office and fired for elder abuse.

The abuse was physical in nature. Joanne caused the breaking of the man's leg. This incident took place in Massachusetts, where the law requires the reporting of each incident of elder abuse. Joanne was worried, when she talked with her lawyer, that she would not be employable as a nurse's aide ever again and that her sole skill for maintaining herself financially would be taken from her because of this "accident." In fact, that is what happened. Her attorney contacted the state registry of abusers and found that Joanne had been reported two previous times for abusing residents in nursing homes. The registry board would not give her another chance.

Legislation and Penalties   Laws regarding reporting and penalties for failure to report abuse vary from state to state. All 50 states have reporting laws as well as agencies designated in one way or another to monitor and investigate allegations of elder abuse. Every state has a hotline for reporting and some procedure for investigating complaints of elder abuse.

Nurses can lose their licenses to practice, be fined from $25 to $1,000, be imprisoned from 10 days to 6 months, and encounter civil liability for damages, for failure to report abuse. Health care professionals may or may not be penalized, depending on the applicable state statute.

For information on your state statute, go to the National Center of Elder Abuse's website, https://ncea.acl.gov.

Domestic Violence

Domestic violence is not simply one partner hitting another. An individual who brutally beats their spouse or intimate partner is committing domestic violence. A person who threatens to harm their spouse or intimate partner is also committing domestic violence. The United States Department of Justice defines domestic violence as follows:

> . . . a pattern of abusive behavior in any relationship that is used by one partner to gain or maintain power and control over another intimate partner. Domestic violence can be physical, sexual, emotional, economic, or psychological actions or threats of actions that influence another person. This includes any behaviors that intimidate, manipulate, humiliate, isolate, frighten, terrorize, coerce, threaten, blame, hurt, injure, or wound someone.

(Continues)

(Continued)

Physical Abuse: Hitting, slapping, shoving, grabbing, pinching, biting, hair pulling, etc. are types of physical abuse. This type of abuse also includes denying a partner medical care or forcing alcohol and/or drug use upon them.

Sexual Abuse: Coercing or attempting to coerce any sexual contact or behavior without consent. Sexual abuse includes, but is certainly not limited to, marital rape, attacks on sexual parts of the body, forcing sex after physical violence has occurred, or treating one in a sexually demeaning manner.

Emotional Abuse: Undermining an individual's sense of self-worth and/or self-esteem is abusive. This may include, but is not limited to constant criticism, diminishing one's abilities, name-calling, or damaging one's relationship with their children.

Economic Abuse: Is defined as making or attempting to make an individual financially dependent by maintaining total control over financial resources, withholding one's access to money, or forbidding one's attendance at school or employment.

Psychological Abuse: Elements of psychological abuse include—but are not limited to—causing fear by intimidation; threatening physical harm to self, partner, children, or partner's family or friends; destruction of pets and property; and forcing isolation from family, friends, or school and/or work.

Domestic violence can happen to anyone regardless of race, age, sexual orientation, religion, or gender. Domestic violence affects people of all socioeconomic backgrounds and education levels. Domestic violence occurs in both opposite-sex and same-sex relationships and can happen to intimate partners who are married, living together, or dating.

Domestic violence not only affects those who are abused, but also has a substantial effect on family members, friends, co-workers, other witnesses, and the community at large. Children, who grow up witnessing domestic violence, are among those seriously affected by this crime. Frequent exposure to violence in the home not only predisposes children to numerous social and physical problems, but also teaches them that violence is a normal way of life—therefore, increasing their risk of becoming society's next generation of victims and abusers.

The United States Department of Justice. (n.d.). What Is Domestic Violence? Retrieved from www.justice.gov/ovw/domestic-violence.

In 2021, the 1994 Violence Against Women Act (VAWA) was reauthorized by Congress. The VAWA provided $1.6 billion to confront the national problem of gender-based violence. The VAWA recognizes that there is no place—home, street, or school—where women are spared the fear of crime. Under Title I, Safe Homes for Women, the bill addresses the right of women to be free from domestic violence specifically through the interstate enforcement of protection orders. Prior to the passing of the VAWA, the majority of states did not give full faith and credit to protection orders issued in other states. According to *Black's Law Dictionary*, the full faith and credit clause of the United States Constitution (Article IV, §1) provides that the various states must recognize, with some exceptions, legislative acts, public records, and judicial decisions of the other states within the United States. Without full faith and credit statutes, a state may only protect victims of domestic violence within its boundaries, limiting the protection afforded victims if they leave the state issuing the protective order.

The passing of the VAWA offered women two avenues of protection from domestic violence: the state courts and the federal courts. The original petition for protection against domestic violence is filed in the state courts and through the state court system. The federal courts enter when there is an interstate violation of a protection order and the matter becomes a federal offense, as is shown in the following:

> In January of 1995, the U.S. Attorney for the Southern District of West Virginia charged a man in the first federal domestic violence case. Christopher Bailey was indicted on January 4, 1995, by a grand jury for interstate domestic violence and federal kidnapping after bringing his unconscious wife to a Kentucky hospital. Bailey faces up to life imprisonment and $500,000 in fines. The FBI has been involved in the investigation and has alleged that Christopher Bailey seriously injured his wife in their home in West Virginia and then travelled through West Virginia, Kentucky and Ohio for six days with his wife sometimes tied up in the trunk. Because the federal domestic violence law is untested, Bailey is also charged with federal kidnapping.
>
> Klein, C. F. (1995, Summer). Full Faith and Credit Interstate Enforcement of Protection Orders Under the Violence Against Women Act of 1994. *Family Law Quarterly, 29*(2), 253–272.

In addition, the Violent Crime Control and Law Enforcement Act of 1994 makes it a federal crime to possess a firearm and/or ammunition while subject to a protection Order or after conviction of a qualifying misdemeanor crime of domestic violence.

The magnitude of the problems rooted in and affected by domestic violence is evidenced in the facts that follow:

In the United States, more than 10 million adults experience domestic violence annually.

- If each of these adults experienced only one incidence of violence, an adult in the US would experience violence every three seconds. However, because domestic violence is a pattern, many experience repeated acts of abuse annually, so an incident of abuse happens far more frequently than every three seconds.
- 1 in 4 women and 1 in 10 men experience sexual violence, physical violence and/or stalking by an intimate partner during their lifetime with 'IPV-related impact' such as being concerned for their safety, PTSD symptoms, injury, or needing victim services.
  - Approximately 1 in 5 female victims and 1 in 20 male victims need medical care.
  - Female victims sustain injuries 3x more often than male victims.
  - 1 in 5 female victims and 1 in 9 male victims need legal services.
  - 23.2% of women and 13.9% of men have experienced severe physical violence by an intimate partner during their lifetime.
- From 2016 through 2018 the number of intimate partner violence victimizations in the United States increased 42%.
- On a typical day, domestic violence hotlines nationwide receive over 19,000 calls.
- An abuser's access to a firearm increases the risk of intimate partner femicide by 400%.
- In 2018, partner violence accounted for 20% of all violent crime.
- Intimate partner violence is most common against women between the ages of 18–24.
- 19% of intimate partner violence involves a weapon.

National Coalition Against Domestic Violence. (2020). Domestic Violence. Retrieved from www.assets.speakcdn.com/assets/2497/domestic _violence-2020080709350855.pdf?1596811079991.

Health care providers' offices, emergency rooms, and ambulatory care clinics offer victims of domestic violence an opportunity to receive help not only in the treatment of current wounds but also in the prevention of future incidents. Recently, the AMA has made provider assistance in the reduction of domestic violence a priority. The AMA Code of Medical Ethics provides guidance on medical care providers' obligation to help patients avoid future abuse.

Sexual Assault

The United States Department of Justice defines sexual assault as "Sexual assault is any type of sexual contact or behavior that occurs without the explicit consent of the recipient. Falling under the definition of sexual assault are sexual activities as forced sexual intercourse, forcible sodomy, child molestation, incest, fondling, and attempted rape." Health care professionals will encounter victims of sexual assault when a victim seeks treatment in medical facilities following a sexual assault or when a patient is sexually assaulted by personnel providing medical care within the facility.

The patient–provider relationship is determined to be a fiduciary relationship, which means that the provider is held to the highest standard of trust. According to *Black's Law Dictionary*, the term *fiduciary* refers to a duty to act for someone else's benefit. It is the highest standard of duty implied by law. Although rape is a crime whenever it is committed, it is a particularly heinous one when committed by a health care provider in the patient–provider relationship. Patients must be able to trust their health care providers. Public policy demands that patients be protected from abuse of power and breach of trust. This policy is intended to cover all persons involved in the care of the ill, children, and older adults.

Although all states require that health care providers report evidence of the rape of a minor child or of older adult, not all states require a health care provider to report treating an adult rape victim. In *Rape and Sexual Assault Reporting Requirements for Competent Adult Victims*, attorney Teresa P. Scalzo reports that not all states have laws that require medical professionals to report that they have treated an adult rape victim. Of the laws that do exist, Ms. Scalzo indicates that laws "requiring medical personnel to report that they have treated a competent, adult rape victim can be broken down into the following categories: (1) laws that specifically require medical professionals to report treatment of a rape victim to law enforcement; (2) laws that require the reporting of injuries that may include rape; (3) laws relating to other crimes or injuries which may impact rape and sexual assault victims; and (4) laws regarding sexual assault forensic examinations which may impact rape and sexual assault reporting."

Fraud

The high cost of fraudulent and abusive claims has given rise to an interagency "Strike Force" led by the U.S. Department of Justice in conjunction with the Department of Health and Human Services. The government has the capacity to do "real time" analysis of Medicare billings to ensure that hospitals, laboratories, health maintenance organizations, and providers' offices are complying with billing and service requirements.

In addition, federal statutes including the Stark Law, Federal False Claims Acts, the Anti-Kickback Statute, as well as statutes that criminalize intentional acts of fraud upon a health care insurance company, support the Strike Force's mission to eradicate insurance fraud and abuse. Insurance fraud and abuse can both result in improper payments being made to health care providers. They differ, however, in that fraud involves an intent to defraud whereas abuse involves business or billing practices that are unsound or unprofessional. See Table 4-1 for definitions and examples of insurance fraud and abuse.

In 2021, the University of Miami (UM) paid $22 million to settle alleged violations of the False Claims Act. The alleged violations included (1) failing to provide the proper notice of higher charges to patient's due to the conversion of doctors' offices to hospital facilities, which allowed UM to bill Medicare at higher rates than at a doctor's office; (2) billing for medically unnecessary tests by requiring a specific set of tests for all transplant patients rather than tailoring them for the individual patient; and, (3) submitting inflated claims based upon rules that govern how

Table 4-1 Definitions and Examples of Insurance Fraud and Abuse

	Fraud	**Abuse**
Definition	Knowingly submitting, or causing to be submitted, false claims or making misrepresentations of fact to obtain a Federal health care payment for which no entitlement would otherwise exist Knowingly soliciting, receiving, offering, or paying remuneration (e.g., kickbacks, bribes, or rebates) to induce or reward referrals for items or services reimbursed by Federal health care programs Making prohibited referrals for certain designated health services	Practices that may directly or indirectly result in unnecessary costs to the Medicare Program Abuse includes any practice that does not provide patients with medically necessary services or meet professionally recognized standards of care
Examples	Knowingly billing for services at a level of complexity higher than services actually provided or documented in the medical records Knowingly billing for services not furnished, supplies not provided, or both, including falsifying records to show delivery of such items Knowingly ordering medically unnecessary items or services for patients Paying for referrals of Federal health care program beneficiaries Billing Medicare for appointments patients fail to keep	Billing for unnecessary medical services Charging excessively for services or supplies Misusing codes on a claim, such as upcoding or unbundling codes Upcoding is when a provider assigns an inaccurate billing code to a medical procedure or treatment to increase reimbursement

Source: Medicare Learning Network. (January 2021). Medicare Fraud & Abuse: Prevent, Detect, Report. U.S. Department of Health & Human Services. Retrieved from www.cms.gov/Outreach-and-Education /Medicare-Learning-Network-MLN/MLNProducts/Downloads/Fraud-Abuse-MLN4649244.pdf.

much related parties can charge for tests. While the settlement included no finding of liability or admission of guilt, the United States Office of the Attorney General's press release made clear the damage caused by fraud in health care:

"Health care providers who charge for medically unnecessary services and knowingly violate billing rules contribute to the soaring cost of health care," said Acting Assistant Attorney General Brian M. Boynton for the Justice Department's Civil Division. "The department will investigate and hold accountable those who seek to profit at the expense of federal health care programs and their beneficiaries."

"Medical providers who submit fraudulent claims to our taxpayer-funded health care programs not only violate the public's trust, they compromise the very integrity of these programs," said Acting U.S. Attorney Juan Antonio Gonzalez for the Southern District of Florida. "Our office will aggressively pursue investigations against all providers who knowingly violate these billing rules no matter their size."

"Bilking the Medicare program and patients by charging for medically unnecessary services will always draw the attention of my office," said Special Agent in Charge Omar Pérez Aybar of the Department of Health and Human Services Office of Inspector General (HHS-OIG). "Working with our law enforcement partners, our agents are committed to investigating alleged billing scams that result in tremendous costs to federal health care programs and its beneficiaries."

Contemporaneous with the civil settlement, UM has also agreed to enter into a corporate integrity agreement with the Department of Health and Human Services.

U.S. Department of Justice, Office of the Attorney General. (2021, 10 May). University of Miami to Pay $22 Million to Settle Claims Involving Medically Unnecessary Laboratory Tests and Fraudulent Billing Practices. Press release. Retrieved from https://www.justice.gov/opa/pr/university-miami-pay-22-million-settle-claims-involving-medically-unnecessary-laboratory.

Fraud can take many forms. It includes "upcoding" procedures to more expensive ones than were actually performed, kickbacks for referrals, filing false information, and billing for services not provided. It can even include "renting patients," in which patients are recruited and paid for procedures they do not need. The government's net is wide when it investigates and prosecutes for fraud.

In addition to following your employer's policy regarding reporting fraud, you can report instances of Medicare or Medicaid fraud by completing the online form found at www.medicaidfraudhotline.com/report-online-form.php or by calling 888-742-7248.

False Billing

A Houston physician was sentenced to five years in prison and ordered to pay $9.5 million in restitution as a result of her participation in a $17 million Medicare fraud scam. Yolanda Hamilton, MD, was found guilty of signing false home health services care plans and other medical documents that were then used to submit fraudulent claims to Medicare. Hamilton received illegal payments in the form of a co-pay from home health care services for certifying and recertifying. Dr. Hamilton and her co-conspirators compensated patients to undergo medically unnecessary home health care services. Prosecutors charged that Dr. Hamilton and her co-conspirators submitted more than 2,500 fraudulent billings to Medicare.

> Hamilton typically would not release the home healthcare paperwork until the home healthcare companies or their marketers paid her the kickback, the evidence showed. The scheme resulted in approximately millions in false and fraudulent claims for home-health services to Medicare and in Hamilton receiving over $300,000 in kickbacks.
>
> . . .
>
> To date, several co-conspirators including marketers, patient recruiters along with doctors, and nurses who purchased plans of care and other signed medical documents from Hamilton have been charged, found guilty, or pleaded guilty to conspiracy to commit health care fraud and/or paying or receiving kickbacks.
>
> U.S. Department of Justice, Office of the Attorney General. (2020, 18 November). Texas Physician Sentenced for Multi-Million Medicare Fraud Scheme. Press release. Retreived from www.justice.gov/opa/pr/texas-physician-sentenced -multi-million-medicare-fraud-scheme.

Billing for Services Not Authorized or Warranted

A recent case of billing fraud involved radiologists providing diagnostic tests not ordered by primary care providers and then billed for procedures not supported by the medical records. These providers entered into a settlement with the government by paying $2 million and agreeing to a 5-year integrity agreement.

Billing for Unnecessary Services

Fraud frequently involves providing unnecessary medical services to patients who are not aware they are healthier than their providers have told them. In a 2007 case, a provider routinely found his patients had skin cancer, performed unnecessary surgeries, and billed Medicare.

Although it may seem that government strike forces are the only ones interested in fraud, that is far from the truth. Many of the cases do come from the government sector because it is such a large payer for so many people. Private insurance companies encounter the same types of fraud as is experienced by Medicare.

Delegation of Duties

Health care delivery by proxy is another area that sets the trap for fraudulent Medicaid and Medicare billings. Even though some health care professionals can legally perform a given service under the terms of a state's medical practice act, it does not mean that Medicare will pay for the service. This is an area that has particular significance for health care professionals. Accuracy in billing is just as important as accuracy in the patient's health records.

Forgiving Copayments

In an August 18, 2015, article entitled "Healthcare Fraud Shield's Latest Article: Patient Cost Forgiveness—Why is it a problem?" providers were warned that "In addition, routinely waiving patient copays could also be construed as fraud . . . Providers who waive copays are exposed to HIPAA risk because, arguably, the provider is misstating their charge to the commercial plan. For example, assume a $100 total charge where the patient has an 80/20 plan. If the provider waives the patient's obligation to pay 20%, then, again arguably, the commercial plan owes only 80% of $80." Notably, each state has different laws and policies regarding insurance fraud. In some states, the waiver of copayments may qualify as fraud. So, be aware of your state's regulations, and review your policies and procedures.

Kickbacks

The Medicare-Medicaid Antifraud and Abuse Amendments contain a provision that makes it illegal for a person or institution to make or receive payment of any kind in return for obtaining or introducing the referral of Medicaid or Medicare patients, as this can be an impermissible conflict of interest. Criminal penalties will be imposed on anyone who knowingly and willfully solicits or receives any kickback, bribe, or rebate in return for referring a patient to a provider, physical therapist, pharmacy, and so on, or for referring to a patient any item or service that may be paid for in full or in part by Medicare or Medicaid.

Conflicts of Interest

The Stark law addresses, among other things, conflict of interest situations and prohibits health care providers and their immediate family members from benefiting financially from Medicare/Medicaid patient referrals. A health care provider who is rewarded financially for patient referrals, patient orders, and so on faces a conflict of interest because the promise of financial reward can result in the overuse of medical services or the ordering of services that are not medically necessary.

The Stark law, the federal Anti-Kickback Statute, and similar state laws address the conflict of interest that arises regarding a provider's acceptance or solicitation of something of value in exchange for something in return. Pharmaceutical representatives bringing the office staff donuts or treating them to lunch may constitute violations of these laws. When faced with a friendly and food or gift-bearing pharmaceutical representative, make sure you understand your employer's policy and obtain approval before you accept anything of value.

If you report a Stark violation, you may be eligible for a whistleblower reward, as explained below. A Stark violation can be reported online in the same way that any Medicaid or Medicare fraud can be reported (i.e., via the online form www.medicaidfraudhotline.com/report-online -form.php).

Penalties

The government has established an office—the Office of the Inspector General (OIG) in the U.S. Department of HHS—to police the entire realm of fraud and abuse. The government no longer needs to show intent— only that the provider knew or should have known that the charges were improper.

For every claim that OIG finds was not provided as reported, the provider may be fined and held liable for as much as double the amount claimed for each item or service. There is also the possibility of criminal prosecution and sanctions involving suspension from the program. Sanctions have a serious impact on a provider who has built a practice at least in part on income from Medicare patients.

Informants

An investigation is usually triggered by a tip. Tips come from Medicare carriers, peer review organizations, state licensing boards, whistle-blowing providers, ex-staff members, and patients. Investigators make their case through beneficiary or patient interviews, documentation within the medical record, and interviews of other providers and nurses. Some cases are easy, as in the following: "We had an ophthalmologist who had his machine repossessed for nonpayment by the manufacturer, and for a year after that he was still billing Medicare for procedures performed by the machine. He pleaded guilty and is serving time."

The government provided an incentive to those who know of fraudulent provider behavior by recognizing their right to bring a lawsuit on behalf of the government in exchange for generous rewards. This

qui tam lawsuit (also known as a "whistleblower lawsuit") has been popular since the mid-1990s and provides significant disincentive to cheat the system because it empowers virtually anyone with knowledge to sue the provider.

Health care professionals may be considered co-conspirators with the provider in fraud. The gist of a conspiracy is to agree to disobey or disregard the law. Two types of intent must be proven: intent to agree and intent to commit the substantive offense. For example, when an assistant prepares bills for a provider and agrees to include any information in the insurance form that does not reflect the true situation, the assistant may be found guilty of conspiring to commit fraud even if the assistant did not profit in any way.

qui tam lawsuit A lawsuit alleging fraud and initiated by a whistleblower who receives a share of any recovery as a reward.

Health Insurance Portability and Accountability Act of 1996

On August 21, 1996, President Clinton signed into law the HIPAA, also known as the Kassenbaum-Kennedy Health Insurance Reform Bill. Included in the HIPAA is a provision requiring every health plan and provider to maintain "reasonable and appropriate" safeguards to ensure the confidentiality of health information. The safeguards are intended to protect the disclosure of "individually identifiable information" that refers to any information that (1) identifies the individual; (2) relates to the individual's physical or mental health—past, present, or future—or payment for health care; or (3) is created or received by a health plan, provider, or employer.

Any health plan provider, or other person, who knowingly obtains or discloses "individually identifiable information" in violation of the Act is subject to a fine of $50,000 and a year in prison. If the information is obtained or disclosed through false pretenses, the fine increases to $100,000 and 5 years in prison. If such information is obtained or disclosed with the intent to sell, transfer, or use it for commercial advantage, personal gain, or malicious harm, the fine becomes $250,000 and 10 years in prison.

Individuals and organizations may request the U.S. HHS Inspector General to issue fraud alerts to inform the public that certain practices are considered suspect or of concern to the Medicare and Medicaid programs. As a requirement of the Act, the HHS, in consultation with the attorney general, will issue advisory opinions, within 60 days of request, to determine whether these activities are prohibited by fraud and abuse provisions.

These decisions are an attempt to address unsettled areas of past law, whether a waiver of coverage or deductibles or the transfer of items or services for free or for less than market value is "remuneration," and other matters of similar concern. Such waivers will be legal only when they are not used to solicit patients, are not routinely waived by the provider, and are waived only because of a patient's financial need.

Under the Act, health care fraud is made an independent federal crime and includes knowing and willful schemes to defraud any health care benefits program, not just Medicaid and Medicare. Penalties include fines and up to 10 years in prison, which may become 20 years if the crime results in serious bodily injury and life imprisonment if the crime results in death.

The Act establishes the Medicare Integrity Program for private investigations and audits, encourages individuals to report fraud, and allows for rewarding individuals who report fraud. In addition, the Act requires the HHS to establish a national data bank to record information about providers and suppliers that have committed health care abuse.

Since the enactment of HIPAA, the HHS has developed a large number of sweeping regulations, especially affecting the privacy of patient information.

Embezzlement

Embezzlement occurs in the medical office when the person handling payments from patients takes the money and uses it for their own purposes. To have embezzlement, (1) there must be a relationship, such as employment, between the individual who embezzles and the owner of the money; (2) the money must come into the hands of the embezzler because of the relationship; and (3) there must be intent to fraudulently misappropriate the money.

Illegal Sale of Prescription Drugs

The number of medical professionals arrested for illegally selling prescription drugs is on the rise. To be found guilty of this offense, the substance in question must be a controlled substance; the individual being charged must have a perceptible amount of the substance on their person or have distributed some perceptible amount of that substance with the intent to distribute it to another person or persons; and the individual must have done so knowingly or intentionally:

Michael Troyan, a physician assistant who operated two urgent care clinics on the east end of Long Island was arrested this morning pursuant to a grand jury indictment with conspiring to illegally distribute oxycodone, a highly addictive prescription pain medication. Also this morning, a search warrant was executed at the East End Urgent and Primary Care in Riverhead by the DEA's Long Island Tactical Diversion Squad which is comprised of agents and officers of the DEA, Nassau County Police Department, Rockville Centre Police Department, and Port Washington Police Department. The Long

Island Tactical Diversion Squad was also assisted by agents and officers of the Department of Health & Human Services, the Southampton Town Police Department, and the Suffolk County District Attorney's East End Drug Taskforce . . .

The indictment and public filings allege that between November 2011 and October 2015, Troyan, a physician assistant with authority to prescribe controlled substances, issued prescriptions for thousands of oxycodone pills to co-conspirators for the purpose of illegally re-selling the pills for cash. Troyan was captured on video in an undercover operation writing phony prescriptions for oxycodone and receiving large quantities of cash at his Riverhead medical office for prior illegal sales. Troyan was receiving half of the profit from the sale of the oxycodone pills . . .

If convicted, the defendant faces a maximum sentence of 20 years' imprisonment and a $1 million fine.

Office of the Attorney General, Eastern District of New York. (2015, November 4). Riverhead Physician Assistant Arrested for Conspiracy to Illegally Prescribe Oxycodone. United States Department of Justice. Retrieved from www.justice.gov/usao-edny /pr/riverhead-physician-assistant-arrested-conspiracy -illegally-prescribe-oxycodone.

One of the defenses available to the defendants in the preceding case charges the investigators with illegal search and seizure, which is discussed in the following section.

Search and Seizure

The Fourth Amendment of the U.S. Constitution protects an individual against unreasonable searches of person, house, office, or vehicle and unreasonable seizure of person, papers, and effects. The amendment further provides that no warrant shall issue except upon probable cause supported by oath or affirmation and, particularly, a description of the place to be searched and the persons or things to be seized. It is generally accepted that police may not enter a person's home without a search warrant.

Individuals who are arrested for driving while intoxicated are asked to take breathalyzer tests and provide blood samples for laboratory analysis. The U.S. Supreme Court has upheld the admissibility of blood tests by a provider using standard medical procedures in which the blood was taken from a conscious person who did not consent but who offered no physical resistance. Other incidents of search and seizure are found in medical treatment situations. For example:

> A gun battle between the police and three armed men occurred following the robbery of a supermarket. One policeman and one robber were killed; another robber was shot but escaped. A few weeks later, the police picked up an individual they suspected was the robber who got away. He was taken to the hospital, where X-rays indicated metallic fragments in his buttocks. The police obtained a search warrant, and a surgeon removed the metal while the suspect was under local anesthesia. The metal fragments were identified as parts of police bullets and used as evidence against the defendant. He was convicted of the policeman's murder. He appealed the conviction and the Indiana Supreme Court held that such an extensive intrusion into his body had constituted a sufficiently unreasonable violation of his constitutional rights to require reversal of his conviction.
>
> *Adams v. State of Indiana*, 229 N.E.2d 834 (Ind. 1973)

Other Reporting

Federal, state, and local statutes, as well as office or hospital protocols, require that you report certain incidents. Some reporting is mandated and some reporting is required to comply with protocols found in your office manual. In all instances, it is imperative that the reporting be accurate, complete, timely, and as detailed as possible.

Every state has statutes that set forth the mandatory reporting of certain health matters, including births and deaths, venereal and other communicable diseases, injuries resulting from violence such as stab and gunshot wounds, child and elder abuse, blindness, immunological proceedings, requests for plastic surgery to change a person's fingerprints, and cases of industrial poisoning, among others. The method for reporting will vary with each state but will generally include the type of information required for suspected child abuse. Health care professionals should be aware of the health matters in their home state that require mandatory reporting and the method for reporting.

In addition, you may encounter a scenario where you observe an illegal or unsafe activity in the health care setting and must report it by following proper protocol. In such an instance, consult your office manual for detailed reporting instructions. Most offices and hospitals will have a written protocol that includes some or all of the following steps:

1. Record facts of the illegal or unsafe activity and the people involved.
2. Follow office protocol in contacting the appropriate person or department (often called Quality Assurance). Identify yourself and the purpose of your call (to report an illegal or unsafe activity).

3. Confirm that you will not be penalized for reporting the illegal activity and request information about protocol should you experience retaliation.

4. Provide detailed information about the illegal or unsafe activity and ask how the process works, what type of response you can expect, and when you can expect it. Ensure you do not violate any patient privacy statutes or rules by disclosing patient information that would otherwise require a patient's authorization. Your state statute should provide guidance as to what you can report, to whom, and when, and your office manual should have this clearly defined for you.

5. Take detailed notes about the questions you ask and the responses provided to you.

6. If you do not receive a response within the time you were told, follow up with the appropriate person or department and make notes about the questions asked and responses given.

7. Retain your notes so you have evidence that you made the report and that you followed protocol in your reporting.

Sometimes an error in patient care requires reporting, as well. In such an instance, consult your office manual for detailed instructions. Most offices and hospitals will have a form for recording an error in patient care (sometimes called a "patient incident report" or "incident report") and a written protocol that includes the following steps:

1. Provide a detailed report to a supervisor or other person as directed by your office manual.

2. On the patient incident report, record the patient's status before the incident and complete the section that discusses the incident with as much detail as possible.

3. Complete all other sections of the patient incident report including all people involved in the incident; how the incident was corrected; any related policies, procedures, or protocols; observations about patient or family reaction to the incident. Sign and date the incident form and obtain any other required signatures. Submit the form as dictated by your office protocol.

When you are making a report of any incident, ensure that you record your detailed notes of the event that required reporting, the people involved, and the steps you took in reporting the event. If your notes include patient information protected by federal or state privacy statutes, ensure your notes are disclosed to third parties only with proper authorization.

Civil Causes of Action—Intentional Torts

Civil law covers all bad acts except criminal actions. Most cases in medical malpractice law fall within the civil law of torts. A tort is a private wrong or injury, other than breach of contract, for which the court will provide a remedy. To have an action in tort, there must exist a legal duty between the plaintiff and the defendant, a breach of that duty, and injury as a result of the breach. Tort liability is classified as intentional, negligent, or liability without fault. An intentional tort differs from negligence. In negligence, injury to the patient occurs because the defendant fails to exercise the degree of care required in doing what is otherwise permissible.

The importance of intentional torts for the patient or plaintiff lies in the ability of the victims to receive damages for injury. In a criminal case of assault and battery, for example, the victim may get back money, if robbed, but cannot sue for emotional distress, pain and suffering, diminished employability, and so on. The criminal complaint functions to punish the perpetrator. In this instance, the victim could also file a civil complaint. The civil complaint functions to make the victim whole by restoring them to their original position before the assault and battery.

Intentional torts against the person include assault, battery, intentional infliction of emotional distress, false imprisonment, invasion of privacy, and defamation of character. Defenses available to defendants include privilege, consent, self-defense, the defense of others, and error.

Assault and Battery

Assault is defined as any willful attempt or threat to injure another person with the apparent ability to do so. Battery is nonconsensual touching. A health care provider can be charged with assault and battery due to the failure to obtain informed consent to treatment.

Invasion of Privacy

The United States Supreme Court has recognized that privacy is a constitutional right. Independence in making certain kinds of important decisions is a privacy interest. For example, *Roe v. Wade*, a case decided by the Supreme Court in 1973, determined that a woman's decision to have an abortion was a right of privacy.

> This right of privacy, whether it be founded in the Fourteenth Amendment's concept of personal liberty and restrictions upon state action . . . or in the Ninth Amendment's reservation of rights to the people, is broad enough to encompass a woman's decision whether or not to terminate her pregnancy.
>
> *Roe v. Wade*, 410 U.S. 113, 93 S. Ct. 705, 35 L.Ed.2d 147 (1973)

The individual's right to expect privacy in situations of medical care must be respected by health care providers and professionals. It has been established for many years that the admission of nonessential persons during treatment without the consent of the patient constitutes a violation of the right of privacy. The following is a case from 1881 that is still good law today:

> A doctor was called to the home of a woman in labor to deliver her baby. He took a friend with him who was not a physician. The friend was present throughout the delivery and held the woman's hand while she was experiencing labor pains. The doctor did not tell the patient that his friend was not another physician. The patient sued for violation of her right to privacy and the court held that she had a legal right to privacy at the time that her child was born.
>
> *DeMay v. Roberts*, 9 N.W. 146 (Mich. 1881)

False Imprisonment

The tort of false imprisonment is defined as intentionally confining a person without the legal right to do so or without their consent. Examples of false imprisonment are found where patients have been kept in a hospital for failing to pay their bills or have been committed to a mental hospital when there was no probable cause to commit.

False Claims Act

The Department of Justice civil fraud section follows provisions of the False Claims Act (FCA) to recover funds in the health care area. The government needs to prove only a deliberate (i.e., reckless but not intentional) false claim and may obtain a fine or penalty of $5,000–$10,000 per claim plus multiple damages. The most difficult aspect of the FCA is to determine the "knowledge" standard, or what one must "know" to be held liable under the act.

The FCA defines *knowing* and *knowingly* to mean that a person "(1) has actual knowledge of the information; (2) acts in deliberate ignorance of the truth or falsity of the information; or (3) acts in reckless disregard of the truth or falsity of the information" (31 U.S.C. §3729[b]). There is "no proof of specific intent to defraud" requirement. The importance of the FCA for health care professionals is involved with billing procedures.

The Affordable Care Act added amendments to the False Claims Act, including, among others, redefining "obligation" under the False Claims Act to include retention of any overpayments and reporting requirements when an overpayment occurs, and the federal Anti-Kickback Statute, which criminalizes the act of soliciting, receiving, offering, or paying for money in exchange for patient referrals for services paid by the government. The Anti-Kickback Statute makes clear that, "a person need not have actual knowledge . . . or specific intent to commit a violation." So, "not knowing" is not a defense.

Defamation of Character

Defamation of character occurs when one person communicates to a second person about a third person in such a manner that the third person's reputation is harmed. Such a written communication is termed libel, whereas spoken defamation is slander. The key points in a defamation case is that the shared information is false and that damages suffered result from the false statement. The following case is an example of truth being an absolute defense to defamation:

A nurse who cared for incapacitated and dependent adults sued her former employer after she was released due to reports of patient abuse that was substantiated by the patient and other staff. The incident that drew attention to the nurse's practices involved a patient who, according to the nurse, used his call bell too often. The nurse took it away from the patient and admonished him. The nurse was unable to prove the needed elements in her case, which included proving the falsity of the statements made about her conduct.

Kathleen Waugh v. Genesis Healthcare LLC et al, 2019 ME179 (December 30, 2019)

In the above case, plaintiff did not produce any evidence that the employer "knew that their statements were untrue, acted in reckless disregard of their truth or falsity, or acted solely out of ill will" (Waugh, 2019 ME179, 10). A defamation case cannot be sustained when the statement at issue is true.

Charges against health care providers for defamation of character are closely interwoven with charges of invasion of privacy or disclosure of confidential information.

Intentional Infliction of Emotional Distress

The intentional infliction of emotional distress is sometimes referred to as the tort of "outrageous conduct." This term distinguishes it from insults, indignities, threats, or annoyances. It is a tort that is usually tried before a jury because conviction depends on whether an average member of the community would consider the conduct outrageous.

A couple underwent infertility treatment at a hospital that more than twenty years later sent them a letter that read: "If you would like WIH to continue to store your embryos/oocytes, please return a copy of this letter, signed and notarized, along with a check in the amount of $500." Otherwise, the hospital indicated it would designate the embryos "legally abandoned," which meant the hospital could discard them.

The couple found this letter to be shocking. Years ago they had been told that they had used all remaining embryos when they tried to have a second child five years after the birth of their first son who was born via in vitro fertilization. Had they known there were more embryos, they could have been used twenty years earlier when they were trying to have a second child. When they called the lab, the lab confirmed that there were two frozen embryos remaining, and they later learned the vial containing the embryos had fallen to the bottom of the holding tank and cracked. They were no longer viable.

During a meeting with the couple and the hospital representatives, the couple learned the hospital knew for several years that the embryos had been missing yet never told the couple. The couple wrote a letter to the hospital and other public health care officials, including the Rhode Island attorney general and the head of the state's department of health, and stated, "As parents who cherished children, we would NOT have forgotten that our embryos were missing," they wrote. "We would not have rested until they were found and cared for." The hospital's risk management director responded to the letter with a call indicating that the situation happened a long time ago and it was time to move on. The risk management director's response was offensive to the couple as the embryos represented potential humans. As of June 2021, the pandemic continued to delay the progress of the case.

Rosman, K. (2021, April 16). The Lost Embryos. *The New York Times*. Retrieved from www.nytimes.com/2021/04/16/style/freezing-eggs-and-embryos.html.

☑ SUMMARY

- Felony crimes are more severe than misdemeanors.
- Felonies include robbery, theft, murder, attempted murder, euthanasia, manslaughter, conspiracy, and larceny.

- Child abuse, elder abuse, and domestic violence have mandatory reporting statutes governed by state law, and in some cases, federal law.
- Insurance fraud and abuse occurs in public and private health care insurance situations, and can include false billing, billing for services not authorized or warranted, billing for unnecessary services, delegation of duties, forgiving co-payments, kickbacks, and embezzlement.
- HIPAA makes health care fraud an independent federal crime.
- Civil law covers all bad acts except criminal actions.
- For a tort to be intentional, the defendant must intend to commit the act.
- Intentional torts include assault and battery, invasion of privacy, false imprisonment, defamation of character, and intentional infliction of emotional distress.

SUGGESTED ACTIVITIES

1. Research the mandatory reporting procedures for child abuse and for older adult (also known as "vulnerable adults") abuse in the state in which you intend to practice. Are the reporting requirements the same? What federal act requires that states have laws or regulations that require mandatory reporting of child abuse and neglect?
2. Using the COVID-19 pandemic as the backdrop, including testing sites, vaccination sites, and hospitals treating patients, create a list of situations where acts of fraud could be committed and consider how a witness to the fraud might report them.
3. You witnessed a co-worker putting medical waste in the regular, non-medical waste basket. Role-play the steps and chain of command for reporting the OSHA violation.
4. Find and read the AMA Code of Medical Ethics Opinion 8.10 on the Internet. How can health care professionals help providers to comply with this opinion?
5. Research the gunshot reporting obligations of the state in which you intend to practice. In your intended area of practice, would you be considered a mandatory reporter of a gunshot wound?

STUDY QUESTIONS

1. Murder is a crime. How does murder differ from euthanasia? Do the courts treat the two differently? If so, why?
2. How is the health care industry affected by statutes and regulations on child and elder abuse?

3. Explain the difference between robbery and larceny.

4. A patient who has not paid a bill has come to the emergency room for medical treatment. While there, a medical assistant notices a large amount of money in her purse. The medical assistant tells the security guard. The guard stands at the patient's room and refuses to let her leave until she pays some money toward her bill. Can the patient file charges against the hospital? If so, what will the proper complaint read?

5. Identify which of the following are examples of insurance fraud and which are examples of insurance abuse:

   a. New patients are pursued with the enticement of waived co-payments.

   b. Bills are submitted to insurance for patients who missed their appointment.

   c. Medical records are falsified to indicate that a procedure is medically necessary.

   d. Unprofessional or problematic billing practices result in unnecessary insurance reimbursement.

   e. Excessive use of health care services (e.g., ordering multiple tests to receive higher reimbursement).

CASES FOR DISCUSSION

1. In most states, physicians are mandated to report suspected or confirmed child abuse. Determine whether you would report either of these hypothetical cases as child abuse:

   • Max's parents brought the 7-year-old to his pediatrician's office for an annual well-child exam. Max's two brothers, Sammy, 5 years old, and Henry, 8 years old, each drew on paper given to them by the staff while they waited quietly just outside the exam room. Neither of them made eye contact with the staff member who brought them the paper. Max's parent's shared that Max was healthy and had no health issues. During the examination, the pediatrician observed two linear bruises on Max's right palm and inside forearm. When the pediatrician asked Max what happened that caused the bruises, Max was silent and his father said that he used a belt to spank his buttocks, and Max had tried to block the belt with his hands. Max had no other bruises or injuries and was otherwise healthy. The pediatrician observed Max's development as age appropriate, but his parents reported that he was performing poorly in school.

   • Felipe and Sue brought their 19-month-old daughter, Alejandra, to the emergency room with burns on her lower torso, legs, and arms.

Sue reported to the ER nurse that they had stepped outside to move a box into their garage, during which time Alejandra found her way into the bathroom, turned on the hot water, and climbed into the tub. During the examination, Sue stepped out of the exam room to check on her son, who was home and being watched by a neighbor. While Sue was out of the exam room, the ER physician came in and asked Felipe what happened. Felipe stated that Alejandra's 3-year-old brother turned on the water and pushed the child into the tub while the parents were moving a dresser to another part of their house. Felipe reported that they did not decide to bring Alejandra to the ER until several hours after Alejandra received the burns because they did not think the injured were serious.

2. A woman went to the provider with severe stomach pains. She was examined by a surgeon who, she stated, told her that her spleen was "hanging by a thread" from her collarbone. The surgeon recommended surgery to "build up ligaments" in her spleen. Following the operation, the surgeon informed her spouse that it had been necessary to remove the spleen. The pathology report revealed no evidence of any disease in the spleen. The woman and her spouse brought a cause of action against the surgeon for fraud. Should the court rule in their favor? What facts are important in your analysis?

3. Charles Venner swallowed 24 or 25 balloons of hashish oil in Morocco, flew to New York, passed 5 balloons, went on to Baltimore, and was brought by friends to the emergency room of Sinai Hospital "euphoric, disoriented, and lethargic, but responding to verbal orders." While under observation, he passed in bedpans the remainder of the balloons, one broken. The hospital staff saved the balloons and turned them over to the Baltimore police without a warrant. Should the police require a search warrant to use the balloons as evidence in a cause of action for possession of an illegal substance with the intent to distribute?

4. A patient went to a plastic surgeon to have repairs made on his nose. The surgeon took pictures before and after the operation. These were published without the patient's consent in a medical journal article titled "The Saddlenose." The patient sued the plastic surgeon, stating that the pictures were being used to advertise the surgeon's work. Should the patient win?

5. Parents took their 13-year-old daughter to the family provider for treatment of a foot infection. He advised the parents that she should stay at home in bed and that they should ask the school for a home teacher. The form the provider signed that went to the superintendent of the school incorrectly stated that the girl was pregnant. The child's parents requested that the provider change the report, but he told them that he had checked his files and found nothing that would

indicate that he had made such a report. He also told them that if they brought the report to his office, he would do what he could to correct any error if he had made one. The school would not release the report. The parents continually called the provider. The office told the parents to stop bothering the provider about the matter and that he would not call the school. The father brought charges against the provider for libel. Do you think the provider had a defense that would convince a jury?

Chapter 5

What Makes a Contract

> " If the maintenance of public credit, then, be truly so important, the next enquiry which suggests itself is, by what means it is to be effected? The ready answer to which question is, by good faith, by a punctual performance of contracts. States, like individuals, who observe their engagements, are respected and trusted: while the reverse is the fate of those, who pursue an opposite conduct. "
>
> Alexander Hamilton

Objectives

After reading this chapter, you should be able to:

1. Explain the elements necessary to make a contract.
2. Differentiate between express and implied contracts.
3. Describe the law of agency.
4. Identify who can and who cannot be a party to a contract.
5. Define advance directives.
6. Identify the various ways to terminate a contract.
7. Identify situations that would be considered a breach of contract in the health care field.
8. Identify the individual responsible for payment of medical fees.
9. Describe basic collection protocol for past due accounts.

Building Your Legal Vocabulary

Abandon
Acceptance
Advance directives
Age of majority
Agent
Breach
Conservator
Consideration
Contract

Duress
Emancipated minors
Express contract
Guardian
Implied contract
Incompetent persons
Injunctive relief
Legal capacity
Legal disability

Mature minor
Mental incompetence
Minors
Mutual agreement
Offer

Principal
Remedies
Specific performance
Undue influence
Warranty

Contracts, In General

offer A proposal to perform or refrain from a certain action.

acceptance An agreement to the terms of an offer.

consideration Something promised that results in making an agreement a lawful, enforceable contract.

contract A voluntary agreement, written or unwritten, between two parties that creates an obligation to do or not to do something.

express contract An explicit agreement between two or more parties.

implied contract An agreement not indicated by direct words but evident from the conduct of the parties.

legal capacity A person's ability to enter into contracts because no legal disabilities exist.

breach To act contrary to a contractual provision or to fail to perform a contractual provision.

remedies Ways to make a nonbreaching party whole after a contracting party has breached.

specific performance The remedy of requiring a party to a contract to perform the contract as specified.

injunctive relief Remedy preventing or requiring someone to perform or to refrain from performing a particular action.

The patient–provider relationship is the foundation of medical practice. That relationship is contractual and can be illustrated in its simplest form as follows: The patient seeks medical care (the **offer**) and the health care provider agrees to provide the medical care (the **acceptance**). The promises made to the other party (the patient's promise to pay a fee and the health care provider's promise to provide health care) are the **consideration** needed to form a legally binding contract.

A **contract** is a voluntary agreement between two or more parties that establishes a legally enforceable obligation. An offer, an acceptance, and consideration are all required to make an enforceable contract. A contract can be written or oral, and it can be an **express contract** or an **implied contract**. The contracting parties must have the **legal capacity** to form a contract. Any party to a contract may appoint an agent to form the contract or to perform some or all of the contractual obligations.

A **breach** of contract occurs when a party to a contract fails to perform one or more terms of the agreement. Contracts are enforceable by the courts, and there are **remedies** for damages that occur as a result of a breach, including money, **specific performance**, and **injunctive relief**.

Contracts are an essential and pervasive part of any health care facility. If there is more than one health care provider in a medical practice, the entire practice is considered to have formed a contract with a patient. Medical practices, insurance companies, hospitals, nursing homes, and other health care facilities are held together through contract law.

Health care providers and professionals may have employment contracts that state that they are employed, at what rate, what the job consists of, and whatever other terms are necessary to define the framework of employment. If there is no employment contract, the employee is deemed to be an employee-at-will, which means that the employer can dismiss the employee at any time, without warning, and for any nondiscriminatory reason.

In addition to contracts related directly to the patient–provider relationship, contracts encountered in a health care facility can include:

- contracts with insurance companies.
- contracts for office or medical supplies.

- contracts to lease office space.
- contracts for employment.
- contracts with other health care facilities.
- contracts for clinical laboratories services, medical record software, or medical equipment lease or purchase.

Elements of a Contract

A contract comes into being when one party makes an offer, the other party accepts, and some form of consideration passes between them. Parties enter into a contractual relationship by mutual agreement, also referred to as assent or "meeting of the minds." By entering into a relationship with a health care provider, the patient makes the offer of a request for treatment. By opening the office doors, scheduling a patient's appointment, or providing a diagnosis or treatment, the health care facility accepts the patient's offer. The consideration is that the patient promises to pay the fee and that the health care provider promises to treat the patient. Once an offer, an acceptance, and consideration exist, the parties have formed a contract. If those three elements are not present, there is no contract.

Consideration

In any contract, each party promises something in exchange for what is received. These promises are referred to as consideration. The promise made must be something that the party is not already obligated to do or to refrain from doing. In a patient–health care provider contract, the patient promises to pay a fee for the medical care received and the health care provider promises to provide the agreed-upon treatment. In a contract for leased medical office space, the health care facility promises to pay the rent and abide by the terms of the lease, and the landlord promises to make the leased space available as described in the lease. In a contract for medical supplies, the medical supply company promises to supply its products at certain prices, and the health care facility promises to pay for the products it orders. All contracts have some form of consideration. Without consideration, a contract is not enforceable.

Mutual Agreement

To form a contract, there must be a clear understanding between the parties, known as **mutual agreement**, assent, or meeting of the minds. Both the party who makes the offer and the party who accepts must be thinking and saying the same thing. In a health care facility, the patient seeks medical treatment for a fee and the health care provider must be offering to treat the patient for a fee. Whether there was mutual agreement, and,

mutual agreement Common agreement and understanding of all parties to a contract.

therefore, a patient–provider relationship, is often implied by the parties' actions. The courts have found that a variety of acts by health care providers can create mutual agreement. Legal duties and obligations exist once a patient–provider relationship exists, so it is important to understand when the relationship begins and ends.

The cases that have decided the issue of whether a patient–provider relationship exists are heavily fact specific and rely upon state law. Generally, the relationship does not exist until the health care provider affirmatively undertakes to diagnose and treat the patient or participates in some manner of the patient's diagnosis and treatment.

The circumstances that create a patient–provider relationship can be simple and clear. For example, a new patient arrives for her first appointment. Often, however, the situation presents additional facts that require consideration to determine when the relationship began. Courts have held that a health care provider need not interact directly with a patient to establish a patient–provider relationship . As a result, the start of the patient–provider relationship can be unclear in situations involving on-call specialists, informal consultations with a colleague (sometimes referred to as "curbside consultations"), or health care providers who are covering for others on vacation, among others.

The patient presented at the emergency room with a three-day headache. After examination and observation, the emergency room health care provider Dr. Boyle decided that the patient should be admitted to the hospital, which based upon the patient's health care plan, required approval from Dr. Tavera. Dr. Boyle briefed Dr. Tavera and recommended hospitalization. Dr. Tavera did not approve the admission and directed that the patient be treated on an outpatient basis. The patient was sent home and suffered a stroke a few hours later. The patient sued and alleged, in part, that his heath care plan created a patient–provider relationship by contract. The court agreed, in part, because the health care plan obligated its contracted doctors to treat the health care plan members as they would treat their other patients and the patient had essentially pre-paid for the medical care of Dr. Tavera, the health care plan's doctor on duty that night.

Hand v. Tavera, 864 S.W.2d 678 (Tex.App.-San Antonio, 1993)

Courts have differed on whether indirect contact between the health care provider and patient, such as telephone communication between a hospital emergency room physician and an on-call physician regarding the treatment of an emergency room patient, can create a patient–provider relationship.

> The patient arrived at the emergency room with back pain, fever, and a history of a recent back surgery. Dr. Suarez, the emergency room physician, examined the patient and telephoned Dr. St. John, the hospital's on-call internist that night. Because Dr. St. John was not a neurologist or neurosurgeon, and the hospital was not able to handle such cases, Dr. St. John recommended that the patient be referred to a hospital with the requisite neurosurgeon or to the physician who had performed the surgery. The patient's wife requested the patient be transferred to a specific hospital closer to their home. The requested hospital refused the transfer. The patient's wife took the patient home. Subsequent complications due to meningitis caused permanent damage to the patient. The patient sued Dr. St. John. The court found that Dr. St. John had not formed a patient–provider relationship by recommending that the patient be transferred to another hospital after hearing the patient's history. Dr. St. John listened to the patient's history, symptoms, and condition to decide if he should accept the case, not to diagnose the condition or offer treatment.
>
> *St. John v. Pope*, 901 S.W.2d 420, 38 Tex.Sup.Ct.J. 723 (Tex., 1995)

Health care providers can refuse to establish a patient–provider relationship provided the refusal is not for a discriminatory reason. Historically, the rule has been that a health care provider has no duty to accept a patient, regardless of the patient's illness. Mutual agreement allows health care providers to limit or to avoid contracts with patients.

A health care provider can refuse:

- to treat patients outside of a particular specialty.
- to make house calls.
- to treat patients via video appointments.
- to have extended office hours or to not take vacation.
- a patient if the practice is not accepting new patients.
- a patient if the health care provider does not have a relationship with the patient's health insurance company.
- a patient if the patient cannot pay for the costs of treatment.
- a patient if the patient or immediate family member is a medical malpractice attorney.

A health care provider's right to refuse to treat a patient is broad provided the refusal is not based upon a discriminatory reason, such as race, gender, sexual orientation, national origin, or religion.

> **E1.1.2 – Prospective Patients**
>
> As professionals dedicated to protecting the well-being of patients, physicians have an ethical obligation to provide care in cases of medical emergency. Physicians must also uphold ethical responsibilities not to discriminate against a prospective patient on the basis of race, gender, sexual orientation or gender identity, or other personal or social characteristics that are not clinically relevant to the individual's care. Nor may physicians decline a patient based solely on the individual's infectious disease status. Physicians should not decline patients for whom they have accepted a contractual obligation to provide care.
>
> American Medical Association. (2017). Code of Medical Ethics Opinion 1.1.2: Prospective Patients. AMA. Retrieved from www.ama-assn.org/delivering-care/ethics/prospective-patients.

Types of Contracts

A contract can either be express or implied. An express contract is an agreement between the parties, the terms of which are openly stated in distinct and explicit language, either orally or in writing. In medicine, it is generally recognized that without an express contract, a health care provider does not **warranty** the results of his or her work or contract to achieve a particular result.

warranty A promise that specifically named results will occur.

An implied contract gives rise to contractual obligations by some action or inaction without specifically stating the terms orally or in writing. For example, if an individual is taken to an emergency room unconscious, it is implied that the patient will accept treatment and that responsibility for payment of the treatment will be assumed by the patient. If a nurse prepares an injection, and the patient rolls up his or her shirtsleeve to receive the injection, it is implied that the patient consents to the treatment.

Agency

When a person agrees to work for and under the direction or control of another, a principal–agent relationship is created. The **principal** is the employer, and the **agent** is the employee. In a health care facility, the principal is usually the health care provider or the medical practice itself, and the agent can be a lab technician, medical assistant, a dental technician, a nurse, a receptionist, or other employee. Special rules, called the law of agency, govern this relationship. When acting within the scope of their employment, agents are performing tasks

principal The employer, or source of authority, of the agent or employee.

agent One who has authority to act on behalf of another.

on behalf of their employers. Business owners, health care providers, hospitals, and other employers—who generally have greater financial resources than employees and for whose benefit the agent is acting— are required to compensate third parties who suffer damages caused by the employers' agents.

The employee answering a health care provider's phone or making the appointment acts as the health care provider's agent in forming an oral contract, as depicted in the telephone conversation below.

> Medical Assistant: "Good morning. Doctor's office."
> Patient: "Hello, this is Mrs. West I would like to make an appointment with the doctor for a flu shot."
> Medical Assistant: "I can schedule you for Thursday morning at 10:00 a.m."
> Patient: "That's fine; I'll see you on Thursday at 10."

A middle-aged man was worried after a consultation with a surgeon. "Looks like I'll have to have a heart bypass," the patient remarked to the assistant at the front desk.

"Don't worry," she assured him, "the doctor is very good at that procedure. You won't have any trouble. I can promise you that."

The operation was prolonged by unexpected complications, and the patient died several weeks later. His family successfully sued the surgeon on the grounds that his assistant had made a promise that amounted to a warranty.

Belli, Melvin M., *Belli for Your Malpractice Defense* (1986).

Capacity of the Parties

Any person or legal entity (such as a corporation) can contract provided that the contracting party does not have a **legal disability** and is authorized to act as represented in the contract. A person with a legal disability cannot form a contract because a contract cannot be made by or enforced against a person who does not have the legal capacity for mutual agreement. **Minors, incompetent persons,** and individuals under the undue influence of a drug that alters their mental state are among those who are considered legally disabled for the purpose of forming a contract. The capacity to contract is also affected when individuals are under **duress** or required to make an agreement while under the undue influence of another person. In some circumstances, an exception to the requirement that both parties have the legal capacity to contract

legal disability Lack of legal capacity for mutual agreement.

minors Persons who are under the age of majority as set forth by state law.

incompetent persons Those who lack the necessary qualifications to perform a duty.

duress Being influenced by threat to do something one would not otherwise do.

for health care services can be made when the contract is for emergency treatment that is reasonably needed to continue life.

Minors

The general, common law rule is that a minor cannot give effective consent for the administration of medical treatment. Therefore, without the consent of the minor's parents or **guardians**, the health care provider can be held liable for assault and battery (a criminal charge) or medical malpractice (a civil matter). A minor is any person under the **age of majority**. In all but three states, the age of majority is 18 years. The age of majority in Alabama and Nebraska is 19 years, and in Mississippi it is 21 years. Exceptions to this rule are made in medical emergencies and for mature and **emancipated minors**. Other exceptions include states that allow minors to obtain birth control, prenatal, and sexually transmitted disease services without parental involvement. Where parents are also minors, most states allow the minor parent to make medical decisions regarding their own children. The majority of states require that one or more parents be advised of or consent to a minor's abortion. State law determines a minor's ability to consent, and these laws have been changing in recent years.

In most, but not all, instances, a minor's emancipation is governed by state law and requires a court order. Common reasons for emancipation are the minor's marriage, enlistment in the military, abandonment by the minor's parent or legal guardian, or express agreement by the minor's parents. Many state statutes set forth the circumstances under which the court will order emancipation either entirely or for a limited purpose (health care, residential leases, insurance, banking, etc.).

guardian A person entrusted to take care of the person, property, and rights of someone too young or otherwise incapable of managing their own affairs.

age of majority The age, as determined by state law, at which a person becomes legally able to contract, vote, and join the military.

emancipated minor A person under the age of majority who is deemed to be completely self-supporting and able to contract.

> A 17-year-old minor lived away from home with a woman who gave her free room and board in exchange for household chores. The girl made her own financial decisions and "managed her own affairs." Even though the minor's parents provided part of her income by paying for her private schooling and certain medical care, [she is] considered . . . [emancipated.]
>
> *Carter v. Cangello*, 164 Cal. Rptr. 361 (1980)

Generally, neither a minor nor a minor's parents may consent to sterilization, transplants, experimental medical care, or refusal or withholding of treatment without a court order. Yet, in the following action for damages from a vasectomy performed without the consent of parents, the court held that the minor could make his own decision:

> A minor and his wife decided to limit their family, and at 18 years of age, a health care provider performed a vasectomy on the husband. The minor was married, completed high school, the head of his own family, earned his own living, and maintained his own home. Because he was afflicted with a progressive and incurable disease that could affect his future earning capacity and ability to support his family, the court held that the minor could make the decision without involving his parents.
>
> *Smith v. Sibley*, 431 P.2d 719 (Wash. 1967)

A **mature minor** is a nonemancipated minor in mid- to late-teens who has the intelligence and emotional maturity to be able to grasp the information necessary to make an informed decision. The complexity of the medical treatment can affect whether the minor is sufficiently mature to give informed consent. The standards determining a minor's maturity and an individual's capacity to give informed consent are closely related and are often governed by state law.

mature minor A person under the age of majority who has the mental capacity to make certain medical decisions without parental consent.

Constitutional Rights and Minors   American citizens, including minors, enjoy Constitutional rights. The Constitutional right of privacy is fundamental but not absolute for minors in matters of abortion. While the Supreme Court has established that abortion is legal, it has also upheld state laws that require some form of parental involvement in a minor's decision to have an abortion. The majority of states now have laws requiring some form of parental consent or notification for minors who seek an abortion.

Mental Incompetence

Mental incompetence exists when a person does not have the mental capacity to understand the nature and consequences of his or her actions. Some individuals are adjudged incompetent by the courts and have an appointed legal guardian. Generally, the guardian will be appointed by the court to make decisions and enter into contracts on behalf of the incompetent. Many of the contract rules that apply to minors also apply to people adjudicated as mentally incompetent.

mental incompetence Lack of reasoning faculties needed to enable someone to contract.

Incompetence is not necessarily adjudicated just for severe mental illness or developmental disability only. In some situations, individuals can be competent to care for themselves but unable to attend to personal finances. For such individuals, a **conservator** can be appointed to oversee financial matters. A conservator differs from a legal guardian in that a legal guardian is responsible for both the person and the person's financial matters.

conservator A court-appointed person given authority to manage the financial affairs of an incompetent person.

Undue Influence

undue influence Any improper persuasion to make someone act differently from his or her own will.

Undue influence occurs when one party to a contract improperly uses personal influence over the other to cause actions not in the second party's best interests. In the patient–provider relationship, health care providers are in a position to influence their patients' decisions. When the health care provider uses their influential position to form an agreement that is more beneficial to the health care provider than to the patient, the health care provider is using undue influence.

> An older woman saw a psychoanalyst for many years before she died. During the period of treatment she gave him $116,050, and left him a large sum of money in her will. Part of the money was for professional fees, part was for a loan that he had never repaid, and $30,000 was a gift. After her death her heirs attempted to recover all the money except legitimate fees on the grounds of undue influence. The court ordered a hearing. The psychoanalyst had to prove that the transfers were "fair, open, voluntary, and well understood."
>
> *Estate of Reiner*, 383 N.Y.S. 2d 504 (1976)

Health Care Advance Directives

advance directives A document signed and witnessed according to state statute authorizing one person to make decisions for another, including the authorization or refusal of medical treatment.

The Patient Self-Determination Act, enacted in 1990, requires health care facilities to provide written information to each adult admission regarding patient rights under state law to make **advance directives** involving the acceptance or refusal of medical or surgical treatment. It also requires documentation of the patient's receipt of this information in the medical record as well as whether a patient has executed an advance directive. Institutions cannot condition care on the provision that the patient execute an advance directive or agree to accept treatment. This act does not apply to individual health care providers or to private medical offices.

Examples of advance directives, discussed in more detail in Chapter 12, are the living will and health care power of attorney (also referred to as a "health care proxy" or a "medical power of attorney"). It is common for these two directives above to be merged into one comprehensive health care advance directive. In addition, a health care advance directive can include choices regarding organ and tissue donation, as well as other instructions. Contact your state bar association or state department of elder affairs for information appropriate to your jurisdiction.

A living will is a written, legal document that identifies treatments you want or do not want if you cannot speak for yourself due to terminal illness or a persistent vegetative state. A living will usually applies only to end-of-life decisions and the instructions tend to be general.

A health care power of attorney is a written, legal document that gives someone the authority to act on another's behalf with regard to specific health care decisions. A health care power of attorney is typically related only to health care decisions, while a durable power of attorney can relate to just about any matter. The document itself will identify the duration and the subject matter it covers.

A "comprehensive health care advance directive" includes the terms of a living will, a health care power of attorney, as well as any other directives, such as location of treatment or organ donation. The comprehensive health care advance directive is the favored form of advance directive because it is inclusive.

Termination of Contracts

A contract between a health care provider and a patient can be terminated in several ways. The most satisfactory outcome is that the health care provider treats the patient, the patient pays the health care provider the required fee or co-payment, both parties are satisfied, and the contract concludes.

Just as the patient–provider relationship requires mutual agreement by the parties to form a contract, the parties can mutually agree to terminate the relationship. When a health care provider enters into a patient–provider relationship, the health care provider is obliged to attend the case as long as it requires attention, unless the patient is given reasonable notice of the health care provider's intention to withdraw or the patient informs the health care provider that the services are no longer desired.

If the health care provider wants to withdraw from a patient's case, the reasonableness of notice becomes an issue that depends on the patient's condition, the availability of other competent health care providers, the manner of notice, and, indirectly, the patient's educational and economic status. If a patient discharges a health care provider and the patient is in need of further medical attention, the responsibility lies with the health care provider for protection from a charge of abandonment by confirming discharge by the patient. A letter to the patient confirming discharge using certified mail will usually protect the health care provider. Some health care providers follow this procedure when a patient does not keep an appointment or fails to follow the health care provider's medical advice.

A health care provider's termination of a patient should be provided by written notice sent by certified mail, return receipt requested and filed in the patient's chart, and it should explain the patient's medical problems. The terminating health care provider must allow time for the patient to find other medical care. The amount of time should be stated, as well as the projected termination date. If a patient relationship is not properly terminated, the health care provider can be sued for a breach of contract, abandonment, or medical malpractice.

Breach of Contract

A breach of contract occurs when one of the parties does not keep a promise—by not performing, not paying for services, not keeping to schedule, or not doing the procedure as had been agreed. Breach of contract also occurs when one party prevents the other party from performing.

Examples of breach of contract can occur in the practice of medicine when the patient does not pay the health care provider's bill or when a health care provider makes a warranty that the health care provider will cure the patient but fails to do so. When the promised cure does not take place, the health care provider becomes liable for breach of contract regardless of whether there was negligence.

When the court determines there is a breach of contract, the objective of the court becomes making the nonbreaching party whole. The most common means for accomplishing this is to award the nonbreaching party monetary damages in an amount sufficient to offset the losses incurred. The amount of damages varies greatly based upon the facts and the relevant state law.

Abandonment

abandon To give up or cease doing.

To **abandon** a patient means that the health care provider gives up completely—deserts the patient—and implicitly indicates that the health care provider intends to terminate the contractual relationship before the contract's obligations are complete. A health care provider is free to withdraw from a case for nonpayment of fees but is liable for abandonment if proper termination procedures are not carried out or if the patient continues to need services.

Statute of Limitations

The statute of limitations is the length of time a person has to file a lawsuit after injury. Included in the statute of limitations is usually a "discovery rule," which maintains that the statute of limitations does not begin to run until the injured party knew, or should have known, that there was injury.

A minor does not have the capacity to sue in court and is dependent on the parent to file lawsuits before the age of majority. For one reason or another, a parent or legal guardian can decide not to pursue a cause of action. To cover this possibility and safeguard the minor's best interest, many states have maintained a statute of limitations extending 2 or more years beyond the age of majority. If a state has this provision, health care providers must keep the records of pediatric patients longer than the time that is legally required for adults or at least until the required number of years after the patient reaches the age of majority.

Who Pays?

Even though managed care has changed some of the relationship between health care provider and patient, the relationship between health care provider and patient still remains contractual in nature. The health care provider provides the service, and the patient pays the fee, usually a co-payment or deductible. The reliability of this arrangement is essential to the fundamental principles of contract law and necessary to continuing commerce. As illustrated in the quotation at the beginning of this chapter, the U.S. economic system is built on the expectation that parties will honor their contracts.

Generally, the patient who receives treatment is responsible for payment even if someone else requests the services. In certain circumstances—for example, in the care of minor children and incompetent persons—others are responsible for payment. In a situation involving minor children or those who are mentally incompetent, the parent or legal guardian is responsible for payment.

Minors lack the legal capacity to contract without a parent or guardian's permission. The interest of the state in this matter is to protect minors from the consequences of their unknowing acts. If a minor contracts for basic necessities, such as food, shelter, and certain life-saving medical services, the policy of protection from unknowing acts is not urgent. When medical care is considered a necessity, however, the court will generally conclude that a fair trade was made and an implied contract will be upheld. The minor, or the person legally responsible for the minor, must pay.

In most instances when you encounter a child patient with divorced parents, the divorce order clearly identifies who is responsible for payment of medical expenses (including co-pay, pre-pay, co-insurance, self-pay, as well as prescriptions, etc.) and the provision of an insurance policy.

In the rare instance where the divorce order does not identify who is to pay for the child's health care, check to see if your office has a protocol in place that provides guidance. In addition, if one or both of the divorced parents have health insurance, work with the health insurance plan's administrators to see if the policy dictates which policies should cover the child and in what order of precedence.

When a minor contracts for plastic surgery for cosmetic purposes, the issue of necessity can be questioned, and the need to protect the minor becomes more urgent. In this situation, the minor may or may not be obligated for the cost. It is reasonably certain that an emancipated or mature minor would be responsible for the fee.

A minor who arranges for medical care can, by statute, invoke the parent's responsibility because parents are responsible for children's necessities. Yet, under certain circumstances, even if a child is living with a parent or guardian, the liability for medical services can rest entirely on the minor if the services were rendered entirely on the credit of the minor. For example, when the expense of treatment was a material and substantial consideration in a judgment recovered by a minor as the result of litigation or settlement, the minor was liable for the medical bills.

When an individual, who is not legally obligated to pay the health care provider's fee, agrees to pay the health care provider's fee, a legal principle called "the statute of frauds" requires that the agreement be in writing. An agreement to pay made by an individual, who is not legally obligated to pay the health care provider's fee, is not legally enforceable unless it is in writing.

Collections

Health care providers and facilities will have their own policies on how payment is collected, and what happens when a patient does not or cannot pay their share of the services rendered. For health care professionals whose job duties include collecting current or past due payments, it can be awkward to discuss financial issues in a health care setting. A simple "how would you like to pay?" is a professional way to request payment of co-pay, pre-pay, co-insurance, or self-pay once you have explained what is due, regardless of whether the payment is currently or past due.

Overdue Accounts

Every business has overdue accounts. Some patients do not pay because they do not have the money, but others are habitual delinquents. Many health care businesses collect payment at check in or check out. Health care offices that are on top of collection problems keep in contact with patients and update addresses and phone numbers. Additional methods to reduce delinquent patient accounts include allowing for online payments through payment processing websites or through the facility's patient portal.

Because the debt is "incurred primarily for family or household purposes," attempting to collect the due amount is subject to a number of federal and state regulations. Health care professionals should know and follow office policy and procedure when trying to collect overdue accounts. In all instances, if your office has a protocol that differs from what is described herein, follow your office protocol.

The first step in collection is to contact the individual and determine whether there is a valid reason for the failure to pay the aging account, which is an account that is past due and categorized by the number of days the account is past due. You may ask whether they received the bill, if they have questions about the bill, or any other question will lead to a discussion of payment. Typically, a phone call may precede a letter to serve as a "friendly reminder," for example when the account has aged to 30 days past due. At 60 days, a letter would be sent; followed by another letter at 90 days.

Remaining professional during discussions with patients about past due payments is key. If a health care provider's staff members or their agents engage in overly vigorous collection activity, they risk being sued for defamation, invasion of privacy, intentional infliction of emotional distress, or other torts.

In addition, the federal Fair Debt Collections Practice Act (FDCPA) and state law govern collections practices. The FDCPA prohibits many different collection practices—for example, threats of violence, use of abusive language when trying to collect the debt, harassment by means of phone calls, and deception and unfair methods of collection (e.g., threatening to deposit a postdated check before the date of the check, intentionally causing the debtor's other checks to be dishonored). Check your state statute on collections to determine if you are in a state where health care offices are deemed debt collectors under the FDCPA. Third-party collection agencies that pursue past due health care debt are governed by the FDCPA.

Bad Checks

A check tendered for services rendered that is returned unpaid by the bank, for whatever reason, is grounds for a criminal complaint. In some states, creditors are allowed to simultaneously pursue both criminal and civil actions to secure payment; in others, the creditor must choose the venue. Threat of a criminal suit cannot be used to settle a civil action.

Collection of health care providers' fees is complicated because of third-party reimbursement. Regardless of the insurance coverage, the patient is responsible for the payment of the fee unless the health care provider has entered into an agreement to accept the insurer's rate of payment as payment in full.

Bankruptcy

Bankruptcy is the process by which a financially troubled individual or business is declared by a bankruptcy court to be incapable of paying his or her debts, the debtor's available assets are distributed to creditors as required by bankruptcy law, and the debtor is granted a discharge from liability for most of the remaining unpaid debts. There are three major kinds of bankruptcy proceedings: liquidation, business reorganization, and repayment plans for debtors with regular income. After an individual initiates bankruptcy proceedings, the creditor (e.g., a health care provider's office) may not seek payment from the debtor patient. The creditor may only communicate with the court-appointed receiver.

Termination of Delinquent Patients

If the provider has decided to terminate the patient–provider relationship due to the patient's failure to pay, the termination must be done according to office policy. An office policy should include written notice to the patient (sent first-class, certified mail, return receipt requested) that the relationship will terminate in 30 days and that during this period the provider will still render emergency care (without this 30-day period, the provider could be charged with patient abandonment). If the nonpaying patient seeks routine or nonemergency care, it is permissible to schedule the appointment after the balance is paid.

☑ SUMMARY

- The patient–provider relationship is contractual.
- To have a contract, there must be an offer, acceptance, and consideration.
- Contracts also require mutual agreement between parties who have the legal capacity to contract.
- Contracts can be express or implied.
- When and whether a patient–provider relationship has been established is fact specific and governed by state law.
- Health care providers can refuse to establish a patient–provider relationship provided the refusal is not for a discriminatory reason.
- It is generally recognized that without an express contract, a health care provider does not warranty the results of his or her work or contract to achieve a particular result. Employees are the agents of their employers (the principals) and, under the law of agency, are able to contract for the principal.
- Minors, incompetent persons, and those under undue influence are able to engage in contracts only on a limited basis.
- Undue influence occurs when one party to a contract improperly uses personal influence over the other to cause actions not in the second party's best interests.

- A comprehensive health care advance directive includes the provisions of a living will and a health care power of attorney, among others.
- Contracts terminate upon completion of the terms or by agreement of the parties.
- If a patient terminates the patient–provider relationship, the health care provider should memorialize the circumstances and conditions of the patient's termination of the relationship in a certified letter sent to the patient.
- If a health care provider terminates the relationship, further provisions must be made for the care of the patient or the health care provider can be found to have abandoned the patient.
- Contracts not performed according to agreement are termed breached.
- A party who sustains a breach of contract is entitled to be made whole by the award of damages. In the medical field, the most common remedy for a breach is monetary damages.
- Interacting with patients regarding issues of who pays and past due accounts requires professionalism.

SUGGESTED ACTIVITIES

1. What is the age of majority in your state?
2. Find an advance health care directive on the Internet that is applicable to your state. How would you complete it?
3. Identify the various contracts you encounter in your personal life. What was the last contract you signed? What was the last contract you signed on behalf of someone else (an employer, a child, a disabled relative, etc.)?
4. Find the state statute regarding collections in the state you intend to practice and research whether, under your state statute, health care providers are deemed debt collectors for purposes of the federal statute on collections.

STUDY QUESTIONS

1. Give examples of implied and express consent to medical treatment in a hospital emergency room situation.
2. A patient has just been informed by the health care provider that she must have a hysterectomy and that there is a question of malignancy.

As she leaves the office and you schedule her for hospital admission, she comments: "The doctor makes me feel so good about this. She says that I will be out of the hospital in four days and on my own within a week. Isn't she a wonderful person? She says that I will be completely cured following my surgery." How would you handle this situation? Did the health care provider give the patient a warranty as to the results? If so, was the warranty express or implied?

3. A 15-year-old girl comes to the office in her first-trimester pregnancy. A year ago, she visited the health care provider twice, and then miscarried. There is an outstanding fee to be collected from the patient. Her parents are also patients of the health care provider but do not know that their daughter is pregnant. It is your job to collect the fees from patients. What would you do as an agent of the health care provider in this situation? Could the health care provider terminate the patient–provider relationship at this point in the pregnancy for failure to pay? If so, how should the relationship be terminated?

4. A woman and a 15-year-old minor present at your office for medical care. The woman declares she is the minor's conservator, and she shows you a court document that confirms this. Can she consent to medical treatment on behalf of the minor? How would you handle this situation?

5. Which federal act governs the collection of past due accounts? What does the act prohibit?

CASES FOR DISCUSSION

1. A 16-year-old female was pregnant and wished to get married. Her mother objected strenuously and took her daughter to a gynecologist to have an abortion. The gynecologist refused to enter into a contract to perform the abortion without a court order. Should the court allow the abortion?

2. The director of a drug treatment center called a physician friend and requested that he admit one of the center's patients to the hospital. The physician friend had been seriously ill and was at home recovering when he received the telephone call. He was in no condition to visit the patient in the hospital and conveyed that information to the director but did allow the patient to be admitted to the hospital under his name. The patient never saw the physician before she died of an undiagnosed brain abscess within a few days after admission. Her father sued the physician, claiming that there was a patient–provider relationship between his daughter and the physician. Should the court agree with the physician or the father?

3. A woman was hit by a car and complained of injuries to her leg, knee, hip, and thigh. She was taken to the nearest hospital, where, on the orders of a physician, she received x-rays of her arm and pelvis. No x-ray was taken of her leg, and she was released from the hospital on crutches. The pain in her leg increased, and she went to another hospital some hours later, where an x-ray was taken and revealed that her leg was fractured. She was admitted to the second hospital and remained an inpatient for a month. Ten days after admission to the second hospital, she received a letter from the first hospital telling her to return for a leg x-ray. She sued the first hospital and the radiologist. Does the radiologist, who never saw her, have a contractual relationship with the patient?

4. A clinic patient was operated on by a hospital resident for removal of his gallbladder. It was later determined that a piece of gauze was left in the patient's abdomen. The defendant in this case was a consultant physician who saw the patient before and after the operation but who was not present at all times during surgery. He was not paid a fee for his services and did not expect payment. Was the consultant physician liable for the gauze in the patient's abdomen?

5. A man had a vasectomy. He and his wife were the parents of two children with developmental disabilities, and the vasectomy was desired to prevent the birth of another child with a disability. After the vasectomy, another child was born who was developmentally and physically disabled. Should the surgeon who performed the vasectomy be liable for breach of contract?

6. A woman went to a plastic surgeon for an operation to improve the appearance of her nose. Before the operation, the woman's nose had been straight but long and prominent. The surgeon undertook, with two operations, to reduce its prominence and shorten it, thus making it more pleasing in relation to the woman's features. Actually, the patient was obliged to undergo three operations, and her appearance worsened. Her nose now had a concave line to about the midpoint, at which it became bulbous; viewed frontally, the nose from bridge to midpoint was flattened and broadened, and the two sides of the tip had lost symmetry. This configuration could not be improved by further surgery. Should the surgeon be liable for breach of contract?

7. The plaintiffs engaged a health care provider to perform a sterilization operation on the wife. Some 17 months later, the wife became pregnant, and nine months later, she was delivered of a child by cesarean section. At the time of this birth, one of her fallopian tubes was found to be intact. This is alleged to have resulted from the negligent manner in which the health care provider performed the sterilization. The plaintiffs alleged a breach of warranty. Should the court allow them to recover damages under a breach of warranty action?

8. A patient was hospitalized for mental illness and as part of the treatment received electroshock therapy. When the psychiatrist realized that the patient could not pay his hospital bill, the health care provider sent the patient home immediately following electroshock treatment. The patient was prescribed a heavy sedative. The patient, confused from the combination of the drug and the effects of the treatment, fell asleep and ignited himself with a cigarette. He suffered nearly fatal third-degree burns over a wide area of his body. Did the health care provider have the right to discharge the patient from the hospital because he could not pay his bill?

9. The plaintiff, a blind person, accompanied by her 4-year-old son and her guide dog, arrived at the defendant's "medical office" on a Saturday to keep an appointment "for treatment of a vaginal infection." She was told that the health care provider would not treat her unless the dog was removed from the waiting room. She insisted that the dog remain because she "was not informed of any steps which would be taken to assure the safety of the guide dog, its care, or availability to her after treatment." The health care provider "evicted" the patient, her son, and her dog; refused to treat her condition; and failed to assist her in finding other medical attention. Because of this conduct on the part of the health care provider, the patient was "humiliated" in the presence of other patients and her young son, and "for another two days while she sought medical assistance from other sources," her infection became "aggravated" and she endured "great pain and suffering." The plaintiff demanded damages resulting from "breach of the health care provider's duty to treat." Should she be awarded damages?

Chapter 6

Medical Malpractice and Other Lawsuits

> ❝ The physician must be able to tell the antecedents, know the present, and foretell the future—must mediate these things, and have two special objects in view with regard to disease, namely, to do good or to do no harm. ❞
>
> Hippocratic Collection, Of the Epidemics, *book I, sect. II (2)*

Objectives

After reading this chapter, you should be able to:

1. Distinguish between a cause of action for negligence and one for malpractice.
2. List the elements of a medical malpractice lawsuit.
3. Identify when there has been a breach of duty to a patient based on an inappropriate standard of care.
4. Analyze the legal cause of a patient's injury and assess accountability of the employee.
5. Identify the legal, moral, and ethical aspects of informed consent.
6. Describe negative consequences of medical malpractice lawsuits.
7. Identify common subjective contributing factors to the patient's choice to litigate.
8. Summarize risk management measures the health care professional can take to avoid lawsuits.
9. Describe defenses available to the defendant in a medical malpractice lawsuit.
10. Analyze emergency situations to determine whether the situation is covered by a Good Samaritan statute.
11. Identify a product liability case of action.
12. Define strict liability in tort.
13. Distinguish between the duty of care owed to invitees, licensees, and trespassers for maintenance of equipment and premises.

Building Your Legal Vocabulary

Adversary
Affirmative duty
Assumption of risk
Burnout
Comparative negligence
Consumer
Contributory negligence
Defensive medicine
Ethical
Expert witness
Good Samaritan
Grossly negligent
Insurance
Invitee

Licensee
Nonverbal communication
Peer review
Product liability
Proximate cause
Reasonable care
Res ipsa loquitur
Sanctioned
Sociological
Statute of limitations
Statutory guidelines
Suit-prone
Trespasser

Practicing Medicine

The practice of medicine is understood to mean diagnosis, treatment, and/or prescribing of medicine or other treatment for prevention or cure of any human disease, ailment, injury, deformity, or physical or mental condition. You must have a license to practice medicine. Traditionally, only medical doctors could practice medicine. With the emergence of new categories of health care professionals such as nurse-practitioners, medical assistants, and lab technicians, among many others, there has been a trend toward allowing professionals other than medical doctors to engage in limited forms of medical practice. The precise limitations of practice vary based upon the state and the specialty.

State legislatures enact laws that govern what duties health care providers and professionals can perform based on the kind of license they have. Each individual who practices medicine in any form is held to professional and/or **statutory guidelines**, as well as accepted standards of care.

statutory guidelines
Legislative laws defining legal rights and responsibilities.

You may very well be the first person a patient encounters during an appointment, as well as the last person they see before they leave. As a result, you are in a key position to positively influence the patient–provider relationship.

If it is unlawful for you to practice medicine that means it is also unlawful to diagnose or suggest treatments over the telephone or during an office visit. This is true even if you know exactly what your supervising health care provider would do. It is similarly unlawful to take or order an x-ray, for example, without a health care provider's directive, even if the bone is obviously broken.

Negligence or Malpractice?

Negligence is failing to act with reasonable and prudent care given the circumstances. Malpractice differs from negligence in that malpractice is the negligence of a professional, such as a doctor, educator, pharmacist, or lawyer. Medical malpractice is a specific type of negligence. Medical malpractice arises from a health care provider's treatment of a patient that causes injury, where the act (or failure to act) does not meet accepted practices within the medical community.

A negligence lawsuit alleges that the defendant did not act in accordance with what a "reasonable person" in similar circumstances would have done. A lawsuit that alleges malpractice involves the misconduct of professionals and implies a greater duty of care to the injured person than the reasonable person standard because of the professional's specialized expertise. The term implies that, in a medical malpractice case, a health care provider, nurse, or other licensed health care professional has special knowledge that raises society's expectations.

For example, a surgeon performing an appendectomy is held to a higher standard of care than a general practitioner performing the same operation. The surgeon has special knowledge, education, training, and experience, which indicates to society that he or she is better qualified to perform an appendectomy.

In a medical malpractice case, each party must have an **expert witness** to testify as to the particular standard of care and whether it was met. Expert witnesses must have experience in the field in which they are testifying. Attorneys will try to find the best qualified expert to testify with the hope that the jury will receive the expert's testimony as credible.

There is no one standard or protocol for establishing a witness as an expert. The witness' experience and background is considered by the court when it is deciding whether the witness qualifies as an expert. Education, number of years in the field, scholarly articles published, and professional affiliations and certifications are just some of what a court may consider when qualifying an expert. Certification and registration with reputable and relevant organizations also support a witness as an expert. The American Association of Medical Assistants (AAMA) and the American Medical Technologists (AMT), for example, maintain national certifying and registration programs. An expert witness who is going to testify about the standard of care of a medical assistant, for example, would likely be a certified member of AAMA and would provide that information to the court as it considers whether the witness qualifies as an expert.

expert witness
A person whose education, profession, or specialized experience qualifies them to testify about their area of expertise as it relates to the lawsuit.

Elements of a Medical Malpractice Lawsuit

To have a medical malpractice lawsuit, the patient must prove the following:

1. There was a patient–provider relationship.
2. This relationship established the duty owed by the health care provider to the patient.
3. The duty had not been upheld at a professional standard of care.
4. The health care provider breached the duty to the patient.
5. The patient had a resulting injury.
6. The health care provider's breach was the **proximate cause** of the patient's injury.

proximate cause
Results as a direct consequence and without which the result would not have happened.

Not only must all these elements be present, but they must be sequential. For example, a health care provider does not have a duty to a patient before there is a patient–provider relationship.

The elements of a medical malpractice case are the same whether the defendant is the health care provider, as in the preceding cases, or a nurse, therapist, technician, medical assistant, or other defendant. For the plaintiff to win in a medical malpractice case, each element must be met by a preponderance of the evidence. This means that the fact finder (the jury or judge) must find that evidence supporting the plaintiff's allegations is more likely than not to be true.

Relationship

The relationship between the health care provider and the patient is established by contract law, which is covered in Chapter 5. If there is no professional relationship between the health care provider and the patient—for example, if the health care provider is at a cocktail party and, during a social conversation with the patient, discusses an illness or some symptoms that the patient reveals—there is no malpractice, even if the patient suffers injury from something that was said during the conversation.

The patient–provider relationship establishes the duty of the health care provider to the patient when it can be shown that the patient consulted the health care provider for medical advice and the elements of a contract were met: offer, acceptance, consideration, and mutual agreement. The specific profession and/or society's expectations establish the duty (also called the "standard of care") required of the health care provider. When a contract is made between a health care provider and a patient for medical care, the health care provider has a duty to the patient that must meet a professional standard of care. Breach of the duty by the health care provider, by action or inaction, is measured against the standard of care. For example:

> Plaintiff brought a medical malpractice suit against her oncologist and alleged that the oncologist failed to follow up on abnormal test results ordered by another doctor, and that the failure resulted in a delay in the diagnosis and treatment of plaintiff's cancer.
>
> The trial resulted in a verdict for the defendants, and the plaintiff appealed. The appellate court's order affirmed the trial court result. The plaintiff's expert witness testified that the oncologist breached the standard of care by failing to follow up with test results and for noting in plaintiff's chart that there was no evidence of disease when the test indicated abnormal findings. The oncologist's expert witness testified that the oncologist met the standard of care because "routine imaging was not necessary where the patient did not complain of new symptoms, and it is not one physician's role to oversee and monitor another doctor's orders. The defense expert stated that the abnormal PET scan report did not trigger any obligation" as it was the responsibility of the doctor who ordered the tests to follow up, and that "doctors would not have expected the cancer to recur less than a year after completing radiation and chemotherapy." The oncologist also had expert testimony of another medical oncologist who testified that the defendant oncologist met the standard of care because "the guidelines for treatment of breast cancer did not call for scans after treatment, as scans were unreliable and would expose the patient to additional radiation. The expert explained that this type of cancer is often incurable when it recurs."
>
> *Ross-Stubblefield v. Weakland*, (Ga. App. 2021) (unpublished)

Duty

In *Ross-Stubblefield v. Weakland*, above, the plaintiff alleged that the health care provider breached their duty of care. Specifically, the plaintiff alleged the first breach of the health care provider's duty occurred when the defendant oncologist failed to follow up with test results and that the second breach of duty was alleged to have occurred when the defendant oncologist failed to note in plaintiff's chart that there was no evidence of disease when the test indicated abnormal findings. The jury found that there was no breach of duty and that the defendants met the applicable standard of care. With slightly different facts, such as test results that conclusively identified the cancer had returned or if the defendant had ordered the test results that had abnormal findings and not followed up, the jury could have found the defendant breached their duty.

Standard of Care

Standard of care is undergoing many changes. In the past, health care providers were held to a local standard of care because of inequities in education and in funding for the latest technology and brightest talent between urban and rural locations. Subsequently, the trend in the court was a shift toward a national standard due in part to advances in communications technology allowing for health care providers at any place in the United States to access training experiences. More recently, standards of care appear to be reverting back to a local standard of care due to health maintenance organization and other managed care organization guidelines used as the basis. Theoretically, health care providers should be protected from malpractice actions by following these recognized practice guidelines because the law sets the standard of care according to accepted medical practices. The guidelines usually set ideal levels of competency, and the law recognizes different medical practices as long as they are generally accepted. There have not been enough cases tried in the courts to accurately assess this trend, but as the managed care networks grow larger and encompass broader areas of the country, the standard of care may again focus on national acceptance.

Injury

To sue for malpractice, the patient must have an injury. Without an injury, there is no case.

Causation

The health care provider's breach of duty must be the cause of the injury. There are two definitions of the legal cause of injury. The first is "but-for" causation. This means that "but for" the action of the health care provider, the injury would not have occurred. In addition to but-for causation, proximate cause must be established. Proximate cause differs in that it takes into consideration any incidents that may have occurred between the original negligent act and the outcome that is the basis for the lawsuit.

Before surgery to reduce a brain tumor, plaintiff's neurosurgeon required that the plaintiff's primary care physician clear plaintiff for surgery. As part of the clearance, the primary care physician ordered an electrocardiogram and a urinalysis both of which showed some abnormalities. The plaintiff was subsequently cleared for surgery. Plaintiff's anesthesiologist was running late, and Dr. Lorenzo, an anesthesiologist, learned that plaintiff's pre-anesthesia evaluation was not complete. To help keep the surgery on schedule, Dr. Lorenzo conducted the evaluation until the assigned anesthesiologist arrived. After losing a large amount of blood and suffering cardiac arrest, the plaintiff did not survive the surgery. Dr. Lorenzo was a named defendant in the lawsuit along with all other treating physicians. The trial court ordered a directed verdict for Dr. Lorenzo because there was "no competent, substantial evidence in the record would allow a reasonable factfinder to conclude Dr. Lorenzo was the 'primary cause' of Espinosa's death."

This case was ultimately appealed to the Supreme Court of Florida—the state's highest court—where the court disagreed with the trial court's ruling and sent the case back to complete the trial with Dr. Lorenzo as a defendant. Florida's Supreme Court stated that the court used the wrong standard to decide if Dr. Lorenzo should remain as a defendant: "An act need not be the exclusive or even the primary cause of an injury . . . rather, it need only be a substantial cause of the injury."

Ruiz v. Tenet Hialeah Healthsystem, Inc., 260 So.3d 977 (Fla. 2018)

In another case that addressed causation, *Holtzclaw v. Ochsner Clinic* (831 So. 2nd 495, La. App. 5th Cir. October 30, 2002), the Court of Appeal of Louisiana found a clinic guilty of malpractice when a nurse answered a phone call after the physicians had left for the day, prescribed aspirin with directions for the patient to "call back in the morning," and did not relay information on the patient's distress to the admitting physician in a timely fashion. The patient had undergone an outpatient colonoscopy and the next day felt intense abdominal pain.

The attending physician rationalized that even if the patient had come to the hospital on the night he began experiencing abdominal pain, the "treatment plan" would not have been different. The court found that an 18-hour delay in administering antibiotics foreseeably caused the patient's injuries. "Since time is critical in arresting any infections the jury could have found that this delay, caused by the nurse's malpractice, denied the plaintiff the opportunity to avoid the [surgical procedure and the hospitalization] by receiving timely treatment."

Sometimes the breach of duty is so obvious, it is not necessary to prove causation. The courts—recognizing that, in certain cases, evidence of what occurred is not available to the injured person—developed the doctrine of **res ipsa loquitur**. Translated from Latin res ipsa loquitur means "the thing speaks for itself." A situation in which a surgeon leaves a sponge or a tool inside the patient is a classic example of res ipsa loquitur. The sponge or the tool would not be inside the patient without an act of negligence, so the elements of duty of care, breach, and causation are assumed to have been proven.

res ipsa loquitur ("the thing speaks for itself") Evidence showing that negligence by the defendant may be reasonably inferred from the nature of the injury occurring to the plaintiff.

> Defendant performed surgery on plaintiff and used sponges to manage the blood flow during the surgery. It was later discovered that one of the sponges was left in the plaintiff post-surgery, which ultimately resulted in infection and required an above-the-knee amputation. Plaintiff brought a medical malpractice claim, and the trial court refused to instruct the jury as to the doctrine of res ipsa loquitor. During trial, the defendant argued that since the nurses performed the post-surgical sponge count, the doctrine of res ipsa loquitor was not applicable because he was not responsible for the error regarding the sponge count. The appellate court reversed and found that the defendant was indeed responsible, and the trial court's failure to instruct the jury on the doctrine warranted a new trial.
>
> *Baumgardner v. Yusuf*, 144 Cal.App.4th 1381 (Cal. Ct. App. 2006)

Informed Consent

Informed consent is an important part of medical practice today. Health care providers are often sued for malpractice because of failure to adequately inform patients of drug reactions, possible adverse surgical results, or alternative forms of treatment.

> Plaintiff sued her obstetrician and alleged medical malpractice and lack of informed consent after her son was born with cerebral palsy. Plaintiff argued that the defendant failed to inform her of risks and available alternative treatments related to material changes in her pregnancy. A jury found in favor of the plaintiff, and the defendant made a motion to set aside the verdict because "it is well established in Maryland that the doctrine of informed consent pertains only to affirmative violations of the patient's physical integrity." On appeal, the court held that an informed consent claim is viable even in cases where there was no "affirmative violation of the patient's physical integrity, because it is the duty of a health care provider to inform a patient of material information, or information that a practitioner knows or ought to know would be significant to a reasonable person in the patient's position in deciding whether or not to submit to a particular medical treatment or procedure."
>
> *McQuitty v. Spangler*, 976 A.2d 1020 (Md. App. 2009)

Analysis of the elements of this case results in the following:

1. *Relationship*: The relationship between the health care provider and patient is established. The health care provider offered services, the patient accepted, consideration was implied, and the fact that hospitalization and delivery took place indicates there was mutual assent.

2. *Duty*: The patient–provider relationship establishes a duty of the health care provider to inform the patient about the procedures to be performed, the associated risks, alternative methods, and the prognosis.

3. *Breach of duty*: The health care provider did not communicate to the patient the alternative methods of treatment once her condition changed, and therefore, the patient could not choose or consent to treatment.

4. *Injury*: The patient's child suffered severe cerebral palsy.

5. *The breach was the cause of the injury*: The cause of action is that the health care provider was negligent for not telling the patient about alternative courses of treatment once the conditions of her pregnancy changed. There was no informed consent; therefore, because the patient would likely have chosen a course of action that would have delivered her baby earlier and without complications, the breach was the cause of the injury.

Informed consent is a legal tightrope on which health care providers must walk. On one side is the health care provider's medical judgment about what information the patient must have to make a decision, and on the other side is the patient's right to know every possible outcome. In the past, the health care provider made the decision about how much information was given to the patient. Today, the patient and society exercise the patient's right to know, often requiring the health care provider to reveal more information than was thought necessary in the past.

Informed consent enters medical practice in many instances. Patients carrying the breast cancer gene have the opportunity to have their own vulnerability to the disease exposed. In a study by the New England Medical Center, 50 percent of patients who had a history of breast cancer in their family refused the test. Of the remaining 50 percent, 47 percent made the decision to receive the results of the testing. The others did not wish to be informed. In addition, under certain circumstances, health care providers may make the judgment that for "therapeutic" reasons, a patient should not be informed about his or her condition.

Another aspect of informed consent occurs when a health care provider has an "impairment" and has to decide whether to inform the patient. For example, the health care provider may have an infectious disease or several malpractice actions may have been brought against the health care provider for whatever reason.

There are ethical and moral implications in informed consent, especially when a drug or procedure is in the research phase and health care providers are experimenting on patients. Health care providers' comments and studies reveal that some patients do not want to hear bad news from the health care provider. In addition, when the risks of a procedure or medication are communicated to a patient, the patient often does not remember what is said. In some situations, a patient may selectively remember comments by the health care provider and selectively forget other important statements. The sicker the patient, the less accurate the memory is for details of pending treatment; the less educated the patient, the less accurate the recall of information. Lawyers develop forms for patients to sign indicating that they have been informed of possible adverse reactions, but these are commonly not understood by the patient.

The Health Care Professional and Informed Consent

Some health care professionals cannot be delegated the responsibility of receiving informed consent from a patient. It is your responsibility as a professional to know the rules that govern what you do. All health care professionals are, however, in a position to protect, or at least warn, the health care provider of potential malpractice actions when the patient's behavior raises doubt as to whether the health care provider adequately informed the patient. Keeping accurate records, providing adequate documentation, and promptly and accurately relaying patient misunderstanding to the health care provider can help prevent such actions.

Health care providers are legally responsible for obtaining informed consent from the patients they treat. Following discussion with the patient, the health care provider should document the fact that the patient has been informed and how.

nonverbal communication
Body language used to communicate something.

Patients often express confusion or ask questions of health care professionals that they will not ask of the health care provider. **Nonverbal communication** from the patient can also tell you that something is amiss. Health care professionals should communicate with the health care provider and document personal observations on a sheet attached to the medical record but not part of the record (unless your office protocol dictates otherwise). This information is for the health care provider and gives the health care provider an opportunity to follow up with the patient and answer any outstanding questions or concerns.

A patient may withdraw consent at any time, even after the authorized treatment has begun.

Impact of Medical Malpractice Suits

It is a devastating experience for health care providers to be sued. Health care providers may feel that everyone is pointing a finger; they may feel disgraced. They may be afraid that one claim of poor treatment will negate all the good performed in a lifetime.

> The trauma of being sued for medical malpractice can linger for many years after a lawsuit is resolved. In a 2015 Medscape survey of physicians who had been sued, 26% of men and 36% of women indicated it was "one of the worst experiences of my life" and another 20% of both sexes said it was a "disruptive and humiliating" experience.
>
> Lawsuits can lumber along for years, putting defendants under constant uncertainty and dread. In the Medscape survey, a physician whose case lasted more than 3 years commented that these were "years of agonizing about the potential for a catastrophic outcome, loss of license, practice, etc."
>
> Keep in mind that most lawsuits will be dropped without any payment at all. Estimates of meritless lawsuits vary widely, but a 2010 analysis by the American Medical Association found that almost two thirds of medical malpractice lawsuits are dropped, dismissed, or withdrawn.
>
> Medscape. (2021). Malpractice: What to Do If You Get Sued: How Plaintiffs Win Their Cases. Medscape.com. Retrieved from www.medscape.com/courses/section/880445.

The fact that the health care provider can be **ethical**, honest, and competent and still be sued is seldom remembered as the defendant proceeds through the lawsuit. Nurses, pharmacists, therapists, and other health care professionals voice the same disbelief when informed that their actions and professional behavior are in dispute.

ethical Conforming to professionally proper conduct.

The emotions of a health care provider who has been sued may fester and potentially poison relations with patients. Embittered health care providers can also have an impact on their colleagues. Health care providers and patients can begin viewing each other as an **adversary** rather than as a partner. The ultimate result is that medical care becomes a business—an impersonal, cold, monetary transaction—rather than a trusting relationship between the patient and the health care provider.

adversary An opponent in a dispute or contest.

Defensive Medicine

Health care providers, concerned that they might be sued for malpractice, may order every known test in search of a definitive diagnosis when presented with specific symptoms. Following the old adage—the best defense is a good offense—they may request more and more laboratory tests, x-rays, assorted diagnostic procedures, hospitalizations, consultations, and referrals. Many hospitals and experienced health care providers, when confronted with an accident victim, cynically "x-ray 'em wherever they hurt."

Advances in medical science and technology have led to increased specialization: general practitioners were no longer willing to deliver babies, and fewer general surgeons were willing to repair broken bones. The increased use of specialists, the development of managed care, and the threat of malpractice allegations all served to increase the psychological distance between health care provider and patient. The gap between the patient and the health care provider began to widen. By continually guarding against litigation, patient hostility—of which health care providers constantly complain—became a self-fulfilling prophecy. Entrepreneurs published lists of patients who were known to have been involved in malpractice actions against health care providers. Medical magazines published articles describing **suit-prone** patient behavior in an attempt to alert health care providers that particular kinds of patients should be avoided. In addition, patients have become more knowledgeable and demanding consumers when it comes to health care. The Internet has contributed to an increased patients' awareness of medicine. Some of the information patients retrieve in this way may be perfectly good; some may be harmful. Once armed with this "knowledge," however, patients have become more assertive when it comes to their care. Likewise, the advent of advertising prescription drugs on television has increased patient demand for certain medications, regardless of whether a patient fully understands the drug's purpose.

suit-prone Likely to sue someone or be sued.

There is some data to suggest ordering more tests may reduce law suits. A study published in The British Medical Journal in 2015 looked at a large number of physicians practicing medicine in Florida from 2000–2009. They found the doctors who ordered the most tests in any given year were substantially less likely to be sued in the following year.

Another aspect of defensive medicine is when a physician or medical practice avoids treating high-risk patients. They cherry-pick patients who are more likely to have good outcomes, or they choose a medical specialty that has less risk of malpractice suits. This can result in the most talented doctors not treating the patients who need their skills the most.

Torrey, T. (2020, February 7). Defensive Medicine and How It Affects Healthcare Costs. VeryWellHealth. Retrieved from www.verywellhealth.com/defensive-medicine-2615160.

Although it is not known for certain whether the practice of **defensive medicine** aids in preventing professional liability suits, health care providers are caught between protecting themselves by ordering tests and being **sanctioned** for ordering unnecessary procedures by professional **peer reviews** or other enforcement entities in a society that is extremely interested in containing medical costs.

The economics of medicine have also changed providers' behavior. When health care providers were getting paid by fee for service, there may have been an incentive to do more than clinically necessary. With the proliferation of capitation, in which a health care provider is paid a set fee per month for each patient covered by an insurance company, there may be an incentive to do too little.

In any event, the circumstances surrounding medical errors, which is the source of malpractice, may be changing. More and more frequently, errors are attributable to the failure of the system of care rather than blaming an individual provider. More commonly now, a health care provider may actually engage in apologizing to a patient; a hospital may work with a patient's family to improve systems of care to benefit individuals beyond the potential malpractice plaintiff.

defensive medicine
The practice of medicine where the main focus is preventing a lawsuit rather than improving the health of the patient.

sanctioned Penalized for violating a law or accepted procedure.

peer review Assessment of academic, professional, or scientific work by others who are experts in the same field.

Economics of Medical Malpractice

Practicing defensive medicine, in short, transformed the malpractice crisis into a vicious circle. Not only did it contribute to the deterioration in the patient–provider relationship, but it contributed to the increased cost of medical care. Health care providers formerly had a stake in selling a lot of health care because they got paid on a fee-for-service basis.

> "
>
> Defensive medicine is a very large contributor to the rise of healthcare costs in the United States. An analysis published in Health Affair in 2018 estimated that defensive medicine adds $25.6 billion annually. It may contribute as much as 34% of the annual healthcare costs in the United States.
>
> Torrey, T. (2020, February 7). Defensive Medicine and How It Affects Healthcare Costs. VeryWellHealth. Retrieved from www.verywellhealth.com/defensive-medicine-2615160.

The excessive number of tests ordered by health care providers to ensure accurate diagnosis is passed on to the patient in the form of dollar cost and lost time and to the American public as a major cause of medical inflation. Health care providers, employers, patients, and insurance companies become paper shufflers, adding to the fixed costs of the medical industry. As inflation spirals upward, the American public succumbs to stress-produced illnesses, anxiety, and despair, which hurts the economy by reducing the nation's productivity.

For the health care provider, one of the immediate effects of the increase in malpractice litigation is seen in higher malpractice insurance premiums and the decline in the number of carriers willing to assume the risk. As the size of awards and number of suits increase, insurance companies suffer losses. Small insurance companies have dropped out of the medical malpractice insurance coverage arena altogether or are selective about who they insure. It is common knowledge that insurance companies are in business to make money and that health care providers are also. Since health care providers cannot absorb the burden of additional insurance premiums, the public again picks up the tab.

Malpractice continues to be a significant concern. Although the issue seems to have a cyclical nature—the "crisis" reappears every 20 years or so—there is also a geographic component to it. In areas of the country where jury verdicts are extraordinarily high relative to the rest of the country, malpractice coverage premiums become a significant barrier to many health care providers continuing in the practice. Some leave and go to another jurisdiction, some retire, and some find new careers in administration with either a provider or a payer organization.

Negative Defensive Medicine

When the penalty for unsuccessfully performing a procedure becomes too high, the thinking person avoids the act. Some health care providers today are shying away from the treatment of difficult cases with a potentially poor result. Fear of malpractice may prevent a health care provider from attempting new procedures or prescribing new drugs. Health care providers have protested the hike of medical malpractice insurance premiums by refusing to treat certain classes of patients, primarily obstetric and orthopedic.

An example of this behavior serves to demonstrate how this limits access to care and contributes to health care provider shortages in certain areas and subspecialties. It is common, for example, for primary care providers in urban areas to no longer perform ECGs, but rather to refer the patient—even one who has no symptoms—to a cardiologist. The cardiologist is then seeing a relatively healthy patient who may have risk factors but no symptoms or history of heart disease. As this volume of patients increases, those who do have heart disease may find it difficult to get in to see the cardiologist. This underscores a perceived shortage of cardiologists, provides a measure of protection against malpractice to the primary care provider, and contributes to the rising costs of health care through what may be overutilization of specialty care.

Analysis of the Problem

A malpractice lawsuit usually arises from two factors: the objective factor, which is the patient's injury, and the subjective factor, which is the patient's alienation, anxiety, frustration, and potential anger. Although medical malpractice as a legal concept requires both injury and negligence, the injury alone does not usually bring about the intense hostility that a lawsuit expresses. Many malpractice suits are brought because of the health care provider's poor communication.

Whether health care providers should apologize to patients if they believe an error caused injury to the patient has been long debated. On one side are those who believe that any admission of error will encourage lawsuits. On the other side are those who believe an apology can help avoid a lawsuit. In recent years, as many as 39 states have enacted laws that prohibit the use of health care providers' apologies or admissions of error as evidence of negligence at trial. However, a Vanderbilt University study suggests that all this "apology legislation" isn't working. Vanderbilt's Owen Graduate School of Management analyzed malpractice claims for 90 percent of the nation's health care providers in a single specialty for a period of eight years.

The study showed that approximately two-thirds of the suits went to court and that the state apology laws made no difference for surgeons. For states with apology laws, however, the claims against non-surgeons were 46 percent more likely to result in a lawsuit. The study suggests the difference is likely due to surgical errors often being more obvious than, for example, a failure to diagnose.

McMichael, B., Van Horn R. L., Viscusi, W. K. (2019 February). 'Sorry' Is Never Enough: How State Apology Laws Fail to Reduce Medical Malpractice Liability Risk. 71 Stanford Law Review 341. Retrieved from www.scholarship.law.vanderbilt.edu/faculty-publications/1086.

The Suit-Prone Health Care Provider

The working habits and personality of a health care provider can make the difference between a vengeful, unhappy patient and a friendly, satisfied one. Bad bedside manners matter when it comes to lawsuits.

If you've ever had a doctor with a terrible bedside manner, it might come as no surprise that rude doctors are sued more often than caring and compassionate ones. Decades of research have shown that how physicians communicate with patients—and how they make patients feel—has a huge impact on whether or not doctors face malpractice lawsuits. . . .

As a whole, medical malpractice is alarmingly rampant. By the time they reach age 65, 75 percent of physicians have been named in a malpractice claim, according to The New England Journal of Medicine—and that's among low-risk specialties. . . .

As horrifying as the medical error rate is, it doesn't mean that doctors everywhere are behaving negligently. In many cases, the same careless physicians are accused of malpractice over and over again. "Approximately 1% of all physicians accounted for 32% of paid claims," according to The New England Journal of Medicine.

And researchers know who those doctors are. Overwhelmingly, they're the ones who don't communicate well with their patients. They don't listen, they don't explain, and they don't inspire confidence. So it's no wonder that their dissatisfied patients often look back and wonder what went wrong. . . .

The patients of frequently sued doctors reported twice as many instances of their doctors shouting at them—an action which, though not malpractice in and of itself, certainly fits the bill of being rude. . . .

"Numerous studies have found that the most common reasons patients sue their doctors for malpractice include:

- The desire to make sure a similar incident doesn't happen to future patients
- Patients' need to understand why and how a negative outcome occurred
- The desire for accountability on the part of health care providers

Perhaps it's no surprise, then, that patients whose doctors presented positive communication behaviors were more likely to see their physicians as competent and less likely to move forward with a lawsuit against either the doctor or the hospital. Even in cases of severe negative outcomes, patients whose doctors were good communicators were more likely to leave their doctors out of the medical malpractice suits they filed against the hospital, *The Western Journal of Medicine* reported.

Console and Associates. (2021, March 25). Bad Bedside Manner or Medical Malpractice? National Law Review. www.natlawreview.com/article/bad-bedside-manner-or-medical-malpractice.

Insults in the Medical Office

It has been said that a malpractice suit is a sort of reverse class action suit—one individual suing the entire medical profession to revenge all the insults of long delays in crowded waiting rooms and health care providers with too little time to give each patient. John A. Appleman, attorney for the plaintiff in *Darling v. Charleston Community Hospital*, has summarized several factors he believes contribute to the problem. First on his list: the health care provider guilty of overbooking the number of patients that can be seen in a day. Many schedule all patients for a given hour. Patients with depression may have a significant wait while being exposed to other patients who are coughing or sneezing.

Lack of Empathy

Empathy is a form of communication that is one level deeper than understanding. Empathy requires vicariously experiencing the feelings or thoughts of another person. Health care professionals cannot identify with each patient but can communicate—through nonverbal communication and listening skills—their recognition of the patient's situation.

Often the health care provider's casual attitude indicates a lack of empathy for his or her patients. Because members of the office staff pick up their cues from the health care provider for acceptable behavior toward patients, too much casualness may lead to a situation that implies contempt for the patient and the patient's complaints. In contrast, too formal an atmosphere may inhibit the staff's freedom to share their observations about the patient with the health care provider, as well as give the office a snobbish, uncaring, cold environment.

Today's practice involves a group of health care providers, with a primary care provider assuming the role of the family physician. The rules of managed care schedule a certain number of minutes for each patient visit with little flexibility to allow for lengthy conversation in any area. Some patients can express their concerns about their health in this time frame, but others require a few minutes to establish or reestablish a trusting relationship in which to reveal troubling problems. It is difficult to exhibit empathy for a patient's situation when the subject causing distress is never broached.

The Effect of a Prescription

Today's health care provider has at hand a pharmacopoeia of pills to address almost every malady known.

The American public is impatient, sees serious illnesses "cured" in 30 minutes on television soaps, and anticipates being back in the swing of things the next day if the proper pill is prescribed. If the prescribed drug does not work against a particular illness, the patient becomes angry at the health care provider. Even worse, if the prescribed drug causes an allergic reaction, it is the health care provider's fault for prescribing the medication. In certain segments of the population, the health care provider is viewed as a dispensing technician and trust is placed in the drug, not the health care provider. One of the challenges of the Internet is the inclination of patients to self-diagnose. The patient's "diagnosis" may be right or wrong, but ultimately the health care provider not only has to deal with the real malady but may need to reeducate the patient as well.

One of the most serious outcomes of the American prescription-conditioned society is that patients do not properly take prescribed medication. Again, the health care provider is battling the time problem. Health care providers may not take, or do not have, the time to explain to patients the importance of properly taking medication.

The changes that have taken place in the delivery of health care have affected pharmacies and the dispensing of medications. Where there used to be a small pharmacy on Main Street in every town, there are businesses, such as CVS, Walgreens, and so on, dispensing pharmaceuticals from megastores strategically situated to draw customers from a defined geographic area. Competition also emerges in the form of discount stores such as Walmart and Target utilizing generic list discounting. A national drug chain has its advantages when the customer is away from home and forgets a prescription, but it also has affected the personal relationship that pharmacist and customer enjoyed in the past.

Risk Management Issues in the Medical Office

Anger is a thread running through the entire medical malpractice saga. The patient is angry, the health care provider is angry, relatives of both are angry, and the American public is angry about the spiraling medical costs, illness, and the inevitability of dependence on others as we age. And, health care providers are angry because they generally feel as if they are wrongly accused.

Within the past 25 years much has been done to prevent injuries and advance medical science, but attention is just beginning to be drawn to the skills and systems necessary to prevent patients from becoming angry and hostile in their relationships with health care professionals. Legally, the first element of the malpractice case that must be proven is that the patient–provider relationship exists. The case, at this point, turns on the health care provider's assertion that the relationship exists or does not exist. Psychologically and **sociologically**, the first element of the malpractice case again involves the patient–provider relationship. Here, the question is not whether a relationship exists but what kind of relationship exists.

sociological Pertaining to human social behavior.

As can be seen from the preceding analysis of the medical malpractice problem, no amount of defensive medicine will aid in reducing the irritants that interfere with a friendly relationship between health care provider and patient. Without a good patient–provider relationship, the patient's inclination to sue skyrockets, and the resulting malpractice situation becomes increasingly destructive to health care provider and patient alike. In an effort to eliminate or reduce the threat of a malpractice lawsuit, health care providers practice assertive preventive medicine.

Fortunately, health care providers are becoming aware of the need for a friendly, professional office environment. A professional office staff can complement the health care provider in all areas. The health care provider's staff stands in the health care provider's corner. Most are working in the health care field because they see themselves as caregivers. A medical assistant or office nurse can alleviate some of the anxiety associated with a visit to the health care provider and fill gaps caused by the health care provider's schedule. Training in the art of making immediate contact with patients and basic skills in good human relations will help health care professionals meet the patient's needs, avoid confrontations, and contribute to a cheerful office environment.

Burnout is both a result and a cause of many problems between people working with the public and the public they are serving. A burned-out health care worker only adds fuel to the fire if a patient is incubating a malpractice action. Burnout can be addressed in an office by staff meetings and training sessions to help the employees support each other.

burnout Exhaustion from overwork.

And so, poor communication still remains the norm. A short while ago, the Annals of Emergency Medicine published a study that examined patient–health care provider communication in the emergency room on the management of acute coronary syndrome, which is chest pain caused by decreased blood flow to the heart, as with a heart attack or angina. About two-thirds of patients left conversations thinking they were having a heart attack, while health care providers believed this to be the case less than half the time. The median estimate of whether a patient might die at home of a heart attack was 80 percent in patients and 10 percent in health care providers. Doctors and patients were reasonably close in their estimates of danger only 36 percent of the time. They clearly weren't hearing each other.

Carroll, A. E. (2015, June 1). To be sued less, doctors should consider talking to patients more. *The New York Times.* Retrieved from www.nytimes.com/2015/06/02 /upshot/to-be-sued-less-doctors-should-talk-to-patients-more.html?_r=1.

A well-educated health care professional can either assist the health care provider in informing a patient or refer the patient to an educational center for instruction. They can tactfully question the patient after the health care provider's explanation to assess the patient's understanding. All areas of health care practice are educating personnel and developing quality assurance systems to improve the quality of care and reduce malpractice claims. Medical societies are educating health care providers in the "art" of practicing medicine. It seems logical to extend this educational process to health care professionals as well.

Defenses to a Medical Malpractice Cause of Action

Common defenses available to a defendant in a medical malpractice cause of action include **statute of limitations**, **contributory negligence**, **comparative negligence**, **assumption of risk**, and emergency.

Statute of Limitations

The statute of limitations sets forth a particular number of years within which one person can sue another. Attorneys representing health care providers who have been sued for malpractice will typically first determine whether the statute of limitations has run out by determining how much time has passed since the time the patient knew or should have known there was an injury and the time the lawsuit was filed. Different causes of action have different statutes of limitations. In medical malpractice actions, the statute of limitations is specified in each state's medical malpractice law. Statutes of limitations are necessary because as the years go by, evidence vanishes, witnesses' memories dim, and witnesses die. By setting a time frame within which a lawsuit may be initiated, there is assurance that relevant evidence is available for the fact finders and the parties.

The statutes of limitations of medical malpractice lawsuits usually give the patient 2 years to sue for damages but can be as long as 10 years depending on the state and the injury. This does not necessarily mean that the medical practitioner is free from concern about malpractice as soon as the statute of limitations expires. In most states, the statute of limitations begins to run when the injured patient becomes aware of the injury. In the case of minors, the statute may not begin to run until the minor reaches the age of majority; therefore, if a child is injured at the age of 1 year, and 18 years is the age of majority, it may be 19 or 20 years before the statute of limitations has expired. If a surgeon leaves a sponge inside a patient, and the patient has no symptoms and does not know the sponge is there, the statute of limitations will likely not start to run until the patient knew or should have known of the surgeon's error.

In some states, the statute of limitations for negligence is longer than that for malpractice. This may be an issue for health care professionals, depending on whether the health care professional is viewed as a layperson or professional. If the health care professional is held to be a layperson, the negligence statute of limitations determines the length of time between the injury and the filing of a cause of action. If the health care professional is held to be a professional, the malpractice time frame will rule.

Contributory Negligence

Contributory negligence is a term used to describe any unreasonable behavior on the part of the patient that contributed, in part, to the cause of injury. In other words, if a patient does anything that contributes to his or her suffering and constitutes behavior that is non-self-preserving, the patient is contributorily negligent. For example:

> Two men, following arrest, were taken to the emergency room following their declaration that they were heroin addicts. The physician on duty observed one of the men writhing, twitching, and moaning, and behaving in a manner that gave the appearance of a person suffering withdrawal symptoms. The physician administered methadone to both men. An hour later one patient stated that he was still having difficulty and the physician gave him an additional dose. The police returned both men to jail. The next morning one of the men was found dead in his cell of an overdose of methadone.
>
> Investigation revealed that one of the men was a drug addict but that the one who died was intoxicated from the combination of Librium, beer, and methadone. The dead man's family brought an action against the emergency room physician. The court held that a patient has a duty to be truthful to a physician, and that failure to do so, in this case, was the sole cause of the death. The dead man had stated he was an addict when he was not an addict. The patient's negligence, or more accurately, his intentional misconduct, barred a malpractice action.
>
> *Rochester v. Katalan, 320 A.2d 704 (Del. 1974)*

The preceding case gives an example of a patient contributing to his own suffering by giving a health care provider false information. What follows is an example of a patient unwilling to follow the health care provider's directions and, as a result, contributing to the injury:

> The patient arrived at the hospital complaining of pain in his lower abdomen, nausea, and vomiting blood for two weeks. Several blood tests were ordered, and the patient's vital signs were recorded as slightly elevated. The doctor ordered a nasogastric tube to be used to check for blood in the patient's stomach. This test required a painful process wherein
>
> *(Continues)*

> *(Continued)*
>
> the tube is inserted through the nose and down the patient's esophagus into his stomach. One nurse tried to insert this tube, but the patient complained that the procedure was painful. A second nurse explained the procedure and why it was necessary. Nevertheless, the patient continued to refuse to have the tube inserted. The nurse then had the patient sign a form indicating that he was refusing medical treatment against medical advice. The nurse then advised the patient that signing out against medical advice could result in dire consequences. The patient died three days later, and the administrator of his estate brought a medical malpractice lawsuit. Because the patient had left the hospital against medical advice, the defense of contributory negligence was appropriate.
>
> *Lyons v. Walker Regional Medical Center, 868 So.2d 1071 (Ala. 2003)*

Comparative Negligence

In states that allow the defense of contributory negligence, the plaintiff is unable to recover any damages for injury if he or she has contributed in any manner to the injury. Under comparative negligence, the plaintiff is allowed to recover damages proportionate to the defendant's fault, at least in a situation in which the plaintiff's negligence is less than that of the defendant.

Assumption of Risk

Assumption of risk is defined as voluntarily accepting a known danger. The consent to assume risk may be express or implied. This is a defense similar to the doctrine of informed consent in that the only way a patient may assume the risk of a procedure is if the patient is informed of it by the health care provider.

Emergency

Good Samaritan A person who helps another person in distress even though there is no duty to do so.

Both common law and the **Good Samaritan** acts protect health care professionals when they respond to an emergency situation. Under common law, the elements of a medical malpractice action are applied to the emergency situation. For example, if a medical assistant witnesses an automobile accident and no one else is available, is the medical assistant liable for what happens to the victim?

1. *Relationship*: No contractual relationship exists between the medical assistant and the victim as long as the medical assistant does not stop to give help. As soon as help is offered—merely stopping a car may prevent someone else from coming to the aid of the victim—a relationship is established with the victim.

2. *Duty*: As long as the medical assistant passes the accident, he or she has no legal duty to assist the victim. After a medical assistant stops, the victim cannot be abandoned unless care is being provided by someone with comparable or better training, or until the first responders arrive on the scene and assume responsibility for the victim. This reasonable person duty applies whether the Good Samaritan is a health care professional or a layperson.

3. *Standard of care*: In an emergency situation, to encourage trained people to stop and assist, states have enacted Good Samaritan statutes to protect the rescuer from liability. The level of training of the Good Samaritan and the standard of care are important to the person being rescued, but the rescuer will only be held liable for reckless behavior.

4. *Breach of duty*: If a person passes an accident, no breach of duty exists because no relationship with the victim from which a duty arises has been established. If a helper stops and assists, he or she will be held to a standard of care appropriate to the individual's training and experience. If the procedures are performed below standard, the usual question of the court is whether the actions increased the victim's injury.

5. *Injury*: The victim is already injured. The Good Samaritan has a responsibility to help the victim, but for the helper to be held liable for the injury, the helper's acts must cause a considerable amount of additional harm.

6. *The breach was the cause of the injury*: Under negligence law, the victim must prove by a preponderance of the evidence that the help offered caused injury. Since the victim is already injured, the helper's behavior would have to be **grossly negligent** to increase the victim's injuries.

grossly negligent
Deliberately failing to perform a necessary duty in extraordinary disregard of the consequences to the person neglected.

As can be seen from the preceding analyses, there is only a slim chance of being charged with malpractice under common law for aiding an accident victim. The reason courts are reluctant to find those who help accident victims guilty is that the public has an interest in encouraging people to stop and aid someone who is injured. Pursuing this reasoning one step further, the states have enacted Good Samaritan laws to encourage trained professionals to provide services at accident scenes.

Good Samaritan statutes provide immunity to volunteers at the scene of an accident as long as they do not intentionally or recklessly cause the patient further injury. It is important to remember that the basis of negligence law is that everyone is responsible for the consequences of his or her own acts.

Office emergencies usually do not fall under the protection of Good Samaritan laws. For example, someone walks into a medical office off the street, obviously ill, and requests medical help. Add to this scene the facts that the potential patient is dirty and has no money, and the health care provider has asked the medical assistant to get rid of this person. It will probably not go well for the health care provider in court if the patient sues for not receiving emergency medical care. It is the public's expectation that emergency care will be provided; therefore, the patient should be treated prior to arranging for transportation to the closest emergency room.

Malpractice Insurance

insurance A contract binding one party to compensate another for specific losses, damages, or injury in exchange for the payment of premiums.

Malpractice **insurance** is a subject that frequently makes headlines because of rising costs to health care providers. In a society in which many are willing to litigate situations that they believe violate their rights and there is the opportunity to do so, it is understandable that the premiums for coverage increase. The subject is complex. Litigation is expensive, and the damages that are awarded to successful plaintiffs are rising. This is an issue that changes over time; sometimes (and in some places) costs become so excessive that malpractice coverage is either prohibitively expensive or simply unavailable.

Most, but not all, states require that health care providers have malpractice insurance. Hospitals, health care facilities, health care providers, nurses, and other health care employees may also have malpractice insurance. Because health care professionals work under the direct supervision of the health care provider, they are often covered by the health care provider's insurance. This is part of the employment benefits package. If the health care provider's office does not offer this as a benefit, health care professionals may need to acquire their own malpractice insurance coverage.

Product Liability

A product liability case is negligence against a manufacturer, a distributor, or some other supplier of goods. Product liability becomes of concern in the medical office when equipment malfunctions, proper instructions are not given for medication, or supplies used in a procedure are defective. The basic theories of recovery are negligence and breach of warranty. Examples of product liability in a health care setting include the following:

> A pediatric nurse checks on a patient, then leaves the room. She returns later to discover that the child has been crushed to death by the automatic lowering device on his electric bed. Several children at other hospitals have been killed by activating such bed-lowering buttons.
>
> A nurse in the post-anesthesia care unit breaks a left-atrial catheter while trying to remove it from a patient's chest after open heart surgery. A piece of it remains permanently embedded.

An ICU patient dies when nurses fail to hear a ventilator disconnect alarm through the plate glass doors. Respiratory therapists rig a remote alarm system. Four more patients die before it's debugged.

A nurse's aid manages to keep a patient from falling when the caster drops off a shower chair, but sustains a disabling injury herself.

Tammelleo, A. D. (1990, October). Who's to Blame for Faulty Equipment? RN, 67.

Product liability cases have surfaced in court when patients have been injured by tampons, pacemakers, wrinkle cream, implant prosthetics, and so on. In the past, common products have become the object of these suits: blood transfusions, Tylenol, silicone breast implants, infant car seats, heart pacemakers, and tobacco. Those who have standing to sue include persons injured by the product, their relatives in certain circumstances, and employees, among others.

Product liability actions that will be faced by workers in medical offices most often include those classified as "failure to warn" suits. Medical office personnel are often responsible for educating patients about the medications that the health care provider has prescribed.

product liability A tort making a manufacturer liable for compensation to anyone using its product if damages or injuries occur from defects in that product.

Duty to Provide Adequate Warnings and Directions for Use

A manufacturer is obligated to provide adequate directions for use of a product. The extensive written material that accompanies a prescription drug is an example of the manufacturer's duty to give directions for use and to warn of any unwanted results. Directions are primarily to secure the efficient use of a product. When a departure from the directions may create a serious problem, a separate duty to warn arises. The following is a case in point:

Heat blocks are used to help revive injured persons. Instructions to wrap the blocks in insulating material before using were given, but there was no statement that if used without insulation, the blocks would cause serious burns. The plaintiff was seriously burned by the blocks. The court, in dictum as to the need for warning, observed that "instructions, not particularly stressed, do not amount to a warning of the risk at all . . ." and found against the defendant.

McLaughlin v. Mine Safety Appliances Co., 11 N.Y.2d 62, 226 N.Y.S.2d 407, 181 N.E.2d 430 (1962)

Strict Liability

consumer A person who uses products or services.

Strict liability is a theory used in product liability cases in which the seller is liable for any and all defective or hazardous products that unduly threaten a **consumer's** personal safety. Plaintiffs who assert claims under a theory of strict liability for manufacturing defects do not need to prove the manufacturer failed to use due care.

They will need to show that there was a defect, that the defect caused the injury, and that the defect made the product unreasonably dangerous.

To prevent the product from being unreasonably dangerous, the seller may be required to give directions or warning, on the container, as to its use. For the most part, actions in strict liability are not applied to health care providers and hospitals because of the requirement that there be a sale of goods. Health care is primarily a sale of services. However, there have been a few exceptions. For example:

> In Texas, a patient was injured when his hospital gown caught fire after the patient dropped a lighted match on it. The court held that where a hospital supplies a product unrelated to the essential professional relationship with the patient, the hospital may be considered the entity to have introduced the harmful product into the stream of commerce for purposes of a strict liability cause of action.
>
> *Thomas v. St. Joseph Hospital*, 618 S.W.2d 791 (Tex. Civ. App. 1981)

Strict liability in health care often arises with regard to drug manufacturing. In such a case, the courts must assess the risk of the drug and whether the health care provider and patient were warned. If the drug has known side effects and the health care provider warns the patient of these, the patient *assumes the risk* of the treatment.

Premises Liability

invitee A person who enters another's property as a result of express or implied invitation.

licensee A person who has express or implied permission to enter another's property.

trespasser Someone who enters another's property without express or implied invitation or permission.

Hospitals, clinics, and individual practitioners are responsible to the public for their offices, laboratories, buildings, and equipment, as shown in the following:

Property owners must observe certain standards of care for the protection of others, regardless of whether they come onto the property legally. People entering another's property are classified as **invitees, licensees,** or **trespassers.**

> Plaintiff was rendered a quadriplegic when he fell on a mat while waiting for an elevator in defendant hospital. Plaintiff contended that the fall was caused by a fold or buckle in the mat and that the hospital was negligent in using and failing to secure the mat. There was a triable issue of fact as to whether the hospital breached its duty of care to plaintiff.
>
> *Caburnay v. Norwegian American Hosp.*, 2011 IL App (1st) 101740 (Ill. App., 2011)

Trespassers

Someone who enters another's property without express or implied invitation or permission is a trespasser. Despite the fact that such a person is not invited and probably not wanted, the owner and the occupier have obligations for the safety of this person. There is a duty to warn of dangers and a duty to reduce and eliminate dangers existing on the property. This duty should be carried out with **reasonable care**. The care necessary to fulfill the duty required, in most cases, is merely giving warning of the activity or condition. There is a stricter responsibility to trespassing children because they are often unable to recognize danger.

reasonable care The amount of care a rational person would use in similar circumstances.

> The house was inherited from the defendants' grandparents and had been unoccupied for some time. There had been a series of intrusions, and the defendants had boarded up the windows and the doors in an attempt to protect the property. They had posted "no trespass" signs on the land, the nearest one being 35 feet from the house. On June 11, 1967, the defendants set a "shotgun trap" in the north bedroom. After Mr. Briney cleaned and oiled his 20-gauge shotgun, defendants took it to the old house, where they secured it to an iron bed with the barrel pointed at the bedroom door. It was rigged with wire from the doorknob to the gun's trigger so it would fire when the door was opened. Briney first pointed the gun so an intruder would be hit in the stomach, but at Mrs. Briney's suggestion it was lowered to hit the legs. He admitted he did so "because I was mad and tired of being tormented," but he did not intend to injure anyone. He gave no explanation of why he used a loaded shell and set it to hit a person already in the house.
>
> The plaintiff entered the old house by removing a board from a porch window which was without glass . . . As he started to open the north bedroom
>
> *(Continues)*

(Continued)

door, the shotgun went off, striking him in the right leg above the ankle bone. Much of his leg, including part of the tibia, was blown away. Only by . . . assistance was the plaintiff able to get out of the house and then to a hospital. He remained in the hospital 40 days.

The trial court held that an owner may not protect personal property in an unoccupied boarded up farmhouse against trespass by use of deadly force. This decision was affirmed by the appeals court.

Katko v. Briney, 183 N.W.2d 657 (Iowa 1971)

Licensees

A licensee differs from a trespasser in that a licensee enters another's property with express or implied permission. Examples of licensees include public servants, such as the police and firefighters, those who may cross property to take a shortcut, social guests, those who come into the office to get out of the rain, traveling salespersons, and charitable solicitors. There is a duty to warn these people about any dangerous conditions that they would not anticipate or easily see.

Invitees

Invitees are persons who enter property for business as a result of express or implied invitation. Store customers; patrons of restaurants, banks, and places of amusement; delivery persons and plumbers; and electricians and carpenters doing work at an owner's request are all invitees. The duty owed to invitees is higher than that owed to trespassers or licensees. Generally, the duty is to make the premises safe by exercising reasonable care to warn the invitee of defects in the property that are known or should be known. This includes an **affirmative duty** to protect the invitee. Reasonable care may include inspection of the premises to discover possible defects.

affirmative duty An obligation to do or to not do something.

A mother took her 5-year-old son to the pediatrician's office. After the visit she left by the back door, stepped into a hole and hurt her ankle. The hole was hidden by some very high grass and neither she nor the pediatrician had noticed it on prior trips through the door. The court found that she was an invitee, even though she was not herself a patient, but held that there was no evidence that the physician had known of the hole.

Goldman v. Kossove, 117 S.E.2d 35 (N.C. 1960)

Premises' owners are increasingly being held liable for injuries intentionally inflicted by third parties unrelated to the victim or the premises owner. For example:

> Plaintiffs who were injured or killed by a fellow patron at a movie theater complex in Aurora, Colorado brought a premises liability claim. The defendant Cinemark sought to have the premises liability claims dismissed and argued that plaintiffs could not show that Cinemark knew or should have known of the danger resulting from the theater's layout and operation. The gunman was able to cause such a tragedy, in part, because he was able to exit the theater via a side door, make at least one trip to his car, and return to the theater through the same side door with assault rifles, handguns, tear gas canisters, body armor, and tear gas canisters. There was no system to survey or monitor the parking areas behind or to the sides of the theaters, and the gunman was undetected by Cinemark personnel. In addition, the side doors to the theaters did not have alarm systems or any other security or alarm features that would alert theater personnel that someone had used the side door. The court held that the plaintiffs had sufficiently stated a claim to survive a motion to dismiss.
>
> *Traynom v. Cinemark USA, Inc.*, 940 F.Supp.2d 1339 (D. Colo. 2013)

While the *Traynom v. Cinemark USA, Inc.* case is an extreme example of premises liability, there are potential premises liability situations you will encounter while at work where you can make a difference. If you see a piece of paper on the floor, pick it up; if you notice a spill on the floor, ensure it is cleaned as soon as possible and prevent others from getting near the spill until it is cleaned; if you see a frayed electrical cord, bring it to the attention of the appropriate person in your office. The saying "if you see something, say something" applies here, as you are on the front line and can prevent injury and lawsuits.

☑ SUMMARY

- Malpractice differs from negligence in that malpractice is the negligence of a professional, such as a doctor, educator, pharmacist, or lawyer.
- The elements of a medical malpractice lawsuit include the following:
  - There was a health care provider–patient relationship.

- This relationship established the duty owed by the health care provider to the patient.
- The duty had not been upheld at a professional standard of care.
- The health care provider breached the duty to the patient.
- The patient had a resulting injury.
- The health care provider's breach was the proximate cause of the patient's injury.

- Breach of the duty by the health care provider, by action or inaction, is measured against the standard of care. Following recognized practice guidelines because the law sets the standard of care according to accepted medical practices.

- The health care provider's breach of duty must be the cause of the injury. There are two legal causes of injury: "but-for" causation and proximate cause.

- Informed consent requires that a health care provider communicate information to a patient regarding the treatment he or she is about to receive. The patient has a right to refuse treatment; therefore, the health care provider must provide enough information to allow the patient to make an informed decision. Only a health care provider can accept consent from a patient.

- There are many negative consequences of medical malpractice lawsuits including providers becoming bitter and emotional, the practice of defensive medicine, higher health and malpractice insurance, lack of specialists in high verdict areas, and higher health care costs.

- Subjective factors that influence a patient's decision to litigate include the patient's alienation, anxiety, frustration, and potential anger. Many malpractice suits are brought simply because of poor communication.

- Risk management measures a health care professional can take to avoid lawsuits include maintaining a friendly relationship with patients, maintaining good human relationship and communication skills, avoiding burnout, helping to ensure the patient understands the information given by the provider.

- Five defenses are available to a defendant in a medical malpractice cause of action: tolling of the statute of limitations, contributory negligence, comparative negligence, assumption of risk, and emergency.

- Good Samaritan statutes provide immunity to volunteers at the scene of an accident as long as they do not intentionally or recklessly cause the patient further injury. It is important to remember that the basis of negligence law is that everyone is responsible for the consequences of his or her own acts.

- Medical malpractice insurance is available to cover monetary awards against a defendant. Health care professionals may or may not be covered under a health care provider's insurance. Insurance is available for the protection of health care professionals not covered by their employer's malpractice insurance.

- A product liability case is negligence against a manufacturer, a distributor, or some other supplier of goods. Product liability becomes of concern in the medical office when equipment malfunctions, proper instructions are not given for medication, or supplies used in a procedure are defective.

- Strict liability is a theory used in product liability cases in which the seller is liable for any and all defective or hazardous products that unduly threaten a consumer's personal safety. Plaintiffs who assert claims under a theory of strict liability for manufacturing defects do not need to prove the manufacturer failed to use due care. They will need to show that there was a defect, that the defect caused the injury, and that the defect made the product unreasonably dangerous.

- Hospitals, clinics, and individual practitioners are responsible to the public for their offices, laboratories, buildings, and equipment. Different standards of responsibility are required for trespassers, licensees, and invitees. The standard of property maintenance for a trespasser is reasonable care. The standard of maintenance increases for licensees. The highest standard of maintenance is due to invitees and requires affirmative behavior on the part of the landlord or occupier to warn the invitee about dangerous conditions or activities that are known or could be discovered with reasonable effort.

SUGGESTED ACTIVITIES

1. Play the childhood game of rumors. Begin by giving directions for taking medication. As the rumor travels around the circle, document the changes. After 15 minutes, try to remember the directions first given. This will give each player an opportunity to learn about some of the confusion a patient experiences in the informed consent process.

2. Role play. Show empathy to a patient who has just learned that he has cancer of the larynx.

3. Watch the TedTalk entitled "Doctors Make Mistakes. Can We Talk About That?" which can be found at www.ted.com.

STUDY QUESTIONS

1. Describe a situation that might place a health care professional in the area you intend to practice in the position of being negligent.

2. Describe a situation that might cause a health care professional to be named as a defendant in a medical malpractice claim.

3. List the possible qualifications for an expert witness in a medical malpractice involving a nurse who works in a pediatrician's office.

4. What relationship is necessary between a health care provider and patient to establish duty of care for the health care provider?

5. List the elements of a medical malpractice cause of action.

6. A newly diagnosed cancer patient approaches you after being informed of two alternatives for treatment, one involving surgery and the second involving chemotherapy. He asks your advice. How do you handle the situation?

7. List, define, and give examples of the five defenses available to a defendant in a medical malpractice suit.

8. An automobile accident occurs in front of your office. You hear the crash and go to the door to see what has happened. One of the passengers in the car is walking around the street in a daze with blood dripping from a facial laceration. Are you obligated to help because you have specialized knowledge as a health care professional? If you do offer emergency assistance, what are obligations?

9. Prepare a question for your future employer to determine whether their malpractice insurance covers a health care professional working in their office.

10. An individual comes onto property owned by the medical office, is drunk, has been told to leave, but remains in the building. There is a floorboard in the front hallway that everyone knew needed to be fixed, but nothing has been done about it. The individual falls when the board gives way and breaks his leg. What is the responsibility of the medical office?

11. While sitting in the waiting room of a medical office, a patient falls when the chair gives way under him. The man is a very heavy person and chose to sit on a regular chair. There was a large chair available for him. The patient ends up in the hospital for observation and later for pneumonia related to his inactivity. Who is responsible for the pneumonia?

12. List equipment you might find in a medical office or hospital that could injure a patient and give rise to a product liability claim.

CASES FOR DISCUSSION

1. A negligence action was brought by a mother on behalf of her minor daughter against a hospital. It alleged that when the mother was 13 years of age, the hospital negligently transfused her with Rh-positive blood. The mother's Rh-negative blood was incompatible with and sensitized by the Rh-positive blood. The mother discovered her condition 8 years later during a routine blood screening ordered by her health care provider in the course of prenatal care. The resulting sensitization of the mother's blood allegedly caused damage to the fetus, resulting in physical defects and premature birth. Did a patient relationship with the transfusing hospital exist?

2. The patient was admitted to the hospital for dilation and curettage. The defendant was an anesthesiologist who injected sodium pentothal into the patient. The patient developed a laryngospasm, which prevented oxygen from entering the lungs and bloodstream. Attempts were made to break and relax the spasm but were unsuccessful. The plaintiff suffered severe and disabling brain damage. Conflicting evidence was submitted with regard to whether the defendant left the operating room to attend another patient before or after an equally qualified health care provider arrived to provide patient care. Was the health care provider at liberty to withdraw from the patient? Should they have obtained informed consent for treatment by second health care provider?

3. A woman was in labor. The nurse on duty refused to call the obstetrician. Instead, the nurse sat and read a magazine, ignoring repeated requests from the patient and her husband to call a physician. The husband informed the nurse when his wife was about to deliver, and the nurse told him to sit down. The woman delivered before the obstetrician arrived, and she was injured during the delivery. Was the hospital liable for the nurse's negligence?

4. A 16-year-old boy was hit by an automobile while riding his bicycle. He was taken to the emergency room by a parent; the physician on call looked him over and sent him home. The boy died a few hours later. Autopsy revealed that he had a massive skull fracture. Was the physician's lack of a thorough examination the cause of the patient's death?

5. The plaintiff was a 21-year-old student who severely injured his right index finger while working in a bakery. He is left-handed. The defendant, a board-certified orthopedist who specializes in hand surgery, testified that the value of the hand had been reduced by some 40 percent. At the plaintiff's request, the defendant took over the

case. There were two operations. The first went well, but after the second, circulation could not be restored to the finger and it had to be amputated at the base. With the amputated finger, the plaintiff had 80 percent use of the hand, which was more than prior to surgery. The plaintiff sued, alleging that the defendant did not inform him of the risks of the operations and that he might lose his finger. Should the court find the defendant guilty of malpractice?

6. The plaintiff, Bonner, was a 16-year-old Washington resident who had a severely burned cousin. The cousin was brought to the defendant, a plastic surgeon, for treatment. The physician advised a skin graft. After many unsuccessful attempts to find a donor, Bonner's aunt asked him to go to the hospital for a test to see if his blood would match with that of his cousin. He went to the hospital, had the test, and his blood matched. The defendant performed the first operation on Bonner's side. Bonner's mother, with whom he lived, was ill and knew nothing of the operation. Bonner later returned to the hospital for a second operation. He told his mother that he was going to have his side "fixed up." Instead, Bonner remained in the hospital, where an unsuccessful graft was attempted. In the course of the operation, Bonner lost a lot of blood and skin and had to remain hospitalized for 2 months. There was sufficient evidence for the jury to believe that Bonner's mother never knew the exact nature of the operations or consented to them. When his mother did learn of the operations, she made no attempt to prevent them but instead allowed Bonner to return to complete them. Bonner was a minor. Must the parents of a minor give consent before an operation for the benefit of another may be performed?

7. Kennedy, the plaintiff, consulted the defendant, a surgeon. The surgeon diagnosed appendicitis and recommended an operation, to which the plaintiff agreed. During the operation, the defendant discovered some enlarged cysts on the plaintiff's left ovary, which he punctured. After the operation, the plaintiff developed phlebitis in her leg, which caused her considerable pain and suffering. The plaintiff alleged that the puncturing of the cysts on her ovary was unauthorized, and she brought an action for damages. Can a surgeon extend an operation without consent?

8. The plaintiff, Anderson, was undergoing a back operation. During surgery, the tip of a forceps-like instrument broke off in Anderson's spinal canal. The surgeon was unable to retrieve the metal, and the patient suffered significant and permanent physical injury caused by the fragment, which lodged in his spine. The plaintiff-patient sued the defendant-surgeon for medical malpractice, the hospital for furnishing a defective instrument, the medical supply distributor for furnishing the defective instrument to the hospital on a warranty theory, and the manufacturer on a strict liability theory for making a defective product. Who can be named as a defendant? Is there a claim for strict liability?

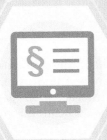

Chapter 7

The Health Record

> 66 Electronic health records are, in a lot of ways, I think the aspect of technology that is going to revolutionize the way we deliver care. And it's not just that we will be able to collect information, it's that everyone involved in the healthcare enterprise will be able to use that information more effectively. 99
>
> Risa Lavizzo-Mourey, M.D., M.B.A.

Objectives

After reading this chapter, you should be able to:

1. Define the Health Information Technology for Economic and Clinical Health (HITECH) Act and Promoting Interoperability.
2. List different types of health records.
3. Identify the owner of a health record.
4. Determine who is allowed access to the health record.
5. Identify the procedures necessary for release of information from the health record.
6. Define the importance of health record credibility.
7. Follow an acceptable method for making corrections to a health record.

Building Your Legal Vocabulary

Data
Premises
Property right

Subpoena
Subpoena duces tecum

Introduction

Despite the changes in the way a health record is kept, the foundational elements remain intact, including privacy, accuracy, timeliness, and reliance. Health care professionals will regularly interact with patient health records, and they should be familiar with the associated issues of privacy, confidentiality, and accuracy, among others.

data Pieces of information.

A medical record, also referred to as a health record, is a recorded collection of **data** on a patient. It includes past history, a statement of the current problem and diagnosis, and the treatment procedures used to solve the problem. Health records are created for many reasons, including the following: Records are often required by licensing authorities; records may contain information required by patient's insurance companies to pay claims; records are essential for communicating important data to all those who participate in a patient's care; records create a legal document to record and substantiate a standard of care; and specific records and pieces of data may be required by health care providers' liability insurance.

The move from paper charts to electronic health records (EHRs) has been one of the most significant changes in health care. Federal legislation that penalizes Medicare providers who continue to use paper charts has accelerated the transition to EHRs. The Health Information Technology for Economic and Clinical Health (HITECH) Act was intended to encourage the use of health information technology. In addition, HITECH has created incentives for using EHRs, as well as penalties for not using them.

Largely due to the data available from EHR, the health record is increasingly being used to determine the necessity for and the quality of health care. This is reflected in the greater use of the health record by health maintenance organization (HMO) peer review teams and insurance company audits. In addition to the fact that insurer reimbursement may depend on adequate documentation of services provided, the quality of a health care provider's health records often tells a lot about the quality of the practice, as well as the people who make the entries in patient health records.

Electronic Health Records

The HITECH Act was enacted as part of the American Recovery and Reinvestment Act of 2009 economic stimulus bill. According to the U.S. Department of Health and Human Services, HITECH Act provides the "authority to establish programs to improve health care quality, safety, and efficiency through the promotion of health IT [information technology], including electronic health records and private and secure electronic health information exchange." Among other changes to the use of information technology in health care, HITECH Act has provided incentives for the promotion of data interoperability (formerly called, "meaningful use") of EHR, and it assesses penalties for noncompliance. Centers for Medicare and Medicaid Services Administrator Seema Verma indicated that "Under Promoting Interoperability, updates to EHR and related technology includes the use of application programming interfaces, or APIs for patients to collect their health information from multiple providers, and to potentially incorporate all of their data into a single portal, application, program, or other software." Complying with the data interoperability requirement relies on accomplishing specific objectives related to the use of information technology.

Objectives that promote data interoperability include computerized provider order entry; writing and transmitting prescriptions electronically; providing patients with an electronic copy of their health record; providing clinical summaries for patients for each office visit; recording patient demographics; maintaining an up-to-date problem list of current and active diagnoses; protecting electronic health information; generating lists of patients by specific conditions; sending reminders to patients per patient preference for preventive/follow-up care; providing electronic syndromic surveillance data to public health agencies; recording electronic notes in patient records; identifying and report specific cases to a specialized registry; and providing structured electronic lab results to ambulatory providers, among many others.

EHR technology includes both computer hardware and software systems that store patient information. Many times, health care providers and hospitals will have similar or identical systems, allowing shared access to the patient's record. Despite the adoption of EHR, there remain several challenges to the universal adoption of EHR systems that can all "talk" to one another. Although there is general agreement that these very expensive systems will help to improve the quality of care, and perhaps the efficiency with which it is provided, the question of "Who pays for it?" looms large. Second, not all forms of EHR "talk" to each other. So the patient who resides in a community and has a health care provider and hospital that use a particular system may not be able to easily access her record if she becomes ill in another location. Interestingly, this need was underscored in the aftermath of Hurricane Katrina in 2005. Patients of the Veterans Administration (VA) hospital found that, because the VA has fully integrated all of its patient record keeping, their records could be accessed from anywhere in the United States.

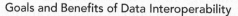

Goals and Benefits of Data Interoperability

To promote data interoperability, the Centers for Medicare & Medicaid Services (CMS) released a set of rules in 2009 to incentivize the use of electronic health records to eligible professionals, critical access hospitals, and eligible hospitals. Formerly called Meaningful Use, Data Interoperability's goal is to improve electronic reporting to public health and ultimately improve patient care. Benefits include:

- Bi-directional communication between state public health departments and clinical care providers
- Standardized data elements for data exchange
- Improved efficiency across the healthcare and public health system

Public Health Registry and Clinical Data Registry Reporting in the Promoting Interoperability Programs include:

- Electronic Case Reporting
- Electronic Reportable Laboratory Test Reporting (for Hospitals only)
- Immunization Registry Reporting
- Syndromic Surveillance Reporting
- Public Health Registries Reporting*
- Clinical Data Registries Reporting

Additional Information:

- Eligible Hospitals and Critical Access Hospitals must attest to at least two measures from 1 through 6 above.
- Eligible Professionals must attest to at least two measures from the Public Health Reporting Objective, measures 1 through 5 above.

Centers for Disease Control and Prevention. (2021, March 26). *Goals and Benefits of Data Interoperability*. Retrieved from www.cdc.gov/datainteroperability/goals-and-benefit.html.

*includes a) Cancer Reporting by Eligible Professionals or Eligible Clinicians only to State Cancer Registries. b) Reporting data by EPs/ECs and Eligible Hospitals/Critical Access Hospitals to CDC/NCHS on Health Care Surveys and c) Reporting data by Eligible Hospitals/Critical Access Hospitals to CDC/NHSN programs on Antibiotic Use & Antibiotic Resistance.

While the majority of health care providers have transitioned to EHR, there are still some who have not. Typically, they are (1) smaller practices who have decided the penalty is less daunting than purchasing, installing, and learning an EHR system or (2) health care providers who just do not want to integrate computers into the way they practice medicine. Some health care providers have even chosen retirement over using EHR.

Professional Confidentiality and EHRs

Professional confidentiality dates back to the time of Hippocrates:

> Whatever in connection with my professional practice, or not in connection with it, I see or hear in the life of men, which ought not to be spoken abroad, I will not divulge as recommending that all should be kept secret.
>
> *Hippocrates*

The federal government, in the form of the Health Insurance Portability and Accountability Act (HIPAA), has weighed in on the issue of patient privacy. See Chapters 2 and 9 for detailed treatment of this important federal law. In the context of EHRs, the challenge is to maintain patient privacy in an era in which electronic storage of records has become commonplace. That method of storage makes access to that data easier—and more easily subject to violation.

Types of Health Records

The typical form of the health record has morphed from a collection of handwritten notes and hard copy test results to an electronic file stored on a network. As with a paper chart, EHR technology is tailored toward the health care provider's type of practice.

In large outpatient clinics associated with teaching hospitals, the integrated health record is common. With an integrated health record, the patient is represented by a single record that includes all outpatient and inpatient activity. Hospitals, HMOs, or private health care providers' offices are completely separate and distinct organizational and legal entities. Cross-indexing of the hospital and outside office records is very limited and usually represented by a copy of the discharge summary from the hospital chart in the office record of the attending health care provider. The hospital record seldom carries any direct report of medical office visits unless the medical office is part of the hospital. And, even then, the technologies of a hospital and one of its practices may not be compatible.

The health record of the nonhospital situation, identified as a record of medical care given in a facility that does not retain the patient overnight, has unique qualities, depending on the specialty of the health care providers and the requirements of the state. The more the outpatient facility resembles a hospital, the more the record resembles a hospital record. The health care professional's management of the health record requires the same attention to detail and confidentiality regardless of whether it is in a hospital setting, a specialist's private office, it is a paper chart, or an EHR.

For most Olympic athletes, the biggest fear is not failing to win a gold medal but falling victim to a last-minute injury that destroys years of hard work and endless hours of practice. But doctors working with big data and cloud-based software are competing to make those heart-breaking injuries less likely.

The 2016 Olympic Games in Rio de Janeiro, for example, is using a cloud-based version of GE Healthcare's Centricity Practice Solutions (CPS) as the official electronic medical records (EMR) keeper. Moving these records into the cloud eliminates the need to ship pallets of paper around the globe in order to monitor athletes' health. The technology is available at all medical posts throughout the games and at the central clinic in the Olympic Village where doctors can deliver more complex care.

"To win the Olympics you have to be the best in the world on a particular day, at a particular time, in your sport," says Bill Moreau, the U.S. Olympic Committee's managing director of sports medicine. "To achieve that is extremely difficult. But, can you imagine training for 20 years and showing up sick or hurt when it could have been prevented? Our goal with electronic medical records is helping to ensure that athletes can deliver their best performance at the right time."

. . .

By drawing on the massive amounts of data, the system also helps the medical team develop new ways to improve the health and performance of all athletes by preventing injuries. Team USA tracks 1,000 data points on each athlete and runs retrospective and forward-looking analytics to spot trends and offer solutions. Using EMR, for example, doctors helped reduce incidence of anemia among women athletes. Using blood tests, doctors can track hemoglobin levels and other lab results and then watch how various nutritional approaches impact stores of hemoglobin in the body, says Dr. Moreau.

Egan, M. (2016, August 9). A Winning Idea: How the Cloud Helps Olympic Athletes Avoid Injury. *GE Reports*. Retrieved from www.gereports.com /a-winning-idea-how-the-cloud-helps-olympic-athletes-avoid-injury/.

Ownership of the Health Record

property right A right of ownership to a certain thing.

premises Physical location, such as an office or building.

State law determines who owns a patient's health record. In the majority of states, the health care provider owns the health record. In at least one state, the patient owns the health record. And, in several other states, there is no express statute that dictates who owns the health record. Although the health care provider and others as owners have a **property right** to the record and can restrict its removal from the **premises**, the patient's interest in the information is protected by law.

Ownership usually carries with it the exclusive right and power to exercise authority and control over the use of the property. In the case of the health record, the owner cannot control the record exclusively. The fact that a hospital or health care provider owns the health record does not prevent other individuals, professionals, corporations, and courts from claiming a right to see and copy the information. There are competing interests in and claims on the contents of a health record. For example, a health care provider is ethically obligated to furnish office records to another health care provider who assumes responsibility for the care of a patient. The following case involves the ownership of a health record.

A dispute occurred between a physician who was employed by a clinic and the estate of a deceased physician, owner of a medical clinic. Following the death of the owner, the employee removed from the clinic the Daily Reference Book, which disclosed the identity of all the persons treated . . ., the receipt book which contained a statement of funds, and all current patient records. The estate accused the physician employee of wrongfully removing the records from the clinic.

The court held that the employee had wrongfully removed the records from the clinic but the importance of the rights and the interests of the patients who elected to receive [the physician employee's] professional services required that he be allowed to retain such of the health records of these patients as might be found necessary to enable him to render them proper care and treatment.

Jones v. Fakehany, 67 Cal. Rptr. 810 (1968)

Another example of the health care provider's inability to absolutely control health records occurs in the disbursement of property at death. Following the death of a health care provider, the records, which are owned by the health care provider, cannot be dispensed with or distributed in the same manner as other property. For example:

The doctor's will directed his executor to burn and destroy all of his office records and files without opening them. The court held that this was against public policy and ordered the executor to make available records and notes pertaining to patients to succeeding physicians upon authorized request.

In re Culbertson's Will, 292 N.Y.S.2d 806 (1968)

Consequently, a health care provider who sought to destroy patient medical records rather than provide patients with an opportunity to transfer their records to new providers would not be acting in accord with the following American Medical Association standards:

3.3.1 Management of Medical Records

Medical records serve important patient interests for present health care and future needs, as well as insurance, employment, and other purposes.

In keeping with the professional responsibility to safeguard the confidentiality of patients' personal information, physicians have an ethical obligation to manage medical records appropriately.

This obligation encompasses not only managing the records of current patients, but also retaining old records against possible future need, and providing copies or transferring records to a third party as requested by the patient or the patient's authorized representative when the physician leaves a practice, sells his or her practice, sells his or her practice, retires, or dies.

To manage medical records responsibly, physicians (or the individual responsible for the practice's medical records) should:

a) Ensure that the practice or institution has and enforces clear policy prohibiting access to patients' medical records by unauthorized staff.
b) Use medical considerations to determine how long to keep records, retaining information that another physician seeing the patient for the first time could reasonably be expected to need or want to know unless otherwise required by law, including:
  i) Immunization records, which should be kept indefinitely
  ii) Records of significant health events or conditions and interventions that could be expected to have a bearing on the patient's future health care needs, such as records of chemotherapy
c) Make the medical record available:
  i) As requested or authorized by the patient (or the patient's authorized representative)
  ii) To the succeeding physician or other authorized person when the physician discontinues his or her practice (whether through departure, sale of the practice, retirement, or death)
  iii) As otherwise required by law
d) Never refuse to transfer the record on request by the patient or the patient's authorized representative, for any reason.
e) Charge a reasonable fee (if any) for the cost of transferring the record.

f) Appropriately store records not transferred to the patient's current physician.

g) Notify the patient about how to access the stored record and for how long the record will be available.

h) Ensure that records that are to be discarded are destroyed to protect confidentiality.

American Medical Association. (2016, June). *Opinions on privacy, confidentiality, and medical records, 3.3.1. Management of medical records.* AMA. Retrieved from www.ama-assn.org/delivering-care/ethics/management-medical-records.

In addition, while HIPAA does have provisions requiring that providers produce their patients' records upon request, the Act does not include provisions about the retention of medical records after a health care provider dies or an office closes. Many states have laws that establish record retention requirements:

An example of some of these state laws:

- In California, physicians must notify patients in advance of closure of the practice and are still responsible for safeguarding records and making sure they are available to patients. The California Medical Association recommends physicians keep records for at least ten years from the last date the patient was seen.

- New York requires that medical records be retained for six years from the date of the most recent entry in the record, and patients are required to [be] informed when a practice closes.

- Virginia prohibits the transfer of medical records as part of the closure or sale of a practice until the provider has first attempted to notify by the patient by mail or by publishing notice in a newspaper of general circulation in the area.

- Texas law requires physicians to keep records for a minimum of seven years after the date of last treatment, and physicians leaving a practice are required to notify patients.

Cordovano, G., McGraw, D., Miri, A. (2020, October 8). How Can Patients Get Medical Records from a Closed Medical Practice? The Health Care Blog. Retrieved from https://thehealthcareblog.com/blog/2020/10/08/how-can-patients-get-medical-records-from-a-closed-medical-practice/.

X-rays, magnetic resonance imaging, electrocardiograms, and the results of other diagnostic tests are a form of health record, and they belong to the health care provider or the hospital where they are taken. Access to x-rays depends on the policy of the owner. Policy is affected by statutes that may require the owner to give the films to another health care provider selected by the patient but may not require the owner to give them to a patient for personal viewing. When a health care provider refers a patient to a radiologist for x-ray studies, the films usually belong to the radiologist and not to the referring health care provider who receives the radiologist's report.

Access to the Health Record

Hospitals and health care providers should have a written policy on file detailing the procedures for releasing patient information. The policy must reflect federal law, and, if applicable, state law as well. In certain states, legislators have given the patient, the patient's health care provider, and/or the authorized agent the right to examine or copy the health record. In other states, judicial precedence has been set for those who base the right to examine the record on the patient's rights.

There is general authorization for the health care provider or hospital to release to insurance companies information about patients submitting third-party payment claims. In addition, office records, as well as hospital records, are subject to inspection by an attorney authorized by the patient to examine them for use in possible litigation against either the health care provider or a third party.

Patients are often required to submit to a physical examination before receiving benefits such as life insurance or welfare or participating in school athletics, for example. In these situations, the patient consents implicitly or expressly to the sending of a truthful record to the third party.

Health Insurance Portability and Accountability Act of 1996

HIPAA is widely known as a set of laws that set standardized guidelines for the protection of a patient's privacy related to health records. To improve efficiency in transferring information about patients within the health care system, HIPAA also directs Health and Human Services to adopt standard "data elements" and "code sets" for electronic coding throughout the entire health care industry. All providers of health care are required to participate in these provisions.

Facsimile (Fax) and Emailed Transmission of Medical Information

There are times when a faxed or emailed message goes astray, either because of error on the part of the sender or imprecise handling by the receiver. In the health care industry, this may cause a breach in the confidential relationship between health care provider and patient. Because of the importance of the timely receipt of information about patients, a fax or secure email may be an appropriate mode for the delivery of medical information. Under other circumstances, either because of the content of the information or the lack of urgency, another method of transferring sensitive information may be more appropriate. Your employer will have a policy as to how to transmit health records, and you should follow that policy.

Physician Revises Faxing Procedures to Safeguard PHI

Covered Entity: Health Care Provider

Issue: Safeguards

A doctor's office disclosed a patient's HIV status when the office mistakenly faxed medical records to the patient's place of employment instead of to the patient's new health care provider. The employee responsible for the disclosure received a written disciplinary warning, and both the employee and the physician apologized to the patient. To resolve this matter, OCR also required the practice to revise the office's fax cover page to underscore a confidential communication for the intended recipient. The office informed all its employees of the incident and counseled staff on proper faxing procedures.

U.S. Department of Health and Human Services. (n.d.). *All Case Examples.*
U.S. Department of Health and Human Services. Retrieved from
www.hhs.gov/hipaa/for-professionals/compliance-enforcement
/examples/all-cases/index.html#case3.

Patient Access to Health Record

HIPAA protects the privacy of patient's medical information, and it also gives patients the right to access much of the information contained in their health records. The U.S. Department of Health and Human Services (HHS) issued two rules in early 2020 to provide further safeguards and support for patients' access to their health records and to enhance interoperability for providers and third parties who use health information technology. The two rules seek to carry out the 21st Century Cures Act (Cures Act) provisions to further the use and interoperability of health care information between insurance companies, providers, patients, and technology vendors. According to the U.S. Food and Drug Administration:

[The Cures Act was] . . . signed into law on December 13, 2016, [and] is designed to help accelerate medical product development and bring new innovations and advances to patients who need them faster and more efficiently.

The law builds on FDA's ongoing work to incorporate the perspectives of patients into the development of drugs, biological products, and devices in FDA's decision-making process. Cures enhances our ability to modernize clinical trial designs, including the use of real-world evidence, and clinical outcome assessments, which will speed the development and review of novel medical products, including medical countermeasures.

U.S. Food and Drug Administration. (2020, January 31). 21st Century Cures Act. U.S. FDA. Retrieved from www.fda.gov/regulatory-information/selected-amendments-fdc-act/21st-century-cures-act.

Health care providers disagree about whether patients should have access to their own records. Some believe that there is the possibility of misinterpretation by the patient; others believe that a little knowledge can be more dangerous than no knowledge at all. Legal commentators view patients' access to their own records cynically, observing that almost everyone except the subject of the records can know what is in them. HIPAA requires that patients have the right to see their records, to obtain copies, and to make corrections in them.

"Based on recent studies and our own enforcement experience, far too often individuals face obstacles to accessing their health information," said Jocelyn Samuels, the director of the Office for Civil Rights at the Department of Health and Human Services, which enforces federal health privacy standards. "This must change."

When patients can see their medical records, the administration said, it is easier for them to participate in their health care. They can, for example, review what they were told by their doctors and, perhaps, consider other options for care.

Pear, R. (2016, January 16). New Guidelines Nudge Doctors to Give Patients Access to Medical Records. *The New York Times.* Retrieved from www.nytimes.com/2016/01/17/us/new-guidelines-nudge-doctors-on-giving-patients-access-to-medical-records.html.

Under certain limited circumstances, a covered entity may deny an individual's request for access to all or a portion of the PHI requested. In some of these circumstances, an individual has a right to have the denial reviewed by a licensed health care professional designated by the covered entity who did not participate in the original decision to deny.

Unreviewable grounds for denial (45 CFR 164.524(a)(2)):

- The request is for psychotherapy notes, or information compiled in reasonable anticipation of, or for use in, a legal proceeding.
- An inmate requests a copy of her PHI held by a covered entity that is a correctional institution, or health care provider acting under the direction of the institution, and providing the copy would jeopardize the health, safety, security, custody, or rehabilitation of the inmate or other inmates, or the safety of correctional officers, employees, or other person at the institution or responsible for the transporting of the inmate. However, in these cases, an inmate retains the right to inspect her PHI.
- The requested PHI is in a designated record set that is part of a research study that includes treatment (e.g., clinical trial) and is still in progress, provided the individual agreed to the temporary suspension of access when consenting to participate in the research. The individual's right of access is reinstated upon completion of the research.
- The requested PHI is in Privacy Act protected records (i.e., certain records under the control of a federal agency, which may be maintained by a federal agency or a contractor to a federal agency), if the denial of access is consistent with the requirements of the Act.
- The requested PHI was obtained by someone other than a health care provider (e.g., a family member of the individual) under a promise of confidentiality, and providing access to the information would be reasonably likely to reveal the source of the information.

Reviewable grounds for denial (45 CFR 164.524(a)(3)). A licensed health care professional has determined in the exercise of professional judgment that:

- The access requested is reasonably likely to endanger the life or physical safety of the individual or another person. This ground for denial does not extend to concerns about psychological or emotional harm (e.g., concerns that the individual will not be able to understand the information or may be upset by it).
- The access requested is reasonably likely to cause substantial harm to a person (other than a health care provider) referenced in the PHI.

(Continues)

(Continued)

- The provision of access to a personal representative of the individual that requests such access is reasonably likely to cause substantial harm to the individual or another person.

Department of Health and Human Services. (n.d.). Individuals' Right Under HIPAA to Access Their Health Information. *45 CFR § 164.524. U.S.* Retrieved from www.hhs.gov/hipaa/for-professionals/privacy/guidance/access/index.html.

Family's Access to Patient Health Records

Health care providers who do not support a patient's direct access to health records comment that there may be information in the records that the patient or members of the family should not see; for example, confidential information on past pregnancies, abortions, sexually transmitted diseases, or mental illness. Artificial insemination presents ethical dilemmas in that the availability of the record to the family affects the woman's privacy regarding conception; on the other side of the issue, there is the responsibility of the provider to maintain an accurate record as well as to preserve information for the future benefit of the child. HIPAA requires, however, that certain health information be provided regardless of the provider's wishes.

Innocent Party in the Health Record

In the case of the mentally ill patient, health records may contain sensitive and private information regarding the patient's family, friends, employers, and associates. A therapist frequently will record intimate aspects of relatives' and associates' lives. This information may contain falsehoods and inaccuracies based on the patient's delusions and misconceptions. The patient's record may also contain the therapist's assessment of the patient's interaction with family members and other patients.

Release of information involving other persons contained in the patient's health record is potentially harmful to all parties involved. Disclosure may damage reputations within the community, affect employment opportunities, cause severe emotional distress, and infringe on the individual privacy of others. If the patient obtains access to the health record and learns about others' opinions, an adverse clinical reaction may occur, and family and social relationships may be severely and permanently disrupted. Information in the health record may be used against people other than the patient in legal proceedings—for example, divorce, child custody, and competency hearings.

At least three courts have held that when family members participate in counseling sessions along with the patient, the health records of the patient may not be disclosed without the consent of the patient and family members.

Release of Information

The best rule to follow, unless instructed otherwise by the law or your employer, is to refuse to disclose information about a patient, which includes not acknowledging whether the individual being asked about is a patient. It is always possible that an enterprising sleuth could figure out the nature of a patient's illness from the specialty of the health care provider.

The most frequently alleged HIPAA release of information issues over the past 15 years are discussed below.

The U.S. Department of Health and Human Services' (HHS) Office for Civil Rights (OCR) is responsible for enforcing compliance with HIPAA privacy rules.

For more than 15 years, the OCR has tracked the most-often alleged compliance issues included in HIPAA complaints.

According to the OCR, they are:

- Impermissible uses and disclosures of protected health information.
- Lack of safeguards of protected health information.
- Lack of patient access to their protected health information.
- Lack of administrative safeguards of electronic protected health information.
- Use or disclosure of more than the minimum necessary protected health information.

Physicians and private practices are alleged to be the second-most common violator of HIPAA privacy regulations, coming in behind hospitals and ahead of outpatient facilities, pharmacies and health plans, the OCR says.

Robeznieks, A. (2021, March 3). Common HIPAA Violations Physicians Should Guard Against. AMA Website. Retrieved from www.ama-assn.org /practice-management/hipaa/common-hipaa-violations -physicians-should-guard-against.

Information should not be released unless the request for that information is specific. The request should have time limits, identify the purposes for which the records will be used, and identify the particular information requested. It is important to check and confirm the credentials of the person and/or organization requesting information from the record. Your office should have a protocol that describes the steps necessary when you have a request for a copy of a health record, and it is highly advisable to follow the protocol.

Notably, health records may not be withheld pending payment of the patient's bill to a health care provider or a hospital.

Capacity to Consent to Release of Information

Any patient who has reached the age of majority can consent to the release of health records. If a former patient is dead, the executor, administrator, or personal representative may release the record. If an adult patient is temporarily unable to consent, a court-appointed guardian will often have authorization to act on behalf of the patient. Under certain circumstances and to the extent necessary in an emergency, HIPAA does allow for release of a patient's medical information without consent.

Minors have particular problems with regard to the release of medical information. In a drug abuse or sexually transmitted disease diagnosis, only the minor involved can release the record, even to his or her parents or guardians. Normally, a parent or guardian can release the minor's records until the minor reaches majority. If one parent has been awarded custody of the minor, it is preferable to get that parent to release the medical information. The mature minor doctrine allows minors to release their records under certain circumstances such as when they are living away from home, self-supporting, or married. Under certain conditions, when a minor knows the nature, quality, and consequences of his or her actions, a minor can authorize the release of a health record.

Release of Information to Attorneys

Attorneys need information from health records under many circumstances. If there is likelihood that medical malpractice charges will be brought against a provider, an attorney will review the patient's medical records before deciding whether to file a lawsuit. By responding indifferently to an attorney's request for records, a health care provider frequently causes unnecessary problems. The attorney may find that it is more efficient to file the lawsuit and engage in formal discovery than to fight with a provider for the records. This attitude hardens feelings between attorneys and health care providers.

Release Forms

A patient's in-person oral request or telephone call is insufficient to properly authorize the release of health records. The request must be in writing. And, when the information requested is disclosed, it must be accompanied by instructions that forbid its re-disclosure to others who are not authorized to receive it.

To compel, or force, the production of health records, a subpoena is necessary. A **subpoena** is a court order for the named person to appear at a certain time and place to give testimony on a certain matter. The particular type of subpoena used for documents or objects is called a **subpoena duces tecum**. Legal subpoenas do not automatically require the release of all requested health information. When sensitive information about patients and other people has been requested without consent of the parties, the issues can be discussed with the judge and attorneys. The judge may then make the decision to review the material privately to determine whether it should be allowed into evidence, and if so, whether it should be separated from the other evidence and sealed by the court for purposes of confidentiality.

subpoena A written order to appear at a specified time and place to give sworn testimony.

subpoena duces tecum A written order to produce documents or things.

Credibility of the Health Record

Credibility of a health record refers to whether the information recorded in the record is believable. An article written for lawyers informing them how to recognize a good medical malpractice case (one they can win) stated the following:

> If you take on a case where the doctor or the hospital changes something in the records, you will need less than the usual quantum of fault to prevail before a jury. The same is true if a record or x-ray is missing. Even a change that the doctor argues was made for a good faith reason or a record lost with the explanation, "fire," "flood" or "robbery," will suggest to the jury that there was a guilty motive afoot—and there probably was.
>
> Gage, S. M. (1981, Spring). Alteration, Falsification and Fabrication of Medical Records in Medical Malpractice Actions. *Medical Trial Quarterly, 27,* 476.

Even though the above article was written well before the widespread use of EHR, the premise remains valid and true today: If a health record has corrections, amendments, modifications, changes, or even misspelled words, it will raise suspicions. The credibility of the health record is crucial in the defense of a health care provider, medical facility, or employee during a medical malpractice case.

Health information is needed to try cases in nearly every area of law. When an attorney meets with a client who has a complaint about medical care, the first step is to obtain all health records available and have them reviewed by an independent health care provider. This independent review may prompt the attorney to further investigate the potential malpractice claim or to explain to the client why there is no evidence of malpractice. Sometimes attorneys find that they can settle with a potential defendant or the insurance company before filing a malpractice suit. One of the reasons for a prelawsuit settlement is when the health record has credibility issues.

The credibility of the record-keeping procedure is subject to question when investigation reveals delayed filing of laboratory test results, incomplete files, illegible records, altered or fabricated records, or the loss or concealment of information. The following sections describe conduct that has caused problems for defendants in a medical malpractice case.

Delayed Filing of Laboratory Tests

Sixty-seven closed claims with a diagnosis of melanoma were reviewed by the Aetna Life and Casualty Company. Failure to diagnose was the most common allegation in the claims, and the health care provider's office was the setting most often identified as the site of the alleged malpractice. The study suggested that the flow of medical reports, such as x-ray readings, may be a factor in malpractice suits involving malignancy. In four cases, the health care provider who ordered an x-ray study did not see the final positive radiology report—the one that probably would have led to earlier diagnosis and treatment. For example:

> A 78-year-old woman was evaluated by an internist for recurrent indigestion. The radiologist's report suggested the presence of a small soft tissue mass below the left diaphragm, but the patient did not call the physician's office to ask about the result as she had been told to. The physician did not see the results until approximately eight weeks later. An upper G.I. series confirmed the diagnosis. Surgical exploration and biopsy disclosed the unresectable reticulum cell sarcoma of the stomach. The patient died within six weeks. The original report may have been placed in the patient's file during the physician's vacation.
>
> Mittleman, M. (1980, February). What Are the Chances When Malignancy Leads to a Malpractice Suit? *Legal Aspects of Medical Practice*, 42.

Incomplete and Error-Filled Records

Health records must be accurate, complete, and correct. In the worst case scenarios, these types of mistakes in health records can have fatal results. In less severe cases, health record mistakes can damage a health care provider's reputation. Consider how you would feel if you were the patient in the following real-life example:

Marilyn Mullins, 62, said she was shocked when she received a note from a chaplain at Sentara Martha Jefferson Hospital that said she had died . . .

A hospital chaplain called Mullins with an apology and explained that a technical error caused the mistake. The hospital said a secretary accidentally checked the box for deceased patient instead of checking discharge to home.

Woman Leaves Hospital, Finds Out She Died. (2016, June 11).
Retrieved from www.nbcwashington.com/news/local/Woman-Leaves
-Hospital-Finds-Out-She-Died-382568031.html.

Altered Health Records

If a record is damaging to a health care provider, they may be strongly tempted to change it. The use of EHR has, however, changed the way someone might alter a health record. With EHR, any changes to a record will be reflected as an amendment and be marked with the user's identification and time and date of the amendment.

For any alteration to be plausible, all other people involved—health care providers, nurses, administrators—must go along with it. Somewhere along the line the chain is almost bound to snap. Altered records demonstrate the defendant's consciousness of wrongdoing, and they can establish liability. If a jury learns that a provider has intentionally altered a health record for improper reasons, they will react, and, for example, award much larger damages. Insurance companies are well aware of this. It is no coincidence that when a medical malpractice case involves altered records, defense lawyers will often advise their clients to settle the case.

As a result of pain in her right breast and family history of cancer, plaintiff Kim Johnson underwent a diagnostic mammogram as well as an ultrasound of her right breast. The studies' results, the doctors' recommendations, and the information Johnson received about the studies are disputed and are at the crux of this case. Johnson received a letter that her "recent mammogram examination . . . revealed no evidence of cancer."

Johnson, however, continued to experience right breast pain. Less than a year later, Johnson was diagnosed with malignant invasive ductal carcinoma which had metastasized. After the lawsuit was filed, the treating physician Amanda Applegate contacted the radiology technician regarding Johnson's mammograms. The

(Continues)

(Continued)

radiologist technician reported that Johnson had been scheduled for a biopsy and provided a screenshot of Johnson's record from the hospital's mammogram, which indicated the record had been modified on that day. Johnson alleges that this screenshot was taken after the radiology technician edited Johnson's medical record to delete references to the "cancer free" diagnosis and letter. In addition, two false mammogram notification letters were included in subpoenaed medical records produced by defendant Fleming County Hospital (FCH).

Johnson's forensic expert showed how two hospital employees altered Johnson's mammogram record several times within six weeks of the lawsuit's filing. The alterations removed records that (1) supported Johnson's claims of medical negligence, and (2) allowed the hospital to produce the fake notification letters that the defendants relied on for their defense.

While some of the defendants have settled with Johnson, the case continues for those few defendants who did not settle.

Johnson v. Wood, 2020-SC-0588_MR (Ky. 2021)

Fabricating Health Records

Altering health records modifies the content of the record, and fabricating health records means inventing facts. The motive is typically to cover up an error or wrongdoing.

Loss or Concealment of Records

Related to the alteration of health records is the destruction, unavailability, or loss of relevant x-rays, laboratory test results, and other physical evidence. Health records may also be summoned in fraud situations in which a provider claims excessive amounts from insurance companies or welfare agencies.

Acceptable Method of Making Changes in Health Records

Although maintaining the record perfectly should always be the goal, it is important to recognize that incorrect entries may happen. Most EHR systems track each entry by user, date, and time. So, if a mistake is made and the record needs to be changed, the original error will remain but there will be an addendum with the correct information.

When an error occurs with a paper chart, cross out the mistake, initial and date it, and then write the correct information. It is highly inadvisable to use correction fluid or some other method to try to hide the mistake.

There are occasions when making a change in a patient's records is necessary. If the changes are made while the patient is under treatment, they may be accepted as rewritten or amended. But if the changes are made beyond a reasonable period of time following discharge, particularly after a health care provider or hospital is on notice of a potential lawsuit, changes in the health record are almost always serious and raise red flags.

It is the responsibility of individuals charged with keeping health records to be accurate. They must bring any error in record keeping to the attention of the health care provider at the time it is discovered, as well as any ambiguous section that may affect the reader's understanding. It is the health care provider's responsibility to correct his or her own error. Keeping good notes is as important to the health care provider as the diagnosis. If the record keeper is in dispute with a health care provider, the facts should be recorded and reviewed by a neutral third party. If your employer has a different policy, follow that policy.

☑ SUMMARY

- The HITECH Act was intended to encourage the use of health information technology.
- EHRs are electronic health records, which are required by the HITECH Act for all health care providers who treat Medicare patients. A provider's failure to use EHRs will result in a monetary penalty.
- Health records and information regarding patients are subject to privacy laws, including HIPAA.
- State law determines the owner of a health record. The owner of a health record is usually the facility that generates the record: A hospital record is owned by a hospital, and an office record by the health care provider or corporation that owns the medical practice. Each facility has a health record that is adequate to meet its own needs.
- Patients often wish to see their records. HIPAA allows patients to see their records and make corrections in them. Health care providers are required to transfer medical information to other health care providers engaged by their patients and to allow attorneys access to records of their clients.
- Contents of a health record should not be transferred or disclosed without the patient's written authorization.

- Records are often required in court and can be ordered by the issuance of a subpoena duces tecum.
- Health records must be credible. This means that there can be no alterations, fabrications, or concealments in a record.
- Corrections to a health record should be made with great care.

SUGGESTED ACTIVITIES

1. There are many HIPAA-compliant health record release forms on the Internet. Find one and complete it so you can obtain a copy of your health record from one of your health care providers.
2. Draft a letter for a fictitious patient who has requested a copy of their health records. Include a copy of the release form you found on the Internet.

STUDY QUESTIONS

1. List the type of information contained in a health record.
2. Discuss the difference between ownership of a health record and ownership of other property.
3. A patient requests his x-rays to take home and show to the family. Role-play how you would handle this matter as an employee of the radiologist.
4. Your office has a relaxed policy with regard to the release of information in health records. A patient asks to see their record. You know that there is information in the record regarding telephone calls from the patient's relatives that would interfere with the family relationship. The health care provider is away for a week. How would you handle the matter?
5. A health record has been subpoenaed and a court order accompanies it. The health care provider has removed important parts of the record. You know that this information is missing. The office sends you to court as the keeper of the record. You must testify about the completeness of the record. What are you going to say?
6. There is an error in a health record that has been subpoenaed. This is a good-faith error and should be corrected. It has to do with the information the plaintiff is interested in and could be damaging to the defendant–health care provider if changed, but also damaging if unchanged. The health care provider asks you to delete the health record and recreate it with the correct information. What do you do?

CASES FOR DISCUSSION

1. The plaintiff's physician received an authorization allowing the release of information to an insurance company following the plaintiff's application for major medical insurance. The physician released the following information: Enclosed is a summary of Mr. Millsaps's recent hospitalization. Physically the man has no notable problems; emotionally, the patient is quite mercurial in his moods. He is a strong-willed man obsessed with faults of others in his family, for which there has been no objective basis. He has completely resisted any constructive advice by his wife, family, minister, or myself. The man needs psychiatric help for his severe obsessions and depression, some of which have suicidal overtones. He is an extremely poor insurance risk.

   The application for major medical insurance was rejected. Did the physician have a right to release this information to the insurance company?

2. The patient alleged that the defendant–physician fraudulently and negligently advised her that she had a brain tumor that required immediate surgery, that the physician negligently performed an unneeded craniotomy on her at the hospital, and that the physician had held staff surgical privileges at the hospital on a continuing basis. The plaintiff–patient further alleged several theories against the hospital. Underlying these was the contention that the hospital had sufficient prior information to be put on notice that the defendant–physician was an incompetent, overaggressive neurosurgeon with a history of performing unnecessary operations, particularly elective craniotomies. The court ordered the hospital to produce copies of all preoperative consultations, operative notes, interpretations of preoperative x-rays, and brain tissue analyses obtained on 140 patients. Included in the order were provisions to ensure the privacy of the patients. The hospital refused the records on the grounds that consent had not been obtained from any of the 140 patients and the production order was in violation of the patient–physician privilege statute. Should the appeals court agree with the hospital?

3. A patient came to the emergency room of the hospital complaining of nausea and chest pains. The nurse on duty refused to call a health care provider, determining that there was no need at that time. The patient died of a myocardial infarction minutes after leaving the hospital. The widow's attorney attempted to review the records during discovery but found that they had been destroyed. Did the hospital have the right to destroy the patient's records?

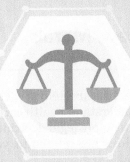

Chapter 8

Introduction to Ethics

 Ethics is the difference between knowing what you have
a right to do and what is right to do.

Potter Stewart, Chief Justice of the U.S. Supreme Court

Objectives

After reading this chapter, you should be able to:

1. Distinguish between ethics, law, morals, and etiquette.
2. Describe the importance of ethics codes in professional organizations.
3. Describe how individual values and morals are developed.
4. Summarize the main concepts of duty-based, utilitarian, and virtue-based ethical theories.
5. Develop a thought process for making ethical decisions.
6. Demonstrate acceptable responses to ethical issues.
7. Distinguish between personal ethics and professional ethics.
8. Describe the relationship between personal ethics and professionalism on the job.
9. Develop a plan for separating personal and professional ethics in the workplace.

Building Your Legal Vocabulary

Amoral
Bioethics
Dilemma
Ethics

Etiquette
Immoral
Philosophy
Values

The Difference Between Ethics, Law, Morals, and Etiquette

dilemma Situation where a challenging decision must be made between two or more options.

ethics Moral principles that guide a person or a society's choices and conduct.

Ethical **dilemmas** are found in every aspect of health care delivery. The study of law in the earlier chapters allows you to understand health care–related laws and regulations, to think legally, and to apply legal doctrines to real-life situations in a health care setting. **Ethics** are related to, yet distinguished from, the study of law in health care.

Both ethics and laws act as rules of personal and societal conduct. A key distinction between law and ethics is that a violation of the law, negligent act, or a breach of contract, for example, may result in prison, fines, or monetary damages, among others. A code of ethics violation in health care may result in license suspension or revocation, or other negative repercussions from your employer, colleagues, patients, family, or friends. Government creates laws. Individuals, professional groups, and employers, among others create codes of ethics. Understanding how ethics applies to the delivery of health care is equally important as understanding how the law applies.

Ethics

philosophy A basic viewpoint of an individual's or a community's value system.

values Principles of thought and conduct that are considered desirable.

Ethics is an area of **philosophy** that focuses on the study of standards that distinguish between acceptable and unacceptable behavior. Studying ethics involves examining emotions, reasoning, and issues of freedom and personal responsibility. Our personal **values** and experiences shape the morals we embrace and how we interpret and solve ethical dilemmas.

When distilled to their essence, ethics are the standardization of conduct through the identification of common morals. The word "ethics" has its roots in the Greek word *ethos*, meaning the character of a society, culture, group, or period of time as evidenced by its beliefs, priorities, and actions. Ethics are collections of established moral principles of right and wrong that provide guidance when there is no applicable law, regulation, or other mandated protocol.

Consider the Following Case Study. Angel, a 62 year old male, has been in an ICU ward for the past 14 weeks. His ICU physician's prognosis is that his condition has not improved, which suggests he will almost certainly not recover. Angel's best case scenario is that he remains in long term acute care hospital for the remainder of his life. He understands the severity of his condition. Angel is able to communicate to his physician that he wants to be administered medicine that will allow him to die. The hospital's ethicist explains to Angel that it is illegal in the state they are in to give a patient something that will hasten death. Angel's family, including his three adult children, objects to his wishes and suggests that Angel does not have the mental capacity to make such a decision. They explain the decision is out of character for the man they know only as being happy and full of life. Angel is examined by a psychiatrist, who concludes he has the capacity to make decisions. Angel pleads to be taken off the ventilator he is on, requests a do not resuscitate order be issued, and declines antibiotics. He makes clear that he wants only palliative care. Angel's family is certain that his decision is wrong and that with more time and care, his condition will improve.

Angel, his family, and his providers all have positions with which we can empathize, but whose direction should be followed? This case study illustrates an ethical dilemma in health care: How much credibility should be given to the family's position that Angel's decision is so far out of character for him, that he cannot be in a position to make life and death decisions? Who should make the final decision? Under what circumstances should the psychiatrist's opinion that Angel has the ability to make decisions be disregarded? If you were the hospital ethicist, how would you resolve this ethical dilemma?

Medical ethics include disputes between theories and positions, to questions involving traditional ethical positions and threats posed by modern medical technology, and to the interaction between ethical constraints and the law. The study of **bioethics** relates to the ethics of biological research and its applications, especially as it relates to medicine. Chapters 10, 11, and 12 raise bioethical issues from reproduction to death.

bioethics Ethical issues and the implications of the application of biological research.

Ethics Codes   Medical associations have their own code of ethics that include standards of conduct that address ethical and moral behavior for that association's specialty. The American Medical Association (AMA) Principles of Medical Ethics include nine standards, also known as tenets, of conduct that define the essentials of health care providers' ethical behavior. The Preamble to the Principles of Medical Ethics states, "The medical profession has long subscribed to a body of ethical statements developed primarily for the benefit of the patient. As a member of this profession, a physician must recognize responsibility to patients first and foremost, as well as to society, to other health professionals, and to self. The following Principles adopted by the American Medical Association are not laws, but standards of conduct that define the essentials of honorable behavior for the physician." See Figure 8-1 for the AMA Principles of Medical Ethics.

Developing a code of ethics is a difficult task. Incorporating the ideals they represent in everyday life is even more difficult. The role of health care professionals involves interpersonal interaction with patients and their families before, during, and after they face difficult decisions.

Principles of Medical Ethics

1. A physician shall be dedicated to providing competent medical care, with compassion and respect for human dignity and rights.

2. A physician shall uphold the standards of professionalism, be honest in all professional interactions, and strive to report physicians deficient in character or competence, or engaging in fraud or deception, to appropriate entities.

3. A physician shall respect the law and also recognize a responsibility to seek changes in those requirements which are contrary to the best interests of the patient.

4. A physician shall respect the rights of patients, colleagues, and other health professionals, and shall safeguard patient confidences and privacy within the constraints of the law.

5. A physician shall continue to study, apply, and advance scientific knowledge, maintain a commitment to medical education, make relevant information available to patients, colleagues, and the public, obtain consultation, and use the talents of other health professionals when indicated.

6. A physician shall, in the provision of appropriate patient care, except in emergencies, be free to choose whom to serve, with whom to associate, and the environment in which to provide medical care.

7. A physician shall recognize a responsibility to participate in activities contributing to the improvement of the community and the betterment of public health.

8. A physician shall, while caring for a patient, regard responsibility to the patient as paramount.

9. A physician shall support access to medical care for all people.

www.ama-assn.org/about/publications-newsletters/ama-principles-medical-ethics

Figure 8-1 AMA Principles of Medical Ethics

Morals

Morals are a collection of principles about what is right. Morals are the foundation for ethics. Personal morals develop and evolve throughout our lifetimes. Our family, friends, mentors, religious leaders, teachers, public figures, culture, and society, among others, expressly or through their actions, teach us what is and what is not acceptable behavior. They teach us morals. We typically develop our personal morals through everyday interactions with those that influence us: your next door neighbor Khalid who you observed treating all people with respect; your Aunt Wanda who showed you, by example, that stealing was wrong when she let the cashier know that she had been given too much change; your seventh grade teacher Ms. Jimenez who clearly explained plagiarism to the class; your childhood friend Matías who frustrated you when he repeatedly cheated when playing board games; your best friend Jean who remained loyal and present during a difficult time; or your co-worker Gunther who falsely claimed to be vaccinated for COVID-19 so he did not have to wear a mask at work. All of these situations teach you about morals and

Table 8-1 Examples of Moral, Immoral, and Amoral Conduct

Behavior	Definition	Example
Moral	principles of and beliefs about what is right	Entering accurate and complete information into a patient's health record in a timely manner
Immoral	not moral	Signing a school vaccine confirmation form for a school-aged child whose health record indicates the parent declined the vaccine
Amoral	without consideration of morals	Logging into your employer's electronic health records system at the beginning of the workday

influence the development of your personal ethics. Behavior that is not aligned with morals is known as **immoral**; behavior that does not take moral principles into consideration is known as **amoral**. Table 8-1 has examples of moral, immoral, and amoral conduct.

immoral Not moral.

amoral Without consideration of morals.

values Principles of thought and conduct that are considered desirable.

When facing ethical dilemmas sometimes moral principles alone can provide the path to resolution. It is more likely, however, that there are several moral paths to resolution. A key part of making ethical decisions is understanding and being able to describe how the decision was made.

Development of Values Morals are the collection of principles people adopt to be accepted in a group, profession, society, or community or to assess whether an action is right or wrong. Values are principles people adopt for their own personal benefit or development. Values allow people to establish priorities for personal growth and to guide their important life decisions.

How do we develop our values? People adopt some values because they appear as self-evident truths. Most values, however, develop as we mature from infancy. There are numerous theories that seek to explain how we develop our values. Lawrence Kohlberg expounded on the theories and research of Jean Piaget, which resulted in one of the more common and controversial theories of value development.

Piaget theorized that value development happens in four stages based upon age and resulting from the thinking process, as well as personal experience. Kohlberg expanded Piaget's theory and studied the evolution of thought process and behavior. Kohlberg identified that the development of moral reasoning can be categorized into three levels:

- Level 1: Preconventional moral reasoning is where decisions are guided by:

    Stage 1: acceptance of authority

    Stage 2: realization that there are multiple perspectives, and some are more advantageous than others.

- Level 2: Conventional moral reasoning is where decisions are guided by:

    Stage 1: following rules and doing what is expected

    Stage 2: duty and respect for rules

- Level 3: Postconventional Moral Reasoning is where decisions are guided by:

    Stage 1: individual thought and rights and how it fits into society

    Stage 2: adoption of principles such as equality, dignity, or respect, as well as other societal rules

Value development both reflects and is part of human development and growth. How we reason and think changes and becomes more complex as we grow and learn.

Professional Etiquette

etiquette Prescribed code of courteous social behavior.

Etiquette is code of well-mannered behavior accepted by a culture, a group, or a profession. Etiquette can change depending on the culture, the times, or the group. It does not require moral understanding or ethical reasoning even though it is based on societal morals, customs, and beliefs. Etiquette requires specific good behavior in a given situation. Professional etiquette is the recognized set of rules to take into account at work.

A code of professional etiquette exists for those working in the health care community. Politeness, proper dress, discretion, and courtesy are at its core. Professional etiquette may, for example, be a provider who instructs staff to put through all calls from other providers. In addition, individual health care offices and facilities have their own etiquette for staff to follow, which may be written in an employee handbook or other office protocol document. Etiquette often has unwritten elements, as well that you may only learn from being observant. It is your responsibility to be familiar with your employer's written and unwritten expectations regarding workplace etiquette.

Workplace telephone etiquette is essential in health care office management. One person's poor telephone etiquette can reflect negatively upon the entire office, including the health care provider, and it can result in dissatisfied patients and patient families. Interpersonal communication etiquette—how you communicate with your colleagues and patients—can define your professional reputation. Interpersonal communication etiquette includes what you say (i.e., the substance of your communication) and how you say it (i.e., the tone and word choice). These details matter. If you are aware of them as you start your career in the health care field, you can adapt a constructive workplace etiquette that will represent the true professional that you are.

Ethical Theories

The term "ethical theories" can initially appear overwhelming and excessively academic, but they are really just decision-making frameworks, or guides, for the resolution of ethical dilemmas. Successfully making, advocating for, and critiquing ethical decisions requires an understanding of the underlying ethical theory.

Western ethical theories can be categorized into two groups: deontological and teleological. Deontological means the study or science of duty. Deontological ethics identifies the morally right action without consideration of the resulting outcomes or consequences. Teleological means the study or science of conduct as it relates to the ends it serves. Teleological ethics identifies the morally right action based upon the outcomes or consequences.

Deontological and teleological ethical theories can be classified according to their focus on the "right" and the "good" and how they interact with one another.

A common deontological theory used in health care is based upon duty, or what is right. Common teleological theories include utilitarianism (also called consequentialism) and virtue-based ethics. Each of these three theories has its own perspective. When health care professionals face ethical dilemmas, being familiar with ethical theories allows for the creation of arguments, the identification of ethical argument flaws and improvements.

All ethical theories have their inherent limitations. For example, duty-based ethics does not consider consequences or results and utilitarian ethics does not consider duty. Table 8-2 has a summary of these common ethical theories.

Deontology

The framework of deontology, or duty-based ethics, focuses on the motives of actions and whether actions were prompted by duty or by something else. The duties that form deontological thinking can require action (duty to look after one's patients) or they can prohibit action (duty not to steal). A deontologist takes the position that we should perform certain actions simply

Table 8-2 Common Ethical Theories

	Deontological	Teleological	
Ethical Theory	**Duty-based**	**Utilitarianism**	**Virtue-based**
Method	identify the actor's duties related to the ethical issue without regard to outcome	identify the action that will result in the most good for the greatest number of people	identify the action that a virtuous person would undertake
Morally right action is dictated by . . .	the actor's duty	the action that produces the most good for the greatest number of people	the action that a virtuous, honorable, and principled person would undertake

because those actions are morally right. Deontological ethics are concerned with what people do, not with the consequences of their actions. When taken to an extreme, deontology requires that the right action be undertaken, even if that action results in more harm than doing the wrong action.

Immanuel Kant, an eighteenth-century Prussian ethicist, developed the duty-based theory, which focused on duty and motivation. Kant presumed that humans could not reliably predict consequences of ethical dilemmas. He believed that the moral value of an action can only be determined by understanding the motivation behind it. Kant believed that we could identify our ethical duty with a high level of certainty if we used our ability to reason and that principles taken from this line of reasoning were universal.

Duty-based ethics holds that there are universal principles that apply to all people in all situations and that an action can only be right or wrong. It cannot be both. A morally right action can be identified when it is aligned with a principle Kant called a categorical imperative, which is a rule that has no exceptions and is true in every situation. According to Kant's theory, we comply with a categorical imperative only because the duty exists, and for no other reason (i.e., the outcome). Categorical imperatives must not only be universally applicable, but they must also not raise any contradictions.

This theory is well-suited for ethical dilemmas that raise the issue of why duty requires or prohibits a given action. Its framework, however, has its drawbacks. It does not have guidance on how to choose when two or more duties are in conflict. Because duty-based ethics does not consider outcomes or consequences, it is possible that a morally right action can produce an unwelcome or bad outcome.

Teleology

The Greek word "Telos" means goal, end, or purpose, and it is the root of the word teleology. A teleological theory studies purposes and objectives in an effort to attain a certain goal. Teleological theory resolves ethical dilemmas by identifying the action that is deemed good or beneficial, and then that action is held to be morally right. Conversely, if the outcome causes harm, then the action is held to be morally wrong. The difference in the two teleological theories discussed below—utilitarianism and virtue based—is how an action is determined to be morally right or wrong.

Utilitarianism

Utilitarianism (also referred to as consequentialism) is a common teleological theory that favors results over rules. Utilitarianism's simplicity is one of its benefits: choose the action that provides the greatest good (pleasure or happiness) for the largest amount of people. Unlike deontological theory that evaluates duty in its search for the morally right action, utilitarianism evaluates consequences or outcomes.

Jeremy Bentham (1748–1832) and John Stuart Mill (1806–1873) both contributed to the development of utilitarianism. They built upon earlier teleological theories to include the notion that not only is an action morally right if it provides the greatest good, but that it must also provide the greatest good for the greatest number of people.

Utilitarian focus on outcomes is considered reasonable, since outcomes or consequences are typically what guide our everyday decision making. This also makes it familiar and easy to implement in an ethical setting. Its credibility is bolstered by the reasonableness of basing moral rights upon the resulting good. Although utilitarianism is favored as a practical approach, it has its weaknesses. There is no crystal ball for ethical dilemmas, so outcomes are not always predictable. While utilitarianism is intended to benefit the most amount of people, it is unlikely that it will benefit all people. So, there will always be a portion of the population that will not benefit. Utilitarianism suggests that an action is acceptable if the end justifies the means, which can create situations that other theories would find unethical.

Virtue Based

Virtue-based ethics can be traced to the work of early philosophers Socrates, Plato, and Aristotle. Unlike deontological (duty or rule based) or utilitarianism (consequence based) ethical theories, virtue-based ethics looks to the ethics of individuals and human nature to determine the morally right action. Its framework presumes that morally right actions should be consistent with the virtuous character of the person performing the action. If a person is virtuous, their actions should be virtuous and morally right, as well. An action is morally right if it is an action that a virtuous person would perform. Aristotle believed that ethics should focus on virtue as demonstrated throughout a person's life as opposed to a single action or incident.

Virtues considered important in using this theory include honesty, loyalty, integrity, and courage, among others. Virtue-based ethics assumes that virtues are morally right and then evaluates actions in relation to the morally right virtues. Virtue-based ethics asks the question, "Are the actions identified as ethical aligned with what a virtuous person would do under the same circumstances?"

Virtue-based ethics use virtue as a barometer, which creates difficulty when there is dispute about what qualifies as a virtuous trait. The theory does not provide much guidance on how to decide what actions to perform. And, virtues may be time or culture specific. For example, a virtue in the eighteenth century may not be considered a virtue today, and, a virtue in one culture may not be a virtue in a different culture.

Ethical Decision Making

An ethical dilemma arises when a path forward is blocked by controversy that emanates from a variety of sources, including religious beliefs, personal values, law, professional ethics codes, and ethical principles. It is essential that health care professionals develop their own awareness and understanding of ethics and ethical decision making, so they are prepared when they come face to face with an ethical dilemma in the workplace.

There are as many factors that influence ethical decision making as there are ethical dilemmas. There is no one universally applied method or approach for making ethical decisions. When the law or governmental or organizational policy does not provide guidance, health care professionals may look, for example, to a professional code of ethics, religious beliefs, ethical theories, or any combination of those or other resources. Ethical decision making may happen with the input of a few people or many.

There are countless models that provide steps for ethical decision making. The models are all very similar and can be distilled into eight steps, as shown in Figure 8-2. Most importantly, when facing ethical dilemmas, a methodical approach will provide credibility and consistency to the resulting decision.

Use the eight steps and each of the ethical theories discussed in the prior section to make decisions about the following case studies. Consider whether the decisions differ based upon the ethical theory used.

1. During the Ebola breakout in 2015, Sierra Leone law required people to call a specialist to dispose of the body of a person who had died from Ebola. Due to the high number of deaths in one remote region, it would take several days for a specialist to arrive. Many felt a duty to bury their deceased loved ones themselves for religious reasons. Dr. Flamant was tasked with improving upon the safety protocol for the disposition of Ebola victims once they have passed because the risk of transmission from bodily fluid exposure was quite high, even with deceased patients. While developing the protocol, he received a report of a confirmed Ebola death nearby and traveled with a specialist to study the current process. The family of the deceased would not allow her to be taken in accordance with the established safety protocol. The family's objection was rooted in their religious belief that the body cannot be buried before the family and a religious leader perform a religious cleaning. Dr. Flamant hoped that the family will change their position once he explained that the risk of transmission was very high. The explanation did not help, and the family still insists that she should not be buried without the religious ritual. How should Dr. Flamant weigh the religious meaning of honoring religious customs with his obligation to prevent the spread of Ebola?

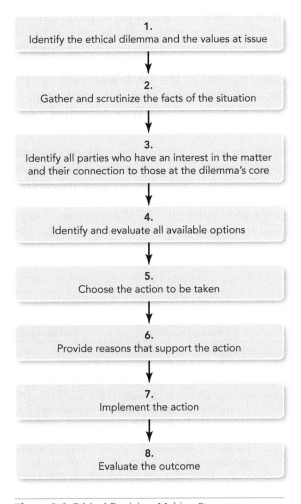

Figure 8-2 Ethical Decision–Making Steps

2. A level 4 trauma unit received a patient that was the victim of a one-car motor vehicle accident. The patient had not been wearing his seatbelt when his SUV hit a utility pole at 50 miles per hour. He was found more than 30 feet away from his crashed vehicle. He had sustained life-threatening injuries and his vital signs confirmed this. He was in respiratory distress and had signs of a head injury and a paralyzing spinal cord injury. The patient's respiratory distress and oxygen saturation levels worsened, and Dr. Armel had the trauma team prepare for intubation and ventilation. Dr. Armel explained the intubation and ventilation plan to the patient, who said, "Don't intubate me." Dr. Armel explained to the patient he is hypoxic and that he will die if the intubation is not performed right away. Given the nature and severity of the injuries, Dr. Armel concluded that the injuries left the patient without decision-making capacity. The patient is intubated, survives, and after much physical therapy returns to his pre-accident condition. Did Dr. Armel make the ethically correct decision? Does your decision change if the patient died of his injuries 3 minutes after being intubated? What if he died 3 hours after being intubated? 3 weeks? 3 months?

See Table 8-3 below for an ethical decision-making case study using each of the three ethical theories discussed earlier in this chapter.

While the application of duty-based, utilitarian, and virtue-based ethical theories to the Table 8-3 case study all resulted in the same action, this will not be true for all ethical dilemmas. Can you expound on each of the ethical theories' reasons that supported the action to disclose

Table 8-3 Ethical Decision-Making Case Study Using Duty-Based, Utilitarian, and Virtue-Based Ethical Theories

	Deontological	Teleological	
Ethical decision-making step	**Duty-based**	**Utilitarianism**	**Virtue-based**
1. Identify the ethical dilemma	Should Nurse Suzanne Angelos tell other health care team members about patient Larry Lee's suicidal intentions without his permission?		
2. Gather and scrutinize the facts	Mr. Lee is a 77-year-old man with aggressive prostate cancer who was told by his oncology health care team that he had 8–12 weeks to live and that any further medical intervention would not be appropriate or fruitful. They recommended only palliative care. Upon receiving this news, Mr. Lee reported to the health care team that he had accepted the fact that he was going to die. Then, Mr. Lee privately told Nurse Suzanne Angelos, who is part of his oncological health care team, that he plans to die by suicide rather than endure the pain of dying with cancer. Mr. Lee adamantly tells Nurse Angelos not to tell anyone else about his plans to die by suicide. Assisted suicide is illegal in the state where the hospital is located.		
3. Identify all stakeholders and their connection to those at the dilemma's core	**Larry Lee**—patient in the oncology department of his local hospital **Mr. Lee's family members**—his wife Emmy, four daughters (Deandra, Wella, Jillian, and Erica), and his sister Mozelle **Nurse Suzanne Angelos**—health care team member with whom Mr. Lee shared his suicidal intentions **Mr. Lee's health care team members**—those at the hospital that are responsible for his treatment and care, including all providers and health care professionals **Hospital's ethicist**—hospital employee paid to provide counsel on ethical dilemmas **Hospital's legal/risk department**—hospital department charged with managing the hospital's legal risks		
4. Identify and evaluate all available options	**Option #1 - Do not disclose the secret.** If Nurse Angelos chooses to keep Mr. Lee's secret, this action will respect the patient's autonomy and confidentiality, but Mr. Lee may then act on his suicidal plans. **Option #2 - Disclose the secret.** If Nurse Angelos chooses not to keep Mr. Lee's secret, this action may result in a violation of the patient's autonomy and confidentiality.		
5. Choose the action to be taken	Nurse Angelos should share Mr. Lee's suicidal intentions with his health care team.		

Table 8-3 (*Continued*)

Ethical decision-making step	Deontological — Duty-based	Teleological — Utilitarianism	Teleological — Virtue-based
6. Provide reasons that support the action	**Duty-based:** Nurses' duty to do no harm, to comply with laws that prohibit assisted suicide, and to prevent a suicidal patient's self-harm supports disclosing Mr. Lee's suicidal intentions to other members of his health care team.	**Utilitarianism:** The best outcome for the greatest number of people supports disclosing Mr. Lee's suicidal intentions because it will extend his life and ensure his safety, which benefits Mr. Lee's family, his health care team, the hospital's risk management team, and, arguably, Mr. Lee. Not disclosing Mr. Lee's intentions would likely result in self harm, which would only benefit Mr. Lee.	**Virtue-based:** The virtues of compassion, integrity, courage, wisdom, and justice support disclosing Mr. Lee's suicidal intentions to other members of his health care team.
7. Implement the action	Alert patient's health care team and initiate hospital's self-harm and suicide protocol, which includes stabilizing Mr. Lee's mental status to prevent self harm, addressing issues of pain and family support, and conducting a psychological evaluation.		
8. Evaluate the outcome	The hospital's self-harm and suicide protocol successfully resolved Mr. Lee's suicidal intentions, and he was transferred to a hospice for palliative care. After 3 months in hospice, he passed away peacefully with his family by his side.		

Mr. Lee's suicidal intentions to other members of the health care team? Are there additional reasons that support disclosure? For each of the ethical theories, what are the arguments against disclosure? Can you craft a defensible argument to not disclose Mr. Lee's suicidal intentions?

Personal Ethics in the Workplace

Personal ethics are a person's value or belief system. It is what guides the decisions they make in their life both personally and professionally. Personal ethics inevitably influence a person's path in life, including personal and professional objectives. Personal ethics can only be chosen by the individual. While each person's ethics will vary, there are common moral principles that run through most people's personal ethics including loyalty, integrity, responsibility, honesty, and respect.

Professional ethics are the standards that professionals must follow in all aspects of their professional lives. Professional ethics are established by your profession, your employer, and accrediting entities. Employees may not choose whether to comply with their employers' or their professions' professional ethics. Compliance is mandatory. Noncompliance may damage professional reputations, jeopardize professional licenses, or cause professionals to be terminated.

There are a few key differences between personal and professional ethics. The principal difference is that personal ethics pertains to a person's values in all aspects of their personal lives, while professional ethics pertains to a person's values within the workplace. For example, a health care professional's personal ethics may not support the medical treatment chosen by a patient. However, the American Medical Association's Principles of Medical Ethics, Figure 8-1, requires "compassion and respect for human dignity and rights." This includes a patient's right to choose whatever available treatment they believe is best for them.

Incorporating personal ethics into a professional setting has its benefits and, if not properly managed, its detriments. Consider the consequences of a provider declining to administer medication that has been tested on animals because of their personal ethics. Is it ethical to allow personal ethics to dictate patient care? Is your answer different depending on which ethical theory you use? How would you feel if, as a patient, your provider's treatment was heavily influenced by their personal ethics? Would it ruin the provider's credibility or trustworthiness? What personal ethics do you possess that if brought into the workplace would cause a conflict? How will you, as a professional, compartmentalize those personal ethics in the workplace?

Health care professionals should take the time to identify and evaluate their own personal ethics, identify any that may be problematic in the workplace, and address how to manage them in advance of any potential controversy. It is important that health care professionals are aware of their role during intense, pressure-filled, decision-making moments. Notably, your workplace is an inappropriate arena for moral debates or the airing of personal moral preferences.

The next four chapters address the ethical issues of confidentiality, allocation of resources, and autonomy versus paternalism under the following headings:

Chapter 9—Laws and Ethics of Patient Confidentiality

Chapter 10—Professional Ethics and the Living

Chapter 11—Reproductive Issues and Early Life

Chapter 12—Death and Dying

As each of these sections is addressed, additional ethical issues emerge. After identifying the issues, the question becomes, "Who is the ultimate decision maker?" Is this a problem for the provider, other health care providers, a lawyer, the courts, the patient (or their family), medical ethicists, or medical office personnel? Indeed, the ultimate decision maker may not be just one person. There are many different types of groups that have ethical decision-making responsibility, including an ethics committee, a hospital's risk department, or a panel composed of different disciplines.

Identifying the ultimate decision maker may shift the ethical perspective. In seeking resolutions to ethical dilemmas in health care, many individuals may have something to say about what is happening: the patient's family members, religious groups, the media, and political interest groups, among others. At some point, the ultimate decision maker must be identified and take the lead.

As you read the remaining four chapters, consider the morals, values, and ethics involved in the various issues presented and how the duty-based, utilitarian, and value-based theories might each resolve them.

☑ SUMMARY

- A violation of the law, negligent act, or a breach of contract, for example, may result in prison, fines, or monetary damages, among others. A code of ethics violation in health care may result in license suspension or revocation, or other negative repercussions from your employer, colleagues, patients, family, or friends. Morals are a collection of principles about what is right, and they are the foundation for ethics. Professional etiquette is the recognized set of rules that defines well-mannered and acceptable social behavior at work.

- Ethical dilemmas are found in every aspect of health care delivery. Ethics are collections of established moral principles of right and wrong that provide guidance when there is no applicable law, regulation, or other mandated protocol.

- Professional associations have their own code of ethics that include standards of conduct, or tenets, that address ethical and moral behavior for that profession's specialty.

- Morals are a collection of principles about what is right. We typically develop our personal morals through everyday interactions with those that influence us. Values are principles people adopt for their own personal benefit or development. People adopt some values because they appear as self-evident truths. Most values, however, develop as we mature from infancy. There are many theories as to how human values develop, most of which are tied to age or life stage.

- Western ethical theories can be categorized into two groups: deontological and teleological. Deontological means the study or science of duty. Deontological ethics identifies the morally right action without consideration of the resulting outcomes or consequences. Teleological means the study or science of conduct as it relates to the ends it serves. Teleological ethics identifies the morally right action based upon the outcomes or consequences.

- There is no one universally applied method or approach for making ethical decisions. When the law or governmental or organizational policy does not provide guidance, health care professionals may look, for example, to a professional code of ethics, religious beliefs, ethical theories, or any combination of those or other resources. There are countless models that provide steps for ethical decision making. The models are all very similar and can be distilled into eight steps.

- The principal difference between personal and professional ethics is that personal ethics pertains to a person's values in all aspects of their personal lives, while professional ethics pertains to a person's values within the workplace. For example, a health care professional's personal ethics may not support the medical treatment chosen by a patient.

- Professional ethics are established by your profession, your employer, and accrediting entities. Noncompliance may damage professional reputations, jeopardize professional licenses, or cause professionals to be terminated.

- Health care professionals should take the time to identify and evaluate their own personal ethics, identify any that may be problematic in the workplace, and address how to manage them in advance of any potential controversy.

SUGGESTED ACTIVITIES

1. There are many categories of ethics, and they can sometimes overlap or come into conflict with each other. Provide an example of a personal ethic that would conflict with professional ethics in health care? What about vice versa? How would you separate your personal ethics from your performance at work?

2. Research an ethical code that applies to your specific area of practice or your specific role and identify the purpose behind each of the code's tenets. Why is it important that we have and respect professional ethical codes?

3. Separating your personal and professional ethics requires that you first identify your personal ethics. Create a list of your top 10 personal priorities and tie each to a specific personal ethic.

   Identify something that happened in your life that required you to make an ethical decision and use each of the ethical theories and the eight decision-making steps to role play making that decision.

4. Find examples of ethics, law, morals, and etiquette in the news. Does their use in news stories further help you to distinguish between them?

STUDY QUESTIONS

1. List three professional ethical dilemmas that you might face at work and identify your personal ethics that may conflict or align with each ethical dilemma. For each of the three professional ethical dilemmas, describe how would you separate your personal ethics from the professional ethical dilemma?

2. Why are ethical codes important in practicing medicine?

3. Why is it important to study ethics as a health care professional?

4. How do duty-based, utilitarianism, and virtue-based ethical theories differ? How are they the same?

5. Compare how morals and values are developed.

CASES FOR DISCUSSION

1. The plaintiff was injured when a tree fell on him. At the hospital, he refused to consent to blood transfusions because of religious beliefs. The plaintiff's wife agreed that he should not be transfused. The hospital petitioned the court for the appointment of a guardian for the plaintiff. The court decided that the plaintiff understood the consequences of refusing the transfusion and that the plaintiff's wife and children would be taken care of and refused to grant the petition. Should he have the right to refuse treatment? Why or why not? Provide an example of acceptable response this ethical issue.

2. An orthopedist licensed to practice medicine in Maine was a member of the Maine Medical Association (MMA) and the American Medical Association (AMA). The MMA's ethics and discipline committee issued charges related to him submitting invoices to the Maine Department of Health and Welfare that showed gross overutilization, malpractice, and unethical practice. The orthopedist can prove that he did nothing illegal, but he cannot prove that he did not violate one or more tenets of the MMA's code of ethics. Should providers lose their licenses for not complying with a professional ethical code? Explain your position.

3. A pharmacy technician held religious beliefs that contraception and abortion are immoral. She did not discuss these personal ethical conflicts with her employer during the interview process or before she started working. After only 2 days on the job, a customer arrived to pick up prescriptions for both the morning after pill and a contraceptive. The prescription was not ready, and the pharmacist asked that the technician complete it. The technician refused to comply with the pharmacist's request without explaining why and was subsequently

terminated. How would you have handled this situation differently? Is there a way in this situation to maintain your personal ethics while also complying with professional ethics?

4. The patient is a 91-year-old man who had been in a long-term care facility for eight months. Before he was admitted, he was living alone and had experienced serious osteoarthritic and osteoporotic pain for a few years. His adult son and daughter arranged for his admission to a long-term care facility because they believed he could not manage his needed medications, and that he was not eating or caring for himself properly. At the time of admission, there was no evidence to suggest the patient had any cognitive deficits. The patient's adult children shared with the facility that he became a constant complainer just a few years ago. The facility staff has branded him a complainer, and they attribute much of his complaints to his disagreeable nature. He currently receives two acetaminophen tablets every 4 hours, which he states does not adequately control his pain. He reports his pain is still too extreme to walk or to remain in a wheelchair for more than a half hour. As a result, he remains in bed a majority of the day and frequently requests help to reposition himself. The patient's daughter registered a complaint with the state regulatory agency that the facility staff is neglecting her father and not taking care of his pain. The patient's son asked the doctor to administer Nalfon, a nonsteroidal anti-inflammatory drug that he read about on the Internet. The doctor agrees to try it. The son also requested that the doctor not administer the same drug that his father received 8 months ago (at the time of admission) that relieved his pain but caused him to be physically and mentally sluggish. The patient, however, has requested that drug because it relieved his pain. After just a few weeks on Nalfon, the patient has dark, tarry stools, began vomiting blood, and he is hospitalized for a severe gastric bleed. Using each a utilitarian, duty-based, and virtue-based ethical theory, perform an ethical decision-making analysis as to whether the doctor's decision to comply with the request of the patient's son to administer Nalfon was ethical.

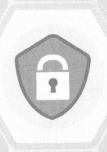

Chapter 9

Laws and Ethics of Patient Confidentiality

> " A secret spoken finds wings. "
>
> Robert Jordan, *The Path of Daggers*

Objectives

After reading this chapter, you should be able to:

1. Distinguish between privacy, confidentiality, and privileged communication.
2. Summarize the Health Insurance Portability and Accountability Act of 1996 (HIPAA).
3. Evaluate health care interactions to determine if they violate HIPAA.
4. Summarize consequences for violating HIPAA.
5. Perform HIPAA compliance reporting.
6. Identify challenges to maintaining patient confidentiality.
7. Identify methods of maintaining confidentiality in medical facilities.
8. Identify situations in which disclosure of health information is legal and necessary.

Building Your Legal Vocabulary

Confidentiality
Patient–provider privilege
Privacy

Privileged communication
Protected health information
Waives

Patient Confidentiality, Privacy, and Privileged Communication

confidentiality Not disclosing information to those who are not authorized to receive it.

privacy Being protected from public scrutiny or having your personal information shared without your permission.

privileged communication A communication (written or verbal) that occurs between two or more people that is protected by law from disclosure in court (see also patient–provider privilege).

protected health information Information held by a covered entity (see Table 9-1 for a definition) related to a patient's health status, their health care, or payment for health care.

Matters tied to patient **confidentiality**, **privacy**, and **privileged communications** can raise both legal and ethical issues. The public's desire to know about a patient's medical condition and the media's mission to provide news people are interested in may conflict with a patient's desire to keep the information private. The Health Insurance Portability and Accountability Act of 1996 (HIPAA) provides the federal privacy protection threshold for **protected health information** (PHI), including who can access it and for what reasons.

Privacy

The U.S. Supreme Court has recognized that various zones of privacy are constitutionally protected. The landmark case of *Griswold v. Connecticut,* 381 U.S. 479 (1965), found a state statute that prohibited the dispensing of contraceptives to a married couple violated a constitutional right of privacy. In *Roe v. Wade*, 410 U.S. 113 (1973), the U.S. Supreme Court held that the patient–provider relationship is protected by constitutional rights of privacy. In health care, this right of privacy (also referred to as the "right to be left alone") has been further interpreted to permit for refusal of medical treatment or the release of one's medical information, among others. While privacy is a right that emanates from the U.S. Constitution and common law, confidentiality is grounded in an ethical duty.

Confidentiality

patient–provider privilege Legal doctrine that protects communications between a patient and a provider from disclosure in court.

The expectation of confidentiality between patient and provider was first documented in 1134 B.C., when Greek physicians recorded case histories on columns in their temples. These primitive recordings included patient names, medical histories, and treatments. Patient confidentiality was protected by restricting temple access to authorized persons. During the Middle Ages, medical information was public, and during the nineteenth century, medical information was secret. A patient's expectation of privacy and the legal doctrine of **patient–provider privilege** have evolved from Hippocrates' (Greek physician, 460 to 370 B.C.) fundamental concept:

> Whatsoever in my practice or not in my practice, I shall see or hear amid the lives of men, which ought not be noised abroad, as to this I will keep silence holding such things unfit to be spoken.
>
> *Hippocrates*

Maintaining confidentiality is a high-priority concern for everyone who has contact with patients and their PHI. The confidentiality of the patient–provider relationship extends to all who have access to patient information. Health care professionals and staff are held to the same standards of confidentiality as providers.

In 1991, Kirk B. Johnson, the American Medical Association general counsel said, "Confidentiality used to be a sacred principle in medicine, but it just isn't as sacred as it used to be ... It is one of the things that got lost in the race to review everything in medicine and get it all computerized." HIPAA revived the sacredness of patient confidentiality. You'll read more about HIPAA later in this chapter.

Privileged Communication

Confidentiality also exists with privileged communications, also referred to as a privilege. Information that has been shared between people who have a special legal relationship is protected by law from disclosure in a legal proceeding. The special legal relationship can be between a husband and a wife; a provider and a patient; an attorney and a client; or religious leaders and those who practice that religion, among others. The privilege is intended to encourage open and honest discussions within those relationships and avoid any concern that others will be able to learn about the content of the discussions.

In a typical patient–provider privilege, a provider cannot reveal confidential patient information in a legal proceeding unless the patient **waives** his or her privilege against disclosure. The patient–provider privilege belongs to the patient, not the provider. So, a provider may not waive the privilege. When a patient files a medical malpractice lawsuit, for example, the nature of the case requires that medical records be available, and the patient–provider privilege is implicitly waived.

waives The act of giving up a claim, privilege, or right.

Health Insurance Portability and Accountability Act of 1996 (HIPAA)

Before the enactment of HIPAA in 1996 and the start of its enforcement in 2003, there was no federal law that governed an individual's health care information. HIPAA provides evolving and complex standards regarding PHI privacy and confidentiality, security of electronic PHI (ePHI), as well as notice of breach and enforcement rules. PHI is "any information held by a covered entity, which concerns health status, the provision of healthcare, or payment for healthcare that can be linked to an individual," and PHI includes all forms of health information, including electronic, written, or verbal. HIPAA has three self-declared major objectives:

1. To protect and enhance the rights of consumers by providing them access to their health information and controlling the inappropriate use of that information;
2. to improve the quality of health care in the U.S. by restoring trust in the health care system among consumers, healthcare professionals, and the multitude of organizations and individuals committed to the delivery of care; and,
3. to improve the efficiency and effectiveness of health care delivery by creating a national framework for health privacy protection that builds on efforts by states, health systems and individual organizations and individuals.

Public Law 104–191

Before HIPAA's enactment, patient information confidentiality was subject to state law, which varied from state to state and was not comprehensive. States may still enact laws regarding patient information, but the laws must be at least as strict as those set forth in HIPAA.

HIPAA's objectives underscore the need for patient confidentiality, as was clearly stated by the U.S. Department of Health and Human Services (HHS):

In short, the entire health care system is built upon the willingness of individuals to share the most intimate details of their lives with their health care providers. The need for privacy of health information, in particular, has long been recognized as critical to the delivery of needed medical care. More than anything else, the relationship between a patient and a clinician is based on trust. The clinician must trust the patient to give full and truthful information about their health, symptoms, and medical history. The patient must trust the clinician to use that information to improve his or her health and to respect the need to keep such information private . . . Individuals cannot be expected to share the most intimate details of their lives unless they have confidence that such information will not be used or shared inappropriately.

Federal Register. (2000, December 28). 65(250), p. 82465. Retrieved from www.gpo.gov/fdsys/pkg/FR-2000-12-28/pdf/00-32678.pdf.

Privacy Rule

HIPAA's Privacy Rule, enacted in 2002, ensures that PHI is protected while also permitting sharing of health information to foster improved health care. Specifically, the Privacy Rule (also referred to as the "Standards for Privacy of Individually Identifiable Health Information") regulates who can have access to PHI, under what circumstances, and to whom the PHI may be disclosed.

According to the HHS, PHI is individually identifiable health information, including demographic information, which relates to:

- the individual's past, present, or future physical or mental health or condition,
- the provision of health care to the individual, or
- the past, present, or future payment for the provision of health care to the individual, and that identifies the individual or for which there is a reasonable basis to believe can be used to identify the individual. Protected health information includes many common identifiers when they can be associated with the health information listed above.

PHI comes in many forms. According to HHS, protected health information includes:

- Information a provider, nurse, or other health care professional put in a medical record
- Conversations a provider has with nurses and other professionals or staff about a patient's care or treatment
- Information about a patient in a health insurer's computer system
- Billing information about a patient at a clinic
- Most other health information about a patient held by those who must follow these laws

The obligations set forth in HIPAA apply only to Covered Entities (CE) and their Business Associates (BA). Table 9-1 defines HIPAA's covered entities. Notably, if a covered entity hires a business associate in furtherance of its health care business, there must be a written contract between the two that, at a minimum, (1) specifies what the business associate is being hired to do and (2) flows down HIPAA's Privacy, Security and Breach Notification Rules to the business associate.

The HHS has an online tool to help identify whether an entity is a HIPAA Covered Entity, and it can be found at www.cms.gov /Regulations-and-Guidance/Administrative-Simplification/HIPAA-ACA /Downloads/CoveredEntitiesChart20160617.pdf.

Table 9-1 Covered Entities Under HIPAA

Health Care Provider	A Health Plan	A Health Care Clearinghouse
This includes providers such as: • Doctors • Clinics • Psychologists • Dentists • Chiropractors • Nursing Homes • Pharmacies ...but only if they transmit any information in an electronic form in connection with a transaction for which HHS has adopted a standard.	This includes: • Health insurance companies • HMOs • Company health plans • Government programs that pay for health care, such as Medicare, Medicaid, and the military and veteran health care programs	This includes entities that process nonstandard* health information they receive from another entity into a standard (i.e., standard electronic format or data content), or vice versa.

*HIPAA requires that covered entities transmit and receive PHI in specific electronic data formats (standard formats). Health Care Clearinghouses translate PHI in "nonstandard" formats to the HIPAA-mandated standard formats.

Source: HHS.gov. (ND). "Covered Entities and Business Associates". U.S. Department of Health and Human Services. Retrieved from www.hhs.gov/hipaa/for-professionals/covered-entities/index.html.

The Security Rule

HIPAA's Security Rule protects PHI that is stored or disclosed electronically. According to the HHS, HIPAA's Security Rule, "...establishes national standards to protect individuals' electronic personal health information that is created, received, used, or maintained by a covered entity. The Security Rule requires appropriate administrative, physical and technical safeguards to ensure the confidentiality, integrity, and security of electronic protected health information." In addition, covered entities that store ePHI are required to have a risk analysis in place to monitor security threats.

The Security Rule expands upon the Privacy Rule's protections and addresses safeguards that CEs must undertake to secure ePHI. Covered entities are required to establish administrative, physical and technical safeguards, to review their security risks to ensure compliance with the Security Rule, and to record all security compliance measures undertaken.

HIPAA's administrative safeguards are defined as "[a]dministrative actions, and policies and procedures, to manage the selection, development, implementation, and maintenance of security measures to protect electronic protected health information and to manage the conduct of the covered entity's workforce in relation to the protection of that information." Administrative safeguards include employee training and protocol, regardless of whether they have direct access to PHI. Physical safeguards include a covered entities physical structure, as well as its electronic equipment and systems. Technical safeguards include the covered entities technology and their policies for its use. See Table 9-2 for examples of administrative, physical, and technical safeguards.

HIPAA's Security Rule also requires that covered entities perform risk assessments, which include the identification of potential areas that may result in the disclosure of ePHI in violation of HIPAA's Rules. The office

Table 9-2 Examples of Administrative, Physical, and Technical Safeguards

Safeguard	Administrative	Physical	Technical
Examples	• Business Associate Agreement • HIPAA training program • Notice of Privacy Practices • Risk management, audit, and analysis • Sanction policy for violations • Review of electronic heath record systems	• Facility access controls • Locked file cabinets • Security of electronic health record systems (software and hardware) • Security officers • Video monitoring • Records of maintenance to physical safeguards	• Electronic health record system unique user identification with security levels based upon user need • Electronic health record system user tracking • Automatic log-off • Encryption and decryption • Emergency access • Antivirus software • Firewalls

of the National Coordinator for Health Information Technology has an online Security Risk Assessment Tool that can be found at www.healthit .gov/topic/privacy-security-and-hipaa/security-risk-assessment-tool.

The Security Rule recognizes that not all covered entities operate the same way, are the same size, or have the same risks. As a result, risk assessments are expected to be adapted to the respective covered entities specific environment and context, which may include factors such as covered entities size, its technical infrastructure (hardware and software), likelihood of potential risks to ePHI, and in some cases, its cost of security.

HIPAA Compliance

HIPAA compliance touches many areas of health care. You may have seen signs in hospitals and provider offices reminding staff members to keep patient conversations confidential. It is now routine procedure for a patient to receive a Notice of Privacy Practices (NPP) once a year while checking in for an appointment. Some provider offices and urgent care facilities use pagers similar to those used in restaurants to avoid mentioning a patient's name when notifying them of their turn to be seen by a provider. Often, for reasons of confidentiality, providers just use a patient's first name when others are within earshot. Files and filing systems have been modified; and electronic systems that manage ePHI with high levels of cybersecurity are omnipresent.

> HIPAA's Privacy Rule requires that health plans and health care providers that qualify as HIPAA covered entities distribute a notice to patients that provides a clear, user friendly explanation of patient rights related to PHI as well as their privacy practices. To help health plans and health care providers that qualify as HIPAA covered entities meet HIPAA's NPP requirement, HHS offers model (NPP) for covered entities, which can be found at www.hhs.gov /hipaa/for-professionals/privacy/guidance/model-notices-privacy-practices.

HIPAA is the basis for providers' adoption of strict policies related to discussing a patient's health care with other professionals, the amount and type of information to be disclosed, and to whom. HIPAA, and similar state statutes, requires written contracts with business associates (e.g., legal, actuarial, accounting, management, administration, accreditation, financial services) before protected information can be shared with them. HIPAA training—for employees and those who do business with the provider—is now commonplace.

The Enforcement Rule

The Enforcement Rule authorizes HHS to investigate complaints that covered entities have violated the Privacy Rule and to fine covered entities for avoidable breaches of ePHI due to lack of compliance with the Security Rule. HHS' Office for Civil Rights (OCR) is also authorized to request that the Department of Justice bring criminal charges when circumstances warrant. Patients who have faced "serious harm" as a result of their PHI being disclosed without authorization, may sue the disclosing covered entity.

Breach Notification Rule

HIPAA's Breach Notification Rule requires that covered entities and their business associates provide notice after a breach of unsecured protected health information. Unsecured protected health information is PHI that has not been protected from disclosure to unauthorized persons. The notice must be sent to the affected individuals and the HHS' Secretary. Where a breach affects more than 500 residents of a State, covered entities are also required to provide notice to the media. And, the rule requires that business associates notify the hiring covered entities if a breach occurs. There are three important exceptions to the Breach Notification Rule:

1. unintentional acquisition, access, or use of protected health information by a workforce member or person acting under the authority of a covered entity or business associate, if such acquisition, access, or use was made in good faith and within the scope of authority.
2. inadvertent disclosure of protected health information by a person authorized to access protected health information at a covered entity or business associate to another person authorized to access protected health information at the covered entity or business associate, or organized

health care arrangement in which the covered entity participates. In both cases, the information cannot be further used or disclosed in a manner not permitted by the Privacy Rule.

3. covered entity or business associate has a good faith belief that the unauthorized person to whom the impermissible disclosure was made, would not have been able to retain the information.

HHS.gov. (nd). Breach Notification Rule. U.S. Department of Health & Human Services. Retrieved from www.hhs.gov/hipaa /for-professionals/breach-notification/index.html.

HIPAA Violations and Penalties

Not being aware of HIPAA Rules is not a valid reason for a covered entity failing to comply. Covered entities are required to ensure that its providers, health care professionals, and staff understand and follow HIPAA's Rules.

A HIPAA violation occurs when a covered entity or a business associate does not comply with one or more of the Privacy, Security, or Breach Notification Rules. There are many ways to violate HIPAA, and a violation may be intentional or accidental. An accidental HIPAA violation can occur, for example, when too much (i.e., more than the minimum necessary requirement) PHI is disclosed. An example of a deliberate violation is failing to notify the media when the breach affects more than 500 residents of a state (a Breach Notification Rule violation).

The minimum necessary requirement is one facet of HIPAA's Privacy Rule, and it captures the practice that PHI should only be used to accomplish a specific objective, and it should not be used or disclosed if it is not needed for that objective.

The Privacy Rule generally requires covered entities to take reasonable steps to limit the use or disclosure of, and requests for, protected health information to the minimum necessary to accomplish the intended purpose. The minimum necessary standard does not apply to the following:

- Disclosures to or requests by a health care provider for treatment purposes.
- Disclosures to the individual who is the subject of the information.
- Uses or disclosures made pursuant to an individual's authorization.

(Continues)

(Continued)

- Uses or disclosures required for compliance with the Health Insurance Portability and Accountability Act (HIPAA) Administrative Simplification Rules.
- Disclosures to the Department of Health and Human Services (HHS) when disclosure of information is required under the Privacy Rule for enforcement purposes.
- Uses or disclosures that are required by other law.

The implementation specifications for this provision require a covered entity to develop and implement policies and procedures appropriate for its own organization, reflecting the entity's business practices and workforce.

Department of Health and Human Services. (2003, April 4). Minimum Necessary Requirement. Department of Health and Human Services. Retrieved from www.hhs.gov/hipaa/for-professionals/privacy/guidance /minimum-necessary-requirement/index.html.

The penalties for violating HIPAA depend upon facts and seriousness of the violation. The HITECH Act (discussed in Chapters 2 and 7), which seeks to further the adoption and meaningful use of health information technology, enhanced the enforcement of criminal and civil HIPAA violations. See Table 9-3 for the structure of HIPAA's violations and penalties.

OCR issues penalties for civil violations of HIPAA Rules and considers several factors when assessing penalties, including the length of time the violation existed, the number of people affected, and the type of PHI disclosed. The amount of a financial penalty may also depend upon the

Table 9-3 HIPAA Violations and Penalty Structure

Tier	Violation Category	Violation Fines
1	A violation that the covered entity was unaware of and could not have realistically avoided, had a reasonable amount of care had been taken to abide by HIPAA Rules	Minimum fine of $100 per violation up to $50,000
2	A violation that the covered entity should have been aware of but could not have avoided even with a reasonable amount of care (but falling short of willful neglect of HIPAA Rules)	Minimum fine of $1,000 per violation up to $50,000
3	A violation suffered as a direct result of "willful neglect" of HIPAA Rules, in cases where an attempt has been made to correct the violation	Minimum fine of $10,000 per violation up to $50,000
4	A violation of HIPAA Rules constituting willful neglect, where no attempt has been made to correct the violation	Minimum fine of $50,000 per violation

Source: Adler, S. (2021, January 15). What Are the Penalties for HIPAA Violations? HIPAA Journal. Retrieved from www .hipaajournal.com/what-are-the-penalties-for-hipaa-violations-7096/.

covered entities prior history of violations, its financial condition, and the harm caused by the violation. A covered entities level of cooperation with an OCR investigation is considered as well. Table 9-4 is a sample of cases investigated and resolved in 2020 by OCR.

In 2019, the OCR began an enforcement initiative to address violations of HIPAA's Privacy Rule standard regarding right of access, which gives patients the right to access and obtain copies of their PHI within 30 days of the request.

OCR Settles Nineteenth Investigation in HIPAA Right of Access Initiative

The Office for Civil Rights (OCR) at the U.S. Department of Health and Human Services announces its nineteenth settlement of an enforcement action in its HIPAA Right of Access Initiative. OCR announced this initiative to support individuals' right to timely access their health records at a reasonable cost under HIPAA's Privacy Rule.

The Diabetes, Endocrinology & Lipidology Center, Inc. ("DELC") has agreed to take corrective actions and pay $5,000 to settle a potential violation of HIPAA Privacy Rule's right of access standard. DELC is a West Virginia based healthcare provider that provides treatment for Endocrine disorders.

In early August 2019, a complaint was filed with OCR alleging that DELC failed to take timely action in response to a parent's records access request made in July 2019, for a copy of her minor child's protected health information. OCR initiated an investigation and determined that DELC's failure to provide timely access to the requested medical records was a potential violation of the HIPAA right of access standard. As a result of OCR's investigation, DELC provided the requested records in May 2021, nearly two years after the parent's request.

"It should not take a federal investigation before a HIPAA covered entity provides a parent with access to their child's medical records," said Acting OCR Director Robinsue Frohboese. "Covered entities owe it to their patients to provide timely access to medical records."

In addition to the monetary settlement, DELC will undertake a corrective action plan that includes two (2) years of monitoring.

Department of Health and Human Services. (2021, June 2). OCR Settles Nineteenth Investigation in HIPAA Right of Access Initiative. Department of Health and Human Services. Retrieved from www.hhs.gov/about/news/2021/06/02 /ocr-settles-nineteenth-investigation-hipaa-right-access -initiative.html?language=en.

HIPAA's criminal violations include intentional theft of PHI for financial gain and unlawful disclosures with intent to cause harm. The illegal sale of PHI, especially the illegal sale of a public figure's PHI, can be

Table 9-4 Sample of Cases Investigated and Resolved in 2020 by OCR

Covered Entity	Violation	Fine
Premera Blue Cross	Failed to: • perform a comprehensive risk analysis • reduce risks to the integrity confidentiality, and availability of ePHI to a realistic and proper level • have enough hardware and software controls	$6,850,000
CHSPSC LLC	Failed to: • conduct a comprehensive risk analysis • perform information system activity evaluations • have enough access controls and security incident response policies • respond immediately to the FBI's cyberattack notification	$2,300,000
Athens Orthopedic Clinic	Failed to: • conduct a comprehensive risk analysis • implement security procedures to minimize risks to ePHI • implement proper hardware, software, and techniques for recording and examining data system activity • implement HIPAA policies up to August 2016 • have business associate agreements with three suppliers • provide timely HIPAA Privacy Rule training to its employees	$1,500,000
Lifespan Health System Affiliated Covered Entity	Failed to: • implement encryption on mobile devices • track the movement of the devices in and out of the facilities • perform an inventory of mobile devices • have a business associate agreement with Lifespan Corporation and Lifespan ACE	$1,040,000
Aetna	Failed to: • undertake regular technical and nontechnical assessments of operational adjustments impacting the security of ePHI • implement procedures to confirm the identity of people or entities with access to ePHI • limit disclosures of ePHI to the minimum required data to accomplish its purpose • have the proper administrative, physical, and technical safeguards to protect ePHI privacy	$1,000,000

lucrative, which may drive some individuals to do so. HIPAA established controls to reduce the chance for individuals to steal and sell PHI and to ensure the prompt identification of unauthorized access to and theft of PHI.

Health care providers and professionals who intentionally use or access PHI for reasons not permitted by the Privacy Rule may face criminal charges pursuant to the Administrative Simplification section of HIPAA's criminal enforcement provision.

Criminal violations of HIPAA are prosecuted by the Department of Justice (DoJ). There have been many criminal violation cases that have resulted in substantial fines and prison sentences. The DoJ criminal penalties for HIPAA violations are categorized into three tiers. The prison sentence and fine assessed for violations in any of the three tiers is decided by a judge after consideration of the facts and circumstances. The three tiers are:

- Tier 1: Reasonable cause or no knowledge of violation—Up to 1 year in jail
- Tier 2: Obtaining PHI under false pretenses—Up to 5 years in jail
- Tier 3: Obtaining PHI for personal gain or with malicious intent—Up to 10 years in jail

Stacey Lavette Hendricks, a former Florida medical clinic adminis- trative worker who accessed patients' PHI impermissibly and sold it to identity thieves was charged and pleaded guilty to wire fraud and aggravated identity theft. The United States Secret Service led the investiga- tion and arrested her after she tried to sell stolen PHI to a law enforcement officer. After the Secret Service obtained a warrant to search her home and car, they found stolen PHI related to 113 different patients.

Hendricks faced a maximum jail term of up to 20 years for the wire fraud charge and a mandatory 2-year consecutive term for aggravated identity theft. She was ultimately sentenced to serve 48 months in federal prison.

Adler, S. (2020, February). Florida Clinic Worker Facing 22 Years in Jail for Wire Fraud and Aggravated Identity Theft. *The HIPAA Journal*. Retrieved from www.hipaajournal.com/florida-clinic-worker-facing -22-years-in-jail-for-wire-fraud-and-aggravated-identity-theft 5/.

Filing a HIPAA Complaint

Anyone who has reason to believe that a covered entity or business asso- ciate violated HIPAA's Privacy, Security, or Breach Notification Rules may file a complaint with the OCR, who investigates complaints. See Figure 9-1 for the HIPAA Privacy and Security Rule Complaint Process. In 2020, the OCR received 27,182 complaints of HIPAA violations.

HHS reports that the most common HIPAA violation complaints are:

- Impermissible uses and disclosures of protected health information;
- Lack of safeguards of protected health information;

(Continues)

(Continued)

- Lack of patient access to their protected health information;
- Lack of administrative safeguards of electronic protected health information; and
- Use or disclosure of more than the minimum necessary protected health information.

According to the OCR, complaints must:

- Be submitted in writing via mail, fax, e-mail, or via the online Complaint Portal (https://ocrportal.hhs.gov/ocr/smartscreen/main.jsf)
- Name the covered entity or business associate involved
- Describe in as much detail as possible the Privacy Rule, Security Rule, or the Breach Notification Rule violation
- Any additional information that may be useful in the complaint's investigation
- Information about the person submitting the complaint
- Be filed within 180 days from the date the complainant learned of the violation

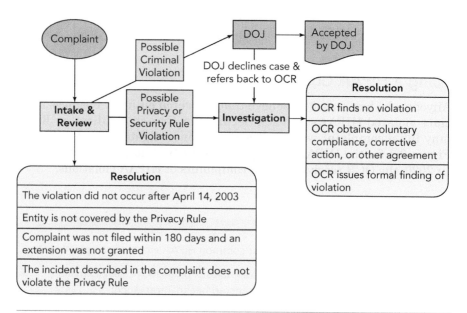

Figure 9-1 HIPAA Privacy and Security Rule Complaint Process

Source: www.hhs.gov/hipaa/for-professionals/compliance-enforcement/enforcement-process/index.html

Challenges to Maintaining Confidentiality

Chapters 2 and 7 discuss HITECH and the integration of the electronic medical record into the everyday practice of medicine. With HIPAA's and the HITECH's requirements to use EHR meaningfully also comes the responsibility of protecting PHI from improper and unauthorized disclosure.

Technology

Use of technology in health care creates an increasing number of ways that patient confidentiality can be compromised. HIPAA's high standards of confidentiality can be breached if, for example, a covered entity places PHI on the Internet without appropriate safeguards to ensure the information remains confidential. By the same token, however, the technology of electronic data storage can sometimes be foiled. One of the ongoing concerns is hackers getting into PHI.

Use of the Internet as a storage point for EHR is commonplace, which permits access to appropriate health care personnel, as well as the patient. It is essential to understand this use and how to protect patient confidentiality in this environment. Internet-based systems that permit different EHR systems to share information create many opportunities for improper disclosure of confidential patient information. Regardless of where the confidential patient information comes from, a key point to remember is that HIPAA applies.

As a part of any medical office staff, you can contribute to the security of ePHI by strictly complying with all computer security policies in your office, not allowing anyone but yourself to use your password, and not opening documents where the sender is unfamiliar, among others.

There have been several incidents where a hacker introduces malware to a health care provider's computer system. The malware allows the hacker to hold the computer system hostage, including patient records, and to demand ransom.

In the fall of 2020, computer services at all 250 of hospital chain Universal Health Services' 250 U.S. facilities experienced a malware attack and had to be shut down. Employees at the UHS hospitals had to keep records manually, experienced very slow lab work and long emergency room delays, all while also managing the overwhelming amount of COVID-19 patients. Employees indicated these conditions compromised patient care.

Bajak, F. (2020, October 1). Hacked Hospital Chain Says All 250 US Facilities Affected. *ABC News.* Retrieved from www.abcnews.go.com/Health /wireStory/hacked-hospital-chain-250-us-facilities-affected-73374804.

The High-Profile Patient

The media is always interested in gathering confidential information about public figures largely because the public is interested in hearing about it. Health care providers are required to keep the information of all patients confidential, even if the patient is the most popular Hollywood actor, the latest Internet celebrity, the highest-paid athlete, or the most disgraced politician. The high-profile patient need not have national or international fame: your local county commissioners, police chiefs, business owners, or corporate executives, among others, also have a right to confidentiality. Breaches of patient confidentiality, including high-profile patients, are very serious matters.

> Actor Jussie Smollett appeared at Northwestern's emergency department saying that two men had attacked him. Later, more than 50 hospital employees were fired for viewing Smollett's PHI. One of the figured employees, a nurse, stated that she did not intend to view Smollett's PHI. Instead, the nurse claimed she only scrolled by his name when searching for another patient and this was likely the case for many of the fired employees. However, the hospital's electronic health record audit log shows exactly who accessed the information, the time of the access and how much time was spent on a given page.
>
> "Breaches such as this are common and provide an example of how the biggest threat to security is often coming from inside an organization. 'Insider' threats, or security risks posed by people who already have access to a provider's system, are a recurring threat, according to the Office for Civil Rights."
>
> Butler, M. (2019, March 12). Hospital Employees Fired for Improperly Viewing Smollett Medical Records. *Journal of AIHMA*. Retrieved from https://journal.ahima .org/hospital-employees-fired-for-improperly-viewing-smollett-medical-records/.

Snooping in a medical record is not the only way high-profile patients might find their confidential information improperly disclosed. A HIPAA Privacy Rule violation occurs when a member of the health care provider's staff improperly discloses the simple fact that a high-profile client is a patient.

HIPAA-Authorized PHI Uses and Disclosures

Tarasoff v. Regents of University of California is a pre-HIPAA landmark case involving conflict between the disclosure of information to a third party and patient–provider confidentiality.

Poddar was undergoing treatment as a voluntary outpatient. He had become obsessed with Tatiana Tarasoff, a student he had met at a dance. He had tape-recorded conversations with her and spent hours replaying the tapes in order to determine her feelings for him. A friend became concerned and suggested that he seek professional help.

Poddar was seen by a psychiatrist, who did not believe that Poddar required hospitalization, but did prescribe medication and arranged weekly outpatient psychotherapy with a staff psychologist. During therapy, Poddar revealed his fantasies of harming, and perhaps even killing, Tarasoff. The friend told the psychologist that Poddar planned to purchase a gun. Poddar stopped therapy. The physicians believed that Poddar should be evaluated for hospitalization and requested help from the campus police.

The campus police went to Poddar's apartment and questioned him about his plans but then left when he denied any intention of harming Tarasoff. Two months later Poddar stabbed Tarasoff to death. He was convicted of second-degree murder, the conviction was overturned on the basis of improper jury instruction, and Poddar returned home to India.

Later, in a civil suit, the Tarasoff family sued the university, including both therapists and the campus police, for negligence. The court held that the therapists had a duty to warn Tarasoff.

Tarasoff v. Regents of University of California, 118 Cal. Rptr. 129 (1974)

The Tarasoff case makes clear that, in some circumstances, there are interests that outweigh a patient's right to confidentiality, and HIPAA recognizes and identifies those circumstances. A covered entity is allowed to use and disclose a patient's PHI without authorization in the following circumstances:

1. Disclosure to the patient.
2. For a covered entities treatment, payment, health care operation activities.
3. Uses and disclosures that give the patient the opportunity to agree or object, which includes asking the patient or by circumstances that clearly give the individual the opportunity to agree, acquiesce, or object.
4. Incidental uses and disclosures, which occur as a result of an otherwise permitted use or disclosure provided the covered entity has adopted reasonable safeguards and it is limited to the minimum necessary pursuant to the Privacy Rule.

5. Public interest and benefit activities, which include 12 national priority purposes:
   a. Required by law.
   b. Public health activities.
   c. PHI of people who have experienced abuse, neglect, or domestic violence.
   d. Health oversight activities.
   e. Judicial and administrative proceedings.
   f. Law enforcement purposes.
   g. Decedents' PHI to identify a deceased person, determine the cause of death, and perform other functions authorized by law
   h. To facilitate organ, eye, or tissue donation from cadavers.
   i. Research, under specific conditions.
   j. Serious threat to health or safety to prevent or lessen a serious and imminent threat to a person, including to law enforcement when the PHI is needed to identify or apprehend an escaped or violent criminal.
   k. Essential government functions, including assuring proper execution of a military mission, conducting intelligence and national security activities that are authorized by law, among others.
   l. Workers' compensation claims.

6. Limited data set, which is PHI from which certain, specified direct identifiers of individuals and their relatives, household members, and employers have been removed.

For more detail on these six permissive uses, visit www.hhs.gov/hipaa/for-professionals/privacy/laws-regulations/index.html.

Permitted uses and disclosures must be identified in a covered entities Notice of Privacy Practices (NPP). Covered entities may rely on professional ethics and best judgments, as discussed later in this chapter, in evaluating the applicability of the six permissive uses and disclosures.

Patient-Authorized PHI Uses and Disclosures

Disclosure of PHI not otherwise authorized by HIPAA must be authorized in writing by the patient. HIPAA-compliant authorizations must be written in plain language and contain specific information. While HIPAA does not mandate that a specific authorization form be used, it does require that authorizations include the following:

1. description of the protected health information to be used and disclosed

2. the person authorized to make the use or disclosure

3. the person to whom the covered entity may make the disclosure

4. an expiration date

5. and (sometimes) the purpose for which the information may be used or disclosed.

An authorization provides covered entities with the needed permission to use and disclose a patient's PHI that is not for treatment, payment, or health care operations. It may authorize the use and disclosure of PHI to the covered entity seeking the authorization or to a third party. Figure 9-2 is a sample HIPAA-compliant Authorization.

AUTHORIZATION FOR RELEASE OF INFORMATION

Section A: Must be completed for all authorizations.

I hereby authorize the use or disclosure of my individually identifiable health information as described below.
I understand that this authorization is voluntary. I understand that if the organization authorized to receive the information is not a health plan or health care provider, the released information may no longer be protected by federal privacy regulations.

Identity of person/organization disclosing protected health information

Patient name: Hilda F. Goodman   **ID Number:** 4309

Persons/organizations providing information:
Practon Medical Group, Inc
4567 Broad Avenue
Woodland Hills, XY 12345-4700

Examples:
• HIV status
• Drug or alcohol use/abuse statements
• Physical or mental abuse statements
• Psychiatric notes

Persons/organizations receiving information:
Jennifer P. Lee, MD
400 North M Street
Anytown, XY 54098-1235

Identity of those authorized to use protected health information

Specific description of information [including from and to date(s)]:
Complete medical records from 4-22-XX to 9-15-XX

Specific description of information to be used or disclosed with dates

Section B: Must be completed only if a health plan or a health care provider has requested the authorization.

1. The health plan or health care provider must complete the following:
   a. What is the purpose of the use or disclosure? Patient relocating to another city

Purpose for disclosure

   b. Will the health plan or health care provider requesting the authorization receive financial or in-kind compensation in exchange for using or disclosing the health information described above? Yes___ No_X_

2. The patient or the patient's representative must read and initial the following statements:
   a. I understand that my health care and the payment for my health care will not be affected if I do not sign this form.

   Initials: _hfg_

   b. I understand that I may see and copy the information described on this form if I ask for it, and that I get a copy of this form after I sign it.

   Initials: _hfg_

Section C: Must be completed for all authorizations.

The patient or the patient's representative must read and initial the following statements:

Expiration date

1. I understand that this authorization will expire on _12_ / _31_ / _20XX_ (DD/MM/YR).
   Initials: _hfg_

Individual's right to revoke this authorization in writing

2. I understand that I may revoke this authorization at any time by notifying the providing organization in writing, but if I do not it will not have any effect on any actions they took before they received the revocation.
   Initials: _hfg_

Rediclosure conditions

3. I understand that any disclosure of information carries with it the potential for an unauthorized rediclosure and the information may not be protected by federal confidentiality rules.
   Initials: _hfg_

Individual's signature

Hilda F. Goodman   September 15, 20XX
Signature of patient or patient's representative   **Date**
(Form MUST be completed before signing)

Date of signature

Printed name of patient's representative:_____

Relationship to the patient:_____

YOU MAY REFUSE TO SIGN THIS AUTHORIZATION
You may not use this form to release information for treatment or payment except
when the information to be released is psychotherapy notes or certain research information.

Figure 9-2 Sample HIPAA-Compliant Authorization Form

Confidentiality as an Ethical Dilemma

In addition to the consequences of violating HIPAA, intentionally disclosing confidential PHI raises issues as to what is ethically right or wrong given the circumstances. For example, is it right or wrong to keep a patient's contagious disease diagnosis confidential, if the patient has stated they will not take precautions from infecting others? Does it matter if the disease is lethal or not lethal? Does it matter if the patient has expressed a desire to infect others? HIPAA and its state law equivalents provide detailed guidance as to the disclosure of PHI, and failure to adhere to these laws can result in significant consequences for the violator. There are many situations in which protecting or releasing protected health information can cause ethical questions or dilemmas, but you must comply with the law and your profession's code of ethics. In all instances, it is wise to keep in mind the separation of personal and professional ethics. An ethical decision-making process that can be used for issues of patient confidentiality and privacy can be found in Chapter 8, Table 8-3. The fourth step in the ethical decision-making process is to "Identify and evaluate all available options." When working with PHI, the choices you make must be aligned with the law, your employer, and society, or you risk being sued or losing your job.

☑ SUMMARY

- Privacy is the "right to be left alone" and to be protected from having personal information shared without permission, while confidentiality is the duty to not disclose information to those not authorized to receive it. Privacy emanates from the U.S. Constitution and common law, whereas confidentiality is grounded in an ethical duty. Privileged communication is information that has been shared between people who have a special legal relationship and is protected by law from disclosure in a legal proceeding.

- HIPAA provides evolving and complex standards regarding PHI privacy and confidentiality, security of electronic PHI (ePHI), as well as notice of breach and enforcement rules.

- HIPAA is the basis for providers' adoption of strict policies related to discussing a patient's health care with other professionals, the amount and type of information to be disclosed, and to whom.

- The penalties for violating HIPAA depend upon facts and seriousness of the violation. The HITECH Act enhanced the enforcement of criminal and civil HIPAA violations.

- Anyone who has reason to believe HIPAA violation may file a complaint with the U.S. Department of Health & Human Services' Office for Civil Rights, who investigates complaints.

- Health care providers are required to keep the information of all patients confidential, even if the patient is the most popular Hollywood actor, the latest Internet celebrity, the highest-paid athlete, or the most disgraced politician.

- As a part of any medical office staff, you can contribute to the security of ePHI by strictly complying with all computer security policies in your office, not allowing anyone but yourself to use your password, and not opening documents where the sender is unfamiliar, among others.

- A HIPAA covered entity is allowed to use and disclose a patient's PHI without authorization in the following circumstances: (1) disclosure to the patient; (2) for treatment, payment, and health care operations; (3) to provide an opportunity to agree or object; (4) use or disclosure incident to an otherwise permitted use and disclosure; (5) for public interest and benefit activities; and (6) limited data set for the purposes of research, public health or health care operations.

- Disclosure of PHI not otherwise authorized by HIPAA must be authorized in writing by the patient. HIPAA-compliant authorizations must be written in plain language and contain specific information.

- For those who believe that it is ethical to follow the rules at any cost, laws about confidentiality solve the ethical dilemma. For individuals who are motivated by other values or ethical thought systems, laws only add conflict to the ethical dilemma. In all instances, it is wise to keep in mind the separation of personal and professional ethics.

SUGGESTED ACTIVITIES

1. Research methods of maintaining the confidentiality of medical records at a local emergency room or hospital.
2. Find out and document the procedure and charges to obtain a copy of your own medical record from a health care provider.
3. Find three HIPAA compliant Notice of Privacy Practices online. How are they the same? How do they differ?

STUDY QUESTIONS

1. Privacy means many different things in a medical setting. Distinguish between the patient's right to privacy and privacy of privileged communication.

2. Explain HIPAA's three main objectives.

3. Explain how a HIPAA covered entity might identify violation that occurred on its electronic health records system.

4. Identify those who are eligible to file a HIPAA complaint.

CASES FOR DISCUSSION

1. A private practice provider denied a patient access to her medical records because she had an outstanding balance for services the provider had provided. Is this permissible under HIPAA? Why or why not?

2. A patient, who was also an employee of the hospital, alleged that her PHI was impermissibly disclosed to her supervisor. The hospital had distributed an Operating Room (OR) schedule to employees via email; the hospital's OR schedule contained information about the complainant's upcoming surgery. While the Privacy Rule may permit the disclosure of an OR schedule containing PHI, in this case, a hospital employee shared the OR schedule with the patient's supervisor, who was not part of the employee's treatment team, and did not need the information for payment, health care operations, or other permissible purposes. Was there a HIPAA violation? Does it matter that the supervisor was not a member of the patient's treatment team since they worked for the same hospital?

3. An HMO sent a patient's entire medical record to a disability insurance company without proper authorization. The authorization form used by the HMO did not comply with HIPAA's requirements. Is an authorization needed in this instance? If you were the investigating officer, what other recommendations might you suggest?

4. As part of the negotiation for a settlement for injuries sustained as the result of a car accident, the defendant's insurance company requested that the plaintiff undergo an independent medical examination (IME) with a specified health care provider. After the examination and at the insurance company's direction, the health care provider who performed the exam denied the plaintiff's request for a copy of the medical record related to the IME. Is the plaintiff entitled to the records given that it was the insurance company who ordered and paid for the IME?

5. A hospital employee called a patient's home number and left a telephone message with the daughter of a patient that detailed both her medical condition and treatment plan. The patient had instructed the practice to leave messages on her work phone only. Was it appropriate to leave the message on the patient's home phone? What requirement is implicated by the message left with the daughter?

6. After treating a patient injured in a rather unusual sporting accident, the hospital released to the local media, copies of the patient's skull x-ray as well as a description of the complainant's medical condition. The local newspaper then featured on its front page the individual's x-ray and an article that included the date of the accident, the location of the accident, the patient's gender, a description of patient's medical condition, and numerous quotes from the hospital about such unusual sporting accidents. The hospital asserted that the disclosures were made to avert a serious threat to health or safety. Was this a permissible disclosure?

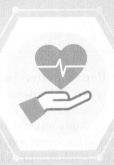

Chapter 10

Professional Ethics and the Living

 In civilized life, law floats in a sea of ethics.

Earl Warren, Chief Justice of the U.S. Supreme Court (1953–1969)

Objectives

After reading this chapter, you should be able to:

1. Identify ethical issues faced by medical professionals in allocating scarce resources.
2. Explain ethical questions associated with medical research and experimentation.
3. Summarize the Tuskegee Study.
4. Summarize the terms of the Nuremberg Code.
5. Summarize the pros and cons of community-based research.
6. Describe what the first transplant operations were and when they occurred.
7. Identify the three categories of transplants.
8. Define the Uniform Anatomical Gift Act.
9. Identify ethical issues related to organ transplants.
10. Explain the importance of balancing autonomy and paternalism in patient care.
11. Explain the reasons for and consequences of medical tourism.
12. Explain ethical dilemmas associated with patient confidentiality.

Building Your Legal Vocabulary

Allocation
Autonomy

Herd immunity
Paternalism

Introduction

allocation The act of distributing something.

In addition to the ethical issues associated with Reproductive Issues and Early Life (Chapter 11) and Death and Dying (Chapter 12), there are many ethical issues tied to the time in between. As a health care professional, you will encounter ethical issues associated with the **allocation** of scarce resources, medical research, transplants, autonomy, paternalism, and influences upon the patient–provider relationship, among many others.

Allocation of Scarce Resources

One of the most pressing issues in health care is the allocation of resources. Scarcity of organs for transplant, limitation of funds for health care delivery systems, and decisions regarding ICU beds all fall under the allocation of resources.

When there needed to be a fair and efficient way to allocate and administer the COVID-19 vaccine, the pandemic provided a contemporary, real-world opportunity to address the allocation of scarce resources.

The National Academies of Sciences, Engineering, and Medicine (NASEM) listed "mitigation of health inequities" as an overarching ethical principle for allocation of COVID-19 vaccines in the United States, noting that in this highly interconnected world, challenges to one group affect us all. However, espousing the goal of equitable vaccine distribution is a far simpler proposition than achieving it. Despite recent improvements, vaccination rates among Black and Hispanic individuals lag behind their share of the general population.

The barriers to equitable uptake of COVID-19 vaccines are varied and deep-seated, including obstacles to accessing care and many patients' lack of vaccine confidence, rooted in decades of racism, discrimination, and reduced access to health care which has inspired mistrust of the government and medical and scientific communities. These hurdles create a formidable challenge to equitable vaccination of the US population.

Fressin, F., Wen, A., Shukla, S., Mok, K., Chaguturu, S. (2021, July 23). How We Achieved More Equitable Vaccine Distribution: Social Vulnerability Analytics Are Necessary, But Not Sufficient. *Health Affairs*. Retrieved from www.healthaffairs.org/do/10.1377/hblog20210721.568098/full/.

The vaccine allocation phase 1B sought to vaccinate health care workers and people aged 65 and older. The Federal Retail Pharmacy Program (FRPP), a partnership between the United States' Centers for Disease Control and Prevention and retail pharmacies, used algorithms—sets of rules used (often by a computer) to calculate something—to identify geographic locations to administer vaccines that best reflected the phase 1B target group. The algorithms' initial results met their stated goals, but the FRPP reported that the "algorithm had not resulted in corresponding proportional vaccination of racial and ethnic minorities, including Black, Hispanic and Indigenous populations." Subsequent modifications to the algorithms coupled with outreach programs resulted in improved, but still not flawless, allocation of the vaccine. The FRPP also identified that the results were not consistent across all locations, which suggested there may be other factors that require consideration. And, the FRPP stated that "[f]rom a numeric standpoint, achieving vaccine distribution that perfectly tracks the population in terms of age, ethnicity, and other criteria would be ideal. However, from a public health and infection control standpoint, distribution that tracks the population in terms of risk of infection, morbidity, and mortality is the preferred goal."

If everyone is provided the same information about the vaccine, including the effectiveness and side effects, as well as locations where it is administered, is it necessary to undertake additional efforts to ensure all have the same opportunity to be vaccinated? Should the vaccine have been made available earlier to those who want to pay for it?

Ethical Conflicts in the Intensive Care Unit

Where there is a shortage of beds in the intensive care unit (ICU), the ethics of health care providers are put to the test. Who gets a bed—an older person or a young person? Someone whose prognosis is limited or one who will probably have many good years if properly treated? The patient who can pay or the one who cannot? The person with five young children or the one with two children? The professor who is on the brink of a discovery that may help society or someone serving a life sentence for a violent crime?

The COVID-19 pandemic provided the opportunity to see how the health care industry responded to this ethical dilemma when, across the country, there were more patients that needed an ICU bed than there were ICU beds.

The devastating pandemic that has stricken the worldwide population induced an unprecedented influx of severe ARDS [acute respiratory distress syndrome] patients dramatically exceeding ICU bed

(Continues)

(Continued)

capacities in several areas of many countries. As a result, four new options never applied to date were considered with the common aim of saving a maximum number of lives: to prioritize ICU beds for patients with the best prognosis; to increase at all costs the number of ICU beds, thereby creating step-down ICUs; to organize transfer to distant ICUs with more beds available, or to accelerate withdrawal of life support in ICUs . . .

In such a crisis, there are ingredients liable to shake up our ethical principles, sharpen our ethical dilemmas, and lead to situations of suffering for caregivers [2]. Faced with these profound changes in patient management, intensivists were caught off guard, forced by the density of work, the lack of immediately available beds and the possibilities of transferring patients to make painfully experienced choices that were contrary to their basic ethical principles and source of immediate burden [3–5].

Robert, R. et al. (2020, June 17). Ethical Dilemmas Due to the Covid-19 Pandemic. *Ann. Intensive Care.* Retrieved from www.ncbi.nlm.nih.gov/pmc/articles/PMC7298921/.

When faced with a shortage of ICU beds, patients usually have a shorter ICU stay than when there is a surplus of beds. This may occur because the patients do not need additional care or because the bed is required for a more seriously ill patient. When hospitals keep patients in the ICU for an extended period, it may be because the hospitals seek to maintain a specific ICU occupancy rate. Alternatively, some providers may find their own workload reduced if a patient receives care in the ICU rather than on a regular medical ward. Allocation of ICU beds is one of the day-to-day ethical judgments faced by the health care industry.

The same question of allocation raised by the COVID-19 pandemic exists in the context of everyday health care. Should everyone who needs expensive life-saving procedures, such as open-heart surgery or organ transplants, have an equal chance to receive them regardless of ability to pay, socioeconomical status, or other nonmedical factors? Is health care for everyone possible? Who will pay? If health care for everyone is not possible, who will receive life-saving services? Managed care is a response to the need to allocate limited health care resources.

Ethical Conflicts Created by Managed Care

Chapter 1 discusses the business of health care and introduces many facets of managed care, and its various models. Today, a majority of the population with insurance is enrolled in some form of managed care, but in less restrictive models such as a preferred provider organization (PPO). This form of insurance is less effective than a health maintenance organization (HMO) in controlling costs; however, it permits the patient greater latitude in choice of providers and is still less costly than the traditional fee-for-service (FFS) model. Ethical and legal conflicts abound for the individuals who operate the system: the providers, nurse-practitioners, triage personnel, case managers, managed care organization administrators, risk managers, utilization reviewers, and corporate executives.

The former FFS system contributed to the rise of health care costs. To contain these costs, a total system change occurred. Because of the shift to managed care, the seriously ill patient needing more services became a burden. From the patient's perspective, the single greatest threat posed by this shift is the potential for managed care systems to cut needed care to save health care dollars. Managed care often obscures the line separating insurers from providers.

Managed care organizations (MCOs) can dictate the specific brands and types of medication prescribed under a certain plan, protocol for diagnostic evaluations, as well as specific providers. While the patient can still choose treatment or providers that are outside their MCO's plan, the patient's contribution will be higher than the treatment or provider that is part of the MCO plan. In some cases, the treatment may not be covered by the plan at all.

MCOs, for example, can dictate the use of medication versus the use of counseling and support therapy for children with suspected mental illnesses. And, the potential consequences of this mandate go beyond parents preferring therapy over medication whose psychological effect may harm the body. It may be years before the medical community knows the effect of certain medications given to children during different stages of development. Because the health care industry is determined to cut costs, MCOs emphasize drug treatment over counseling. Is it ethical that this policy dictates the care that today's children receive?

In addition, health care providers, who are paid on a capitation basis, who realize bonuses for fiscal restraint or who have portions of their salary withheld to control costs, make less money with a seriously ill patient. Does this dynamic create an incentive to decline to accept seriously ill patients? Is it ethical to reward providers who make conservative decisions on patient care? Inherent in the managed care system is this major conflict:

Many physicians' bonuses, 73% per data from 2019–2020, are tied to relative value units (RVUs), which measure time, skill and effort for each patient a physician sees. Fewer physician bonuses are tied to quality-of-care measures, or protocols and processes that encourage increased patient safety measures and decreased death rates.

(Continues)

(Continued)

It is an ages-old quantity vs. quality debate, but with lives in the balance.

To be sure, RVUs are an important measure of physician work and expertise. However, these units alone do not account for the true quality and value of care physicians provide to patients.

For measurement of RVUs to be the most frequent financial incentives method for physicians is wrong. Incentives based on these units can and will increase patient costs, as physicians will be incentivized to see more patients, potentially even those without true medical indications for their physician care, instead of focusing solely on improving patient health and outcomes. This structure leads some physicians to intentionally see patients who medically do not need to be seen.

Piscitello, G. (2021, June 9). These Bonuses for Doctors Create an Immoral Conflict. CNN. Retrieved from www.cnn.com/2021/06/09/opinions/financial -incentives-doctors-ethical-concerns-piscitello/index.html.

Negotiations between medical providers and insurers can raise more ethical issues than the service provided. A *Boston Globe* Spotlight Team series highlighted such a case in Massachusetts:

As his patient lies waiting in an adjacent exam room, Dr. James D. Alderman watches while an assistant reaches into a white envelope and pulls out a piece of paper that will determine where the man will be treated. Big money is on the line . . .

Usually he does the procedure . . . in Framingham. But he sometimes operates in Boston as part of a research program. One time of every four, by the luck of the draw, Alderman and his patient go to a big teaching hospital in the city.

If the white slip of paper directs him to do the procedure in Framingham, the insurance company will pay the hospital about $17,000, not counting the physician's fee. If Alderman is sent to . . . Boston, that hospital will get about $24,500—44 percent more—even though the patient's care will be the same in both places.

"It's the exact same doctor doing the procedure," said Andrei Soran, MetroWest's chief executive. "But the cost? It's unjustifiably higher."

Call it the best-kept secret in Massachusetts medicine: Health insurance companies pay a handful of hospitals far more for the same work even when there is no evidence that the higher-priced care produces healthier patients.

In fact, sometimes the opposite is true: Massachusetts General Hospital, for example, earns 15 percent more than Beth Israel Deaconess Medical Center for treating heart-failure patients even though government figures show that Beth Israel has for years reported lower patient death rates.

Allen, S., Bombardieri, M., Rezendes, M. (2008, November 16). A Healthcare System Badly Out Of Balance. *Boston Globe*. Retrieved from www.bostonglobe.com/specials /2008/11/16/healthcare-system-badly-out-balance/j2ushYtZTBiCSxxUtQegbN/story.html.

In managed care, primary care physicians (PCPs) act as gatekeepers to control the cost-effectiveness of services offered to members and control access to specialists. In addition, many MCOs have adopted authorization requirements, where the MCO must approve certain procedures before the PCP orders them. These MCO payers are controlling access to health care by denying approval for certain procedures and allowing payment for others. They make decisions that reduce the number of hospital admissions, shorten the time until discharge, control the number of expensive diagnostic procedures, and, in the mental health field, substitute medication for therapeutic counseling treatment. Ethical questions arise when gatekeepers have a financial incentive to deny referrals to specialists, limit diagnostic treatments, shorten hospital stays, or recommend medication over counseling. And, when managed care organizations make the decision to allow or deny diagnostic testing and hospital admissions, the well-being of the patient becomes an issue and ethical issues are front and center.

Ethics in Medical Research

The mandates of the Tuskegee Study and the Nuremberg Code are the result of past unethical behavior in medical research. Today, all medical research in the United States, whether in an academic university or in a medical office, must abide by the rules created to ensure such research is ethical.

The Tuskegee Study

In 1972, a public health official objected to the "morality of an ongoing study being sponsored by the Public Health Service—a study compiling information about the course and effects of syphilis in human beings" based upon medical examinations of Black men who lived in Macon County, Alabama and whose incomes were below the federal poverty threshold. The study continued for more than 40 years. The men, however, "were not receiving standard therapy for syphilis . . . [This] has been called the longest running nontherapeutic experiment on human beings in medical history and the most notorious case of prolonged and knowing violation of subjects' rights—the Tuskegee study" (Arthur L. Caplan, "When Evil Intrudes," Hastings Center Report, 22, no. 6 (November–December 1992, p. 29). Public anger over the immorality of the Study spurred Congress to create a panel to review both the Tuskegee Study and the adequacy of existing protections for subjects in all federally sponsored research.

The Centers for Disease Control and Prevention indicate that:

The study initially involved 600 Black men—399 with syphilis, 201 subjects without the disease. The study was conducted without the benefit of patients' informed consent. Researchers told the men they were being treated for 'bad blood,' a local term used to describe several ailments, including syphilis, anemia, and fatigue. In truth, they did not receive the proper treatment needed to cure their illness. In exchange for taking part in the study, the men received free medical exams, free meals, and burial insurance. Although originally projected to last 6 months, the study went on for 40 years.

In July 1972, an Associated Press story about the Tuskegee Study caused a public outcry that led the Assistant Secretary for Health and Scientific Affairs to appoint an Ad Hoc Advisory Panel to review the study. The panel had nine members from the fields of medicine, law, religion, labor, education, health administration, and public affairs.

The panel found that the men had agreed freely to be examined and treated. However, there was no evidence that researchers had informed them of the study or its real purpose. In fact, the men had been misled and had not been given all the facts required to provide informed consent.

The men were never given adequate treatment for their disease. Even when penicillin became the drug of choice for syphilis in 1947, researchers did not offer it to the subjects. The advisory panel found nothing to show that subjects were ever given the choice of quitting the study, even when this new, highly effective treatment became widely used.

The advisory panel concluded that the Tuskegee Study was "ethically unjustified"—the knowledge gained was sparse when compared with the risks the study posed for its subjects. In October 1972, the panel advised stopping the study at once. A month later, the Assistant Secretary for Health and Scientific Affairs announced the end of the Tuskegee Study.

In the summer of 1973, a class-action lawsuit was filed on behalf of the study participants and their families. In 1974, a $10 million out-of-court settlement was reached. As part of the settlement, the U.S. government promised to give lifetime medical benefits and burial services to all living participants. The Tuskegee Health Benefit Program (THBP) was established to provide these services. In 1975, wives, widows and offspring were added to the program. In 1995, the program was expanded to include health as well as medical benefits. The Centers for Disease Control and Prevention was given responsibility for the program, where it remains today in the National Center for HIV/AIDS, Viral Hepatitis, STD, and TB Prevention. In 1997, President Bill Clinton issued a formal Presidential Apology for the study.

The last Study participant died in January 2004. The last widow receiving THBP benefits died in January 2009. There are 10 offspring currently receiving medical and health benefits.

Centers for Disease Control and Prevention. (2021, April 22). The Tuskegee Timeline. National Center for HIV/AIDS, Viral Hepatitis, STD, and TB Prevention, Centers for Disease Control and Prevention. Retrieved from www.cdc.gov/tuskegee/timeline.html.

In 1974, Congress created the National Commission for the Protection of Human Subjects of Biomedical and Behavior Research, which was replaced in 1978 by the President's Commission for the Study of Ethical Problems in Medicine and Biomedical and Behavioral Research. Since then, there have been several commissions that have "differed in their composition, methods, and areas of focus, but they have shared a common commitment to the careful examination and analysis of ethical considerations that underlie our nation's activities in science, medicine, and technology," according to the current Presidential Commission for the Study of Bioethical Issues.

Nuremberg Code

Society has developed guidelines to deal with experimental medical research. This includes the Nuremberg Code, which is the result of criminal trials related to experimentation conducted on prisoners by Nazi physicians during World War II.

On August 19, 1947, the judges of the American military tribunal in the case of the USA vs. Karl Brandt et. al. delivered their verdict. Before announcing the guilt or innocence of each defendant, they confronted the difficult question of medical experimentation on human beings. Several German doctors had argued in their own defense that their

(Continues)

(Continued)

experiments differed little from previous American or German ones. Further-more, they showed that no international law or informal statement differenti-ated between legal and illegal human experimentation. This argument worried Drs. Andrew Ivy and Leo Alexander, American doctors who had worked with the prosecution during the trial. On April 17, 1947, Dr. Alexander submitted a memorandum to the United States Counsel for War Crimes which outlined six points defining legitimate research. The verdict of August 19 reiterated almost all of these points in a section entitled "Permissible Medical Experiments" and revised the original six points into ten. Subsequently, the ten points became known as the "Nuremberg Code." Although the code addressed the defense arguments in general, remarkably none of the specific findings against Brandt and his codefendants mentioned the code. Thus, the legal force of the docu-ment was not well established. The uncertain use of the code continued in the half century following the trial when it informed numerous international ethics statements but failed to find a place in either the American or German national law codes. Nevertheless, it remains a landmark document on medical ethics.

United States Holocaust Memorial. (n.d.). United States Holocaust Memorial Museum
Note: Nuremberg Code. Retrieved from www.ushmm.org/information/exhibitions/
online-exhibitions/special-focus/doctors-trial/nuremberg-code.

Today, research in the United States that includes human subjects must adhere to the terms of the Nuremberg Code, which are largely reflected in the Code of Federal Regulations. Even college students researching the opinions of classmates and asking for confidential information (or the instructors who assign the project) are required to obtain clearance from an institutional review board to proceed. Given the potential for harm, research on human subjects is very carefully reviewed and regulated.

Clinical Trials

An increasing number of Americans are traveling outside the United States to seek medical treatment. They are not alone. *Scientific American* reports that drug companies are also increasingly globalizing their clini-cal trials, raising several medical and ethical issues along the way.

i

The clinical trial for a herpes vaccine flouted just about every norm in the book: American patients were flown into the Caribbean island of St. Kitts for experimental injections. Local authorities didn't give per-mission. Nor did the Food and Drug Administration. Nor did a safety panel.

That's why the trial—run by a startup that has since received funding from billionaire investor Peter Thiel—prompted widespread alarm and censure when it was reported last week by Kaiser Health News.

But in some respects, the herpes vaccine trial isn't all that unusual. Nearly all drug makers seeking U.S. approval today rely in part on overseas locations and populations to test their drugs, the result of a decades-long push by industry to try to cut costs and speed recruitment of patients. In fact, a STAT analysis found that 90 percent of new drugs approved this year were tested at least in part outside the U.S. and Canada.

Robbins, R. (2017, September 17). Most Experimental Drugs Are Tested Offshore—Raising Concerns About Data. *Scientific American.* Retrieved from www.scientificamerican.com/article/most-experimental-drugs-are-tested-offshore-raising-concerns-about-data/.

Studies have shown that data collected in developing countries reflect more positive results of the drug trials than those conducted in developed countries. As a result, conducting drug trials in locations outside the United States with weak or no regulation has resulted in scrutiny of the data collected. Varying standards of medical care, issues of translation, inadequately trained researchers, and fraud are some of the factors that raise concerns about data collected outside the United States. Should the FDA approve drugs exclusively based upon data from outside the United States? Is it ethical to approve a drug based upon data that may not be accurate if it will speed the approval process and potentially save lives that would have otherwise been lost during a longer approval process?

Clinical trials are sometimes halted because the mid-research results prove so conclusive that all patients should be given the option of going on the drug rather than potentially receiving a placebo. This happened during the trials for remdesivir, an antiviral drug used to treat COVID-19. The National Institute of Health reported that the study for remdesivir was stopped early because the drug's benefit was so undeniable that it would be unethical to continue the study.

i

The drug maker Gilead Sciences released a bombshell two weeks ago: A study conducted by a U.S. government agency had found that the company's experimental drug, remdesivir, was the first treatment shown to have even a small effect against Covid-19.

(Continues)

(Continued)

Behind that ray of hope, though, was one of the toughest quandaries in medicine: how to balance the need to rigorously test a new medicine for safety and effectiveness with the moral imperative to get patients a treatment that works as quickly as possible. At the heart of the decision about when to end the trial was a process that was—as is often in the case in clinical trials—by turns secretive and bureaucratic.

. . .

While study enrollment was incomplete and the trial had not demonstrated any significant improvement of the initial primary outcome—clinical improvement, the decision to stop the trial was made because the new primary outcome—median observation time in hospital—was seen to be significant.

Herper, M. (2020, May 11). Inside the NIH's Controversial Decision to Stop Its Big Remdesivir Study. StatNews. Retrieved from www.statnews.com/2020/05/11 /inside-the-nihs-controversial-decision-to-stop-its-big-remdesivir-study/.

Private Office Medical Research

Many health care provider offices are now engaged in clinical trials with pharmaceutical companies, as this has become a new revenue source. Offices engaged in this kind of research must take special care in documenting administration of the medicine and the results. The trend of moving clinical trial research away from academic medical centers began in the early 1990s. The costs of conducting "community-based" research are lower than those for the same trials in an academic medical center. In addition, the research organizations conducting the trials for the pharmaceutical companies can produce results more quickly than an academic medical center. Although this trend raises ethical questions about the objectivity of the research and the treatment of people who serve as subjects for experimental testing, the practice continues to flourish.

Ethical questions arise regarding the motives of privately practicing providers largely because they follow clinical plans designed by the pharmaceutical company rather than their own medical judgment. There is an inherent conflict of interest when faced with balancing the best interest of the patient against satisfying the pharmaceutical company's demands and the need to be paid for the experiments.

On one side of the conflict is the best interest of the patient; and on the other are the pharmaceutical demands for protocol fulfillment. In addition, some contend there are benefits to the arrangement: (1) adding a level of continuity and personal contact to the process; (2) providing an enormous pool of potential research subjects; and (3) allowing patients and their health care providers access to current and scientifically advanced therapies.

Transplants

The allocation of resources related to transplants gives rise to many ethical problems. Medical transplants are divided into three categories, depending on the tissue used. An *autograft* is the transplantation of a person's own tissue from one part of the body to another. This term also describes transplants between genetically identical children. A *homograft* is a transplant from one person to another, and the transplant of animal tissue into a human is a *heterograft*.

The first successful human-to-human organ transplant was a kidney transplant in 1954, and it is now the most commonly transplanted organ. Liver and lung transplants began, with the first recorded heart transplant to a human being attempted in 1964 with a chimpanzee's heart. In 2005, whole face transplants began in France, and in 2016, surgeons in Cleveland, Ohio, performed the first uterus transplant. Figure 10-1 is a timeline of significant transplant milestones.

The rise in the number of transplants has increased competition for organs and blood. In an attempt to control the process, California was the first state to pass statutes allowing a citizen to dispose of their own body or to separate parts of it on death through a will or another written document. The Uniform Anatomical Gift Act was first drafted in 1968 and has been revised several times since then. The Act is intended to be adopted by states and used as a template to simplify the process of allowing individuals to specify their wishes. The main provisions of the Act are as follows:

1. Any individual of sound mind and 18 years of age or more may give all or any part of their body . . . the gift to take effect upon death.

2. In the absence of a gift by the deceased, and of any objection by the deceased, their relatives, in a stated order of priority (spouse, adult children, parents, adult siblings, etc.), have the power to give the body or any of its contents.

3. The recipients of a gift are restricted to hospitals, health care providers, medical and dental schools, universities, tissue banks, and a specified individual in need of treatment. The purposes are restricted to transplantation, therapy, research, education, and the advancement of medical or dental science.

4. A gift may be made by will (to be effective immediately upon death without waiting for probate), or by a card or other document.

5. A gift may be revoked at any time.

6. A donee may accept or reject a gift.

All states use some form of the Act, and many allow individuals to indicate their choice to donate on their drivers' licenses. The use of organs from the dead and, later, from animals presented one set of ethical

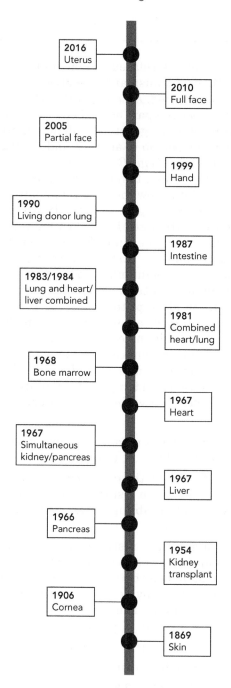

Figure 10-1 First Successful Transplant Timeline

Source: Health Resources & Services Administration. (2021, April). Timeline of Historical Events and Significant Milestones. HRSA. Retrieved from www.organdonor.gov/learn/history.

problems. The use of organs from the living presents even greater ethical dilemmas. Procedures that regulate living donor transplants have been developed through the courts.

Using live donors to obtain organs presents many problems. One is the discomfort of the provider. Many surgeons will not take skin from a donor because of the pain inflicted. The removal of internal organs for transplant, in addition to the ethics involved with inflicting pain on one person for another's benefit, involves multiple dilemmas.

There is a high demand for donor organs. There are also strict protocols that govern organ harvesting, which do not always provide the needed protection for the prospective donor. For example:

An 8-year-old boy died in a California hospital after a near drowning that, although he was not brain dead, caused so much damage that doctors determined he would never wake from the coma he was in. His family chose to remove life support and to donate his liver and kidneys for transplant. Thereafter, local police were called to investigate how he died at the hospital.

After life support was removed, the attending physician administered a dose of fentanyl to ease his suffering. The county coroner, who autopsied the deceased boy, determined that the fentanyl killed him. This conclusion raised the question of whether the fentanyl dose administered was intended to speed his death and improve the chances that his organs would be useable for donation.

As noted, "[t]his unusual case casts light on a once-controversial but increasingly common protocol called 'organ donation after circulatory death,' which occurs after the heart has stopped. (Also sometimes called 'donation after cardiac death,' or DCD.) In contrast, the vast majority of organs in the U.S. come from donors who are brain dead."

. . ."Patients taken off ventilators will often gasp for air. To alleviate the pain from "air hunger," doctors will administer painkillers, though the medical profession establishes a bright line: The dose cannot be so big as to intentionally kill the patient. (Medical experts said it was difficult to determine whether the dosage was appropriate in the L.A. case based on the few publicly available details.)"

Zhang, S. (2017, June 16). The Disputed Death of an 8-Year-Old Whose Organs Were Donated. *The Atlantic*. Retrieved from www.theatlantic.com/health/archive/2017/06/organ-donation-death/530511/.

For centuries, human hair has been used by wig makers, and teeth have been implanted into the jaws of wealthy dental patients. As the number and kind of transplants increase, the demand for organs will also increase. Worldwide, there is consensus that dealing in human organs for profit is illegal, but consensus does not always make law. The trafficking of human organs for profit is lucrative.

The trafficking of human beings for the purpose of organ removal (THBOR) is not a new phenomenon. With a shortage of legally sourced organs around the world, it is estimated that the illegal trade of human organs generates about 1.5 billion dollars each year from roughly 12,000 illegal transplants. THBOR has serious consequences for human security, particularly for the most vulnerable populations, such as the unemployed, homeless people and migrants.

In 2018, the International Labor Organization (ILO) asserted that about 40 million people were victims of Human Trafficking . . . About 90 percent of all detected cases were for sexual exploitation or forced labour purposes. The remaining 10 percent of cases are often lumped together in the "other forms" category—including organ removal. Organ trafficking is a broad concept that includes several illegal activities, of which the main goal is to profit from human organs and tissue, for the sole purpose of transplantation. These activities include THBOR, transplant tourism and trafficking in organs and tissues. Despite international and domestic efforts, about 10 percent of all transplants worldwide are believed to be illegal—approximately 12,000 organs per year. While the number of reports on victims of trafficking in people has increased, only 700 victims of THBOR were detected from 25 countries for the 2006–2019 period.

Gonzalez, J., Garijo, I., Sanchez, A. (2020, May 5). Organ Trafficking and Migration: A Bibliometric Analysis of an Untold Story. *International Journal of Environmental Research and Public Health*, 17(9), 3204. Retrieved from www.doi.org/10.3390/ijerph17093204.

Funding

Financial resources for health care are limited. What is an adequate level of health care? Should everyone have the opportunity to get a transplant, if needed? Should everyone have the opportunity to get proper nutrition, exercise, and inoculations to prevent disease?

On the one hand, it is costly to fund transplant operations; on the other hand, it is costly to fund school lunch programs for undernourished children. Values and ethics become involved in this discussion. The artificial heart, for example, might bring four years of extended life to each of the 25,000 patients annually at a cost $100,000 per life extended. The school lunch program might ensure the improved physical development of hundreds of thousands of children, enabling each child to live healthier lives for 60 years or more and require less medical care. The appeal of the artificial heart is that it rescues people from certain death. The school lunch program does not provide that same level of excitement or emotional appeal. Would the money spent on the development of better artificial hearts be better spent to upgrade the standard of health for a larger segment of the population? All of these factors contribute to the health of the nation, but because society does not have unlimited funds for health care, ethical choices dictate the outcome.

Autonomy Versus Paternalism

Being a patient often means being dependent on your health care provider. Both the health care provider and the patient have the same goal but perhaps different perspectives on how to reach that goal. One of the major issues that generate conflict between persons with different perspectives or different roles is the tension between **autonomy** and **paternalism**.

autonomy Allowing individuals control over themselves.

American culture highly values the autonomy of individuals, which includes their independence and self-reliance. Paternalism can be interpreted as interference with an individual's independence to benefit that individual. The principal goal of obtaining health care is for the patient to benefit from the providers' care. Those administering health care are obligated to take actions that benefit patients, even if those actions interfere with or neglect the patient's autonomy. Yet, others would argue that autonomy should take precedence. These conflicting positions produce ethical dilemmas in health care.

paternalism Providing for people's needs but giving them no responsibility or control over their destiny.

Billy Best, 16 years of age, was a patient at Dana-Farber Cancer Institute in Boston when he was informed that he needed 4 more months of treatments to wipe out the remaining cancer around his windpipe. He was given an ultimatum by his health care providers: continue chemotherapy treatments for Hodgkin's disease or face a painful death. His parents agreed with the health care providers and required Billy to continue the treatments at the Dana-Farber Cancer Institute. At 16 years, he was considered a minor without the capacity to make this decision for himself.

Billy determined he was no longer going to accept chemotherapy and ran away from home, crossing the United States from Boston to Texas. He claimed that the painful treatments were killing him and chose instead homeopathic drug treatment. His parents, after studying the alternative treatments, agreed with his decision, and Billy returned home. A year later tests revealed that the cancer had disappeared. Legally, Billy was unable to make the treatment decision in Massachusetts. It is ethical to force him to undergo treatment against his will. Would your position change if Billy was 8 years old? What about 14 years old?

In addition to health care providers being put in a paternalistic position, government also has plenty of situations in which to be paternalistic. This raises the ethical question: "To what degree is society responsible for its citizens?" Plenty of resources and money, for example, have been put into research showing that cigarettes are harmful to one's health.

The CDC reports: "[Tobacco] [s]moking-related illness in the United States costs more than $300 billion each year, including:

- More than $225 billion for direct medical care for adults
- More than $156 billion in lost productivity, including $5.6 billion in lost productivity due to secondhand smoke exposure." Yet people still smoke.

Use of seat belts and motorcycle helmets is mandatory in many states, yet many refuse to wear them. Should the government be responsible for the health care of people who choose not to wear a seat belt or a helmet and then sustain life-threatening injuries that would have been prevented or reduced had they worn a seat belt or helmet?

The involvement of the state can infringe on the privacy rights when it uses its power to regulate personal behavior. At what point does the balance of the public's interest outweigh an individual's right of privacy? Many states now prohibit smoking in public places or require that businesses have designated smoking areas. The smoking advocate may argue that this infringes on their right to enjoy a cigarette. Public health advocates argue that secondhand smoke endangers the health of those who have chosen not to smoke, thereby not only invading their privacy but injuring them as well. Who is right? People often reach conflicting conclusions for these types of ethical issues that apply to the public's well-being. This was well illustrated during the COVID-19 pandemic.

Once effective vaccines were made available to the public, the debate began as to who, if anyone, has the authority to mandate that people receive it. Can your employer require it? Can your local restaurant refuse to serve you if you cannot show proof of vaccination? How is a restaurant requiring that you wear shoes and a shirt similar to or different from requiring proof of vaccination?

herd immunity The eradication or slowing of the spread of a disease that occurs when a high enough percentage of the population is immune to the disease and it can no longer spread.

Must all health care workers receive the vaccine? Can the federal, state, or local government require all people have the vaccine? What if the government's objective is to acquire **herd immunity** through vaccination? Is the public welfare an ethical reason to require the vaccine? Is the success of the polio and smallpox vaccines reason enough to mandate that all people obtain the vaccine? Why or why not?

In each of these areas, the autonomy of the individual must be weighed against the danger of the individual to self or to others. In restraining a person's liberty, the need for such restraint must be acceptable to society. When freedom is denied to an individual, the freedom of every individual is endangered.

Medical Tourism

Concerns about cost and allocation of resources have resulted in medical tourism, where patients travel—domestically or internationally—solely to seek medical care that is priced lower or otherwise not available locally.

Often those who travel outside the United States for medical treatment do not have health insurance. Others travel for treatments that are not covered under their health insurance planes such as dentistry, cosmetic surgery, and in vitro fertility.

Even before the pandemic, millions of Americans traveled to other countries for savings of between 40 to 80 percent on medical treatments, according to the global medical tourism guide Patients Beyond Borders. Mexico and Costa Rica have become the most popular destinations for dental care, cosmetic surgery and prescription medicines while Thailand, India and South Korea draw in patients for more complex procedures including orthopedics, cardiovascular, cancer and fertility treatment.

In 2019, 1.1 percent of Americans traveling internationally did so for health treatments, according to the National Travel and Tourism Office, although that figure only accounts for those who traveled by air and does not include the thousands of travelers who crossed the United States-Mexico border. Definitive statistics on medical tourism are hard to come by because countries have different recording methods and definitions of the sector.

"Our market has always been what I call the 'working poor' and they just keep getting poorer," said Josef Woodman, the chief executive of Patients Beyond Borders. "The pandemic has gutted low-income and middle-class people around the world and for many of them the reality is that they have to travel to access affordable health care."

Yeginsu, C. (2021, January 19). Why Medical Tourism Is Drawing Patients, Even in a Pandemic. *The New York Times.* Retrieved from www.nytimes .com/2021/01/19/travel/medical-tourism-coronavirus-pandemic.html.

Medical tourism has shown that traveling to a different state, different region of your home state, or even to a different local hospital can make a difference in the cost or availability of a medical procedure.

I assumed that palm trees or streets teeming with foreign humanity were in my future as I began a quest to find a hip replacement at a price I could afford.

Because my severe osteoarthritis was deemed a preexisting condition, my insurance carrier would not pay for the surgery, so money was definitely an object.

(Continues)

(Continued)

Yet, after exploring so-called medical tourism options in Thailand, India, Hungary and Dubai, I settled on nothing so exotic. With rates that rival overseas alternatives, Oklahoma City beckoned me. It seems it has become a medical tourism hot spot.

Granted, I wasn't able to lounge on exotic beaches during my recuperation; instead, I toured a cowboy museum and the livestock market at Stockyards City. But the price was right.

Lytel, J. (2012, October 29). Medical Tourism Doesn't Necessarily Mean Leaving the Country to Get Treatment. *The Washington Post*. Retrieved from www.washingtonpost.com /national/health-science/medical-tourism-doesnt-necessarily-mean-leaving-the-country -to-get-treatment/2012/10/29/8d1bf5ce-d6710-11e1-b2d5-2419d227d8b0_story.html.

Some employers have jumped on the medical tourism bandwagon by negotiating bulk rates for procedures in locations that require the patient to travel:

The patient from Mississippi was staying in a Sheraton in Cancun, which was but a few steps away from the Galenia Hospital where she would soon have knee surgery.

The orthopedic surgeon flew in from Wisconsin the day before.

Health care costs in the United States are so high that it was unquestionably economical for both a highly trained orthopedist from Milwaukee and a patient from Mississippi to perform the procedure in a private Mexican hospital.

The patient's health insurance was provided by her husband's employer, Ashley Furniture Industries, who saved more than half of what it would have cost in the United States. Ashley Furniture's savings are high enough that its employees and dependents who use undertake medical tourism have no out-of-pocket copayments or deductibles, they receive a $5,000 payment from the company, and all their travel costs are covered.

The orthopedist spent fewer than 24 hours in Cancun. He was paid three times Medicare's reimbursement rate—or $2,700. The reimbursement rate is used as a floor by private health care plans when negotiating payment schedules with hospitals.

Galewitz, P. (2019, August 12). Medical Tourism Can Save Employers, Patients Money. *Kaiser Health News*. Retrieved from www.khn.org/news/to -save-money-american-patients-and-surgeons-meet-in-cancun/.

The American Medical Association has issued the following ethics opinion on Medical Tourism:

Medical tourism

Code of Medical Ethics Opinion 1.2.13

Medical tourists travel to address what they deem to be unmet personal medical needs, prompted by issues of cost, timely access to services, higher quality of care or perceived superior services, or to access services that are not available in their country of residence. In many instances, patients travel on their own initiative, with or without consulting their physician, and with or without utilizing the services of commercial medical tourism companies. The care medical tourists seek may be elective procedures, medically necessary standard care, or care that is unapproved or legally or ethically prohibited in their home system.

Many medical tourists receive excellent care, but issues of safety and quality can loom large. Substandard surgical care, poor infection control, inadequate screening of blood products, and falsified or outdated medications in lower income settings of care can pose greater risks than patients would face at home. Medical tourists also face heightened travel-related risks. Patients who develop complications may need extensive follow-up care when they return home. They may pose public health risks to their home communities as well.

Medical tourism can leave home country physicians in problematic positions: Faced with the reality that medical tourists often need follow-up when they return, even if only to monitor the course of an uneventful recovery; confronted with the fact that returning medical tourists often do not have records of the procedures they underwent and the medications they received, or contact information for the foreign health care professionals who provided services, asked to make right what went wrong when patients experience complications as a result of medical travel, often having not been informed about, let alone part of the patient's decision to seek health care abroad.

Physicians need to be aware of the implications of medical tourism for individual patients and the community.

Collectively, through their specialty societies and other professional organizations, physicians should:

(a) Support collection of and access to outcomes data from medical tourists to enhance informed decision making.
(b) Advocate for education for health care professionals about medical tourism.

(Continues)

(Continued)

(c) Advocate for appropriate oversight of medical tourism and companies that facilitate it to protect patient safety and promote high quality care.

(d) Advocate against policies that would require patients to accept care abroad as a condition of access to needed services.

Individually, physicians should:

(e) Be alert to indications that a patient may be contemplating seeking care abroad and explore with the patient the individual's concerns and wishes about care.

(f) Seek to familiarize themselves with issues in medical tourism to enable them to support informed decision making when patients approach them about getting care abroad.

(g) Help patients understand the special nature of risk and limited likelihood of benefit when they desire an unapproved therapy. Physicians should help patients frame realistic goals for care and encourage a plan of care based on scientifically recognized interventions.

(h) Advise patients who inform them in advance of a decision to seek care abroad whether the physician is or is not willing to provide follow-up care for the procedure(s), and refer the patient to other options for care.

(i) Offer their best professional guidance about a patient's decision to become a medical tourist, just as they would any other decision about care. This includes being candid when they deem a decision to obtain specific care abroad not to be in the patient's best interests. Physicians should encourage patients who seek unapproved therapy to enroll in an appropriate clinical trial.

(j) Physicians should respond compassionately when a patient who has undergone treatment abroad without the physician's prior knowledge seeks nonemergent follow-up care. Those who are reluctant to provide such care should carefully consider:

the nature and duration of the patient-physician relationship;
the likely impact on the individual patient's well-being;
the burden declining to provide follow-up care may impose on fellow professionals;
the likely impact on the health and resources of the community.

Physicians who are unable or unwilling to provide care in these circumstances have a responsibility to refer the patient to [an] appropriate [provider].

AMA. (n.d.). Medical Tourism: Code of Medical Ethics Opinion 1.2.13. AMA. Retrieved from www.ama-assn.org/delivering-care/ethics/medical-tourism.

Influences on the Patient–Provider Relationship

The allocation of time, as well as other resources, along with one's relative power influence the patient–provider relationship and raise ethical considerations. The economic environment in medicine has increased the pressure to be more cost conscious and profitable. Weekends and evening hours have become additional opportunities to care for patients and increase revenue. Who, then, must work on evenings and weekends? Is it the chief of staff, the resident, or the intern? Is it the head of a department or the last one to join the organization? Who can change a weekend or evening assignment easily—the head of the department or the last one in? The answer to all these questions is usually "The person with the most power." Is it ethical to base these decisions on one's power within the organization?

The influence of time upon the patient–provider relationship is evident in waiting rooms across the country. A constant sore spot in the patient–provider relationship is the amount of time patients spend waiting in reception and exam rooms. Is it ethical to keep all patients waiting the same amount of time, or do the most influential patients get in first? Are there different standards of care in attending to the needs of waiting patients? Does priority depend on the urgency of each case—for example, should a patient with a broken leg take precedence over a patient with the flu? Do office ethics take into consideration the importance of time for everyone waiting? Is the provider's time more valuable than the patient's time? Time is a limited resource, and it is valuable. Is time equally valuable for the retired person as it is for the person who earns an hourly wage working at a restaurant?

☑ SUMMARY

- As a health care professional, you will encounter ethical issues including how to make decisions about resource allocations. The COVID-19 pandemic provided real-life ethical issues as to the allocation of vaccines and ICU beds.
- Managed care is a response to the need to allocate limited health care resources. It does, however, create an inherent conflict between cost savings and providing the best patient care.
- The mandates of the Tuskegee Study and the Nuremberg Code are the result of past unethical behavior in medical research. Today,

all medical research in the United States, whether in an academic university or in a medical office, must abide by the rules created to ensure such research is ethical.

- Pharmaceutical companies are increasingly globalizing their clinical trials and raising several medical and ethical issues along the way.

- Medical transplants are divided into three categories, depending on the tissue used. An *autograft* is the transplantation of a person's own tissue from one part of the body to another. This term also describes transplants between genetically identical children. A *homograft* is a transplant from one person to another, and the transplant of animal tissue into a human is a *heterograft*.

- The first successful human-to-human organ transplant was a kidney transplant in 1954, and it is now the most commonly transplanted organ. Many other successful transplants followed.

- One of the major issues that generates conflict between persons with different perspectives or different roles, such as the provider and the patient, is the tension between autonomy and paternalism.

- Concerns about cost and allocation of resources have resulted in medical tourism, where patients travel—domestically or internationally—solely to seek medical care that is priced lower or otherwise not available locally.

- The allocation of time, as well as other resources, along with one's relative power influence the patient–provider relationship and raise ethical considerations.

SUGGESTED ACTIVITIES

1. View the movie *Miss Evers' Boys*, based upon the true story of the Tuskegee Study.

2. Visit a local nursing home (with permission, of course) and listen to what the residents and the staff think about matters involving the autonomy of decision making. Ask the residents what matters they find most difficult to allow someone else to decide. Then talk with the social worker to gain another perspective on issues of autonomy and paternalism with older adults.

3. View one of the many documentaries available on the Nuremberg Trials.

4. Research a news article that discusses one area of resource allocation associated with the pandemic (e.g., access to the vaccine, covid testing, ICU beds, ventilators, experimental treatments). Is the allocation fair? How could it be improved? What groups of people did the allocation help or hurt?

5. Research the Uniform Anatomical Gift Act as it applies to the state in which you live or work.

6. Find a recent example in the news for each of the three categories of transplants: autograft, homograft, and heterograft.

STUDY QUESTIONS

1. One of your patients is providing a kidney for transplant to her son. All the tests have been performed, and it has been determined that her tissue is compatible. She confides to you that she is frightened about the operation and living the remainder of her days with only one kidney. How do you handle the situation?

2. How is the government requiring a COVID-19 vaccination different or the same from the annual requirement that school-age children show proof of vaccination before starting school?

3. You are a medical assistant in a pediatrician's office. One of the patients needs a liver transplant. The matter has been in the newspaper, and additional newspapers are seeking interviews with the physician, the staff, and the patient. The newspapers will help advertise the need for an organ, but the family is too upset to handle the publicity. The pediatrician has told you to handle the press. What do you do?

4. A long-time patient calls for follow-up care for an incision infection after travelling abroad for knee surgery. The provider you work for refuses to see the patient or offer alternative care providers. What would be a reason to suggest to the provider you work for that their position is inadvisable? What is the minimum action you would suggest?

5. A person comes into the office and says that he is in a time of financial hardship and wants to sell one of his kidneys. He is not a patient, and you know nothing about him, but one of your patients is waiting for a kidney. Your patient is wealthy and can afford to purchase a kidney. What do you do?

CASES FOR DISCUSSION

1. A prisoner in Florida was sentenced to die. A young child in Denver needed a kidney, and the prisoner asked to be taken to Denver to be tested to determine whether he was a suitable donor. Should the court allow him to go to Denver?

2. A wife told her husband that she wanted a divorce. The following day, a psychiatrist whom she had never met before arrived at her home

but did not tell her that he was there to examine her. A few days later, the psychiatrist and another physician signed commitment papers for her, and she was forcibly removed from her home and taken to the hospital. She refused food and medication for 6 days and was refused permission to mail letters, use the telephone, or call her attorney. She finally was able to contact her relatives by telephone. Should she be released?

3. There is one ICU bed left. There are three patients with COVID-19 who should be admitted to the ICU due to the severity of their symptoms. All three patients require a ventilator. What issues would be ethical to consider when deciding which patient is admitted to the ICU? What issues would not be ethical to consider when deciding which patient is admitted to the ICU?

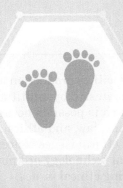

Chapter 11
Reproductive Issues and Early Life

 The two most important days in your life are the day you are born and the day you find out why.

Mark Twain

Objectives

After reading this chapter, you should be able to:

1. Analyze ethical questions associated with artificial insemination and assisted reproductive technology.
2. Summarize the decision of *Roman v. Roman*.
3. Identify examples of genetic disorders.
4. Explain how genetic testing is performed.
5. Analyze ethical questions surrounding genetic research.
6. Identify regulations on cloning.
7. Explain the dilemma of sanctity versus quality of life.
8. Summarize key legal decisions related to abortion.
9. Explain the medicolegal rights of a fetus.
10. Explain the medicolegal rights of a newborn.

Building Your Legal Vocabulary

Amniocentesis
Chemotherapy
Cloning
DNA
Embryonic stem cell
Embryos
Fetus
Genetic

Heterologous artificial insemination
Homologous artificial insemination
Pluralistic
Preimplantation genetic diagnosis
Sanctity
Survival action
Wrongful death

Introduction

There are a wide array of ethical issues associated with reproduction and life's early stages. Many of these issues are hotly contested by multitudes of groups with diverse positions and agendas, which is possible because the United States is a **pluralistic** society. Medicine, law, and ethics are tightly intertwined when considering the complex ethical issues concerning life's early stages. And, each advance in medical technology or knowledge provides additional fodder for these challenging ethical issues.

pluralistic Political philosophy wherein people of different beliefs, political parties, and lifestyles coexist and take part equally in the political process.

Artificial Insemination and Assisted Reproductive Technology

The path to parenthood can vary greatly. Consider the ethical issues raised by the following scenarios: A couple had been married for 6 years and wanted to have a child. After several months of trying, they visited a fertility specialist, who made the diagnosis that the husband did not have enough active sperm to fertilize the wife's egg. They were offered the following options:

1. Adoption.
2. **Homologous artificial insemination.**
3. **Heterologous artificial insemination.**

Now change the facts. The husband is able to donate the sperm, but the wife is unable to conceive. She has healthy eggs and can consider the following options. Which of the following would you find personally preferable?

1. Her sister volunteers to allow an embryo to be implanted and to carry the child to term for the couple.
2. A stranger, a female who will become pregnant with the couple's embryo (sperm and egg), will carry the child to term for a fee.

homologous artificial insemination An artificial insemination procedure wherein a sperm sample is taken from a donor who is the partner of the woman seeking to become pregnant.

heterologous artificial insemination An artificial insemination procedure wherein a sperm sample is taken from a donor who is not the partner of the woman seeking to become pregnant.

Let's change the facts again: The husband, at the age of 22 years, discovers that he has prostate cancer. He has the option, prior to surgery and **chemotherapy**, to have his sperm frozen. His wife could then be artificially inseminated with the sperm at a later date. The control of the cancer is successful, and the couple plans a child. It is determined that the wife cannot conceive because of scarred fallopian tubes. Eggs are surgically removed from the wife's ovaries, and conception takes place in a laboratory petri dish. Some of the embryos are frozen for future implantation. The first attempts to impregnate the wife are unsuccessful. The husband dies. Which of the following seems reasonable?

chemotherapy Drug treatment, most often used in the treatment of cancer, that uses potent chemicals to kill fast-growing cells.

1. Continue to artificially implant the wife with the remaining embryos.
2. Impregnate a surrogate mother.
3. Discard the embryos.

All of these scenarios play out in everyday life, and the associated ethical issues are complex. For example, Randy and Augusta Roman spent 2 years of infertility treatments trying to become pregnant. Ms. Roman's doctor retrieved 13 eggs from her ovaries and fertilized 6 with her husband's sperm. Hours before the embryos were going to be implanted, Mr. Roman said he couldn't go through with it. The couple divorced 16 months later. During the separation of marital property, they could not agree on the disposition of the 3 remaining embryos that had survived the freezing process.

> Augusta wanted to take possession and have [the embryos] implanted, agreeing to release Randy from any financial or parental obligation. Randy wanted the embryos destroyed, or at least frozen indefinitely. He argued that even though he did not want to raise children with Augusta, he would never disavow his genetic offspring. As he would point out in court, the couple had initialed a cryopreservation consent form stipulating that should they divorce, any frozen embryos "shall be discarded."
>
> *Roman v. Roman* is one of an increasing number of divorce cases nationwide in which the custody dispute has revolved around microscopic clumps of cells that are considered—by most states, at least—to be property and not human life.
>
> Advances in assisted reproduction have created a legal landscape that judges and lawmakers could hardly have envisioned before 1984, when an Australian baby became the first created from a frozen embryo (the first U.S. birth came two years later). Since then, in vitro fertilization, or IVF, has become an immensely popular solution to fertility problems worldwide.
>
> Sack, K. (2007, May 30). Her Embryos or His? *Los Angeles Times*. Retrieved from www.articles.latimes.com/2007/may/30/nation/na-embryo30.

The *Roman v. Roman*, 193 S.W.3d 40 (Tex. App., 2006), appellate court ultimately upheld the terms of the written IVF consent agreement that included a provision to discard the embryos should the parties divorce.

The repercussions of the disposition of frozen embryos affect other areas of society. Social security refused to pay benefits to Arizona twins

Juliet and Piers Netting, conceived from their father Robert Netting's frozen sperm 10 months after he died of cancer. An administrative law judge ruled that the children were not entitled to benefits because they were not dependent on the father at the time of his death. A district court upheld the decision. However, a U.S. District Court of Appeals ruled differently and held the children were entitled to social security benefits.

> Because the twins were Netting's legitimate children, the court held they were conclusively deemed dependent on Netting for purposes of Social Security and were entitled to benefits based upon his earnings.
>
> The Court noted, however, that not "every posthumously-conceived child in Arizona would be eligible for survivorship benefits . . . If the sperm donor had not been married to the mother, Arizona would not treat him as the child's natural parent, and he likely would have no obligation to support the child if he were alive." In this type of situation, "no eligibility for benefits would exist unless the Commissioner made a determination that the claimant was the dependent child of the deceased wage earner . . ."
>
> *Gillett-Netting ex rel. Netting v. Barnhart*, 371 F.3d 593 (9th Cir. 2004)

A person must have a license to drive a car and display a sense of financial responsibility to own a home, but is not required to demonstrate an ability to parent before conceiving a child. When the state plans adoptions, potential adoptive parents are placed under intense scrutiny. Should potential biological parents be subject to similar inquiry? For generations, society has discouraged, criminalized, and even prohibited marriages between relatives to prevent the passing of undesirable traits. Now that scientists can identify disease predispositions through genetic testing, should society allow these marriages but require premarital gene mapping or embryonic testing?

On the other side of the issue, does a couple have the right to have a child? Should the financial expense of a child born with a serious genetic disease be shared through insurance premiums? Should there be any criteria for becoming a parent via in vitro fertilization? Should there be an age limit as to when a man or a woman can become a parent? Assisted reproductive technology introduces further questions about parenthood and ethics. Consider the following:

73-year-old Mangayamma Yaramati gave birth to twin girls who were born in India following IVF treatment. Doctors delivered the twins via cesarean section. Yaramati and Sitarama Rajaraoher, her then 82 year old husband, had always wanted children but were unable to conceive. Having children was important to the couple, who also said that they felt stigmatized in their community. "They would call me a childless lady," Yaramati said.

"A day after the babies were born, Rajarao suffered a sudden stroke. . . . 'Nothing is in our hands. Whatever should happen will happen. It is all in the hands of God,' Rajarao had said when asked who would care for the children in case anything were to happen to the couple due to their advanced age.'"

BBC. (2019, September 6). Indian Woman, 73, Gives Birth to Twin Girls. BBC. Retrieved from www.bbc.com/news/uk-49575735.

In vitro fertilization can be cost prohibitive for those whose insurance does not provide coverage. Is it ethical to offer in vitro fertilization only to those who can afford it? Is it ethical to allow anyone regardless of age to undergo IVF?

The average cost of IVF in the U.S. is $10,000 to $15,000, according to the Society for Assisted Reproductive Technology. But the average fertility patient undergoes more than two cycles, so the cumulative IVF costs fall into the $40,000 to $60,000 range, according to data from more than 23,000 fertility patients from FertilityIQ, an online database and fertility information resource.

Snider, S. (2019, August 27). How Much Does IVF Cost and How Can I Pay for It? U.S. World News and Report. Retrieved from www.money.usnews.com/money/personal-finance/spending/articles/how-much-does-ivf-cost-and-how-can-i-pay-for-it.

Genetics

There are more than 6,000 known human **genetic** disorders. At least 500 of these genetic disorders are linked to a defect in just a single gene, and many of the disorders are extremely rare. They include cystic fibrosis, a disorder that occurs in one in 3,000 White people with

genetic Resulting from genes or attributable to them.

often fatal chronic lung problems; sickle cell anemia, a blood disorder found in one in 365 Black people (1 in 13 Black babies is born with the sickle cell trait); hemophilia, a blood clotting disorder that occurs most often in males, has an estimated incidence of 1 for every 5,617 male births (hemophilia A) and 1 for every 19,283 male births (hemophilia B); and Tay-Sachs disease, which causes blindness, paralysis, and early death in one of 3,500 persons of Ashkenazic (Eastern European) Jewish ancestry.

Investigating an individual's genetic makeup can have both positive and negative effects. Genetic information can be used for inappropriate purposes: to discriminate with regard to insurance, to reveal possible future medical issues, to expose information about family members, among many others. Genetic information can also be used for valuable and necessary purposes, including treatments for disorders and diseases.

Testing for genetic information is relatively simple and requires a **DNA** sample from solid tissues, blood, saliva, or other nucleated cells. Genetic data banks are found in both the public and private sectors of society and are usually developed for clinical research and public health programs.

DNA Molecule within cells that holds genetic information responsible for the development and performance of an organism.

Genetic Testing Before Birth

amniocentesis Test used during pregnancy to diagnose a fetus' genetic disorders and other health issues.

fetus Unborn, developing offspring from the period beginning 8 weeks (when the major structures have formed) after fertilization of an egg by a sperm until the time of birth.

sanctity The quality of being sacred.

embryos Fertilized eggs in the early stages of development.

preimplantation genetic diagnosis Genetic testing used to identify whether a parent's known genetic defect is present in an embryo produced by in vitro fertilization.

Amniocentesis allows health care providers to perform genetic tests for defects during pregnancy. Some disorders and diseases that produce dysfunction in humans later in life, such as Alzheimer's disease, have been found to have a genetic basis. Should government mandate abortion when a **fetus** exhibits certain genetic traits? Will society use genetic information to determine who will be educated and to what degree, what profession people must undertake, or who will receive what medical resources? Consider the **sanctity** and quality of life as you read the following.

The New York Times, for example, featured an article on the preimplantation testing of **embryos**. A woman in her late 20s was told that she carries the gene for a fatal neurological disease. She wanted to have children but did not want to pass the gene for the fatal disease on to her children. She and her husband chose to have in vitro fertilization so the embryos could be tested for the gene before implantation. They are now the parents of three children who do not carry the gene for the fatal disease. What are the ethical issues associated with creating embryos that will be discarded if they carry the gene for a fatal disease? What ethical issues are raised if parents use in **preimplantation genetic diagnosis** (PGD) to ensure their child does not carry a specific disease?

Genetic testing of embryos has been around for more than a decade, but its use has soared in recent years as methods have improved and more disease-causing genes have been discovered.

But the procedure also raises unsettling ethical questions that trouble advocates for the disabled and have left some doctors struggling with what they should tell their patients. When are prospective parents justified in discarding embryos? Is it acceptable, for example, for diseases like Alzheimer's, that develop in adulthood? What if a gene only increases the risk of a disease but does not guarantee it will surface? And should people be able to use genetic testing to choose whether they have a boy or girl? A recent international survey found that 2 percent of more than 27,000 uses of preimplantation diagnosis were made to choose a child's sex.

In the United States, there are no regulations that limit the method's use. The Society for Assisted Reproductive Technology, whose members provide preimplantation diagnosis, says it is "ethically justified" to prevent serious adult diseases for which "no safe, effective interventions are available." The method is "ethically allowed" for conditions "of lesser severity" or for which the gene increases risk but does not guarantee a disease . . .

Preimplantation diagnosis often goes unmentioned by doctors. In a recent national survey, Dr. Robert Klitzman, a professor of clinical psychiatry and bioethicist at Columbia University, found that most internists were unsure about whether they would suggest the method to couples with genes for diseases like cystic fibrosis or breast cancer. Only about 6 percent had ever mentioned it to patients and only 7 percent said they felt qualified to answer patients' questions about it . . .

Janet Malek, a bioethicist at the Brody School of Medicine at East Carolina University, said that people who carry a gene for a debilitating disorder have a moral duty to use preimplantation diagnosis—if they can afford it—to spare the next generation.

Kolata, G. (2014, February 3). Ethics Questions Arise As Genetic Testing of Embryos Increases. *The New York Times.* Retrieved from www.nytimes.com/2014/02/04 /health/ethics-questions-arise-as-genetic-testing-of-embryos-increases.html.

What are the ethical issues associated with people who carry genes with disease but who cannot afford the cost of in vitro fertilization and preimplantation embryonic testing? When it comes to procedures covered by insurance, how is covering testing for a disease at the embryonic stage different than covering the cost of care for that disease after birth?

A California-based start-up called Orchid Biosciences provides preimplantation diagnosis for those who can afford it and takes a different approach to reproductive technology.

Orchid "offers prospective parents genetic testing prior to conception to calculate risk scores estimating their own likelihood of confronting common illnesses such as heart disease, diabetes, and schizophrenia and the likelihood that they will pass such risks along to a future child. Parents-to-be can then use IVF, along with Orchid's upcoming embryo screening package, to identify the healthiest of their embryos for a pregnancy."

Orchid sells a "Couple Report," detailing both parent's genetic makeup at a cost of $1,100 and an IVF embryo analysis that allows the parents to choose from the various IVF embryos. Orchid's use of polygenic risk scores to assess an embryo's risk of common diseases and disorders has created skepticism amongst geneticists. For example, "[h]eart disease runs in families just like musical ability or height, but only in exceptional cases can the inherited risk be traced to a single gene. Hundreds or even thousands of genes each contribute in a small way. Polygenic risk scores attempt to sum up the overall likelihood of a particular outcome—such as getting a disease—by simply observing which patterns of variation in a genome are associated with a higher or lower probability of having the condition." Using Polygenic risk scores provides the probability as to who might have a disorder or disease without providing information to understand why, and the data taken from the population at whole may not be relevant to an individual parent. Orchid CEO Noor Siddiqui indicated that, ". . . everyone who wants to have a baby should be able to, and we want our technology to be as accessible to everyone who wants it," and considers the lack of insurance coverage for IVF "a major problem that needs to be addressed in the U.S." Siddiqui further suggested that the parents should be making the decisions, "I think at the end of the day, you have to respect patient autonomy." She also warned that those who stand in the way of providing parents with this autonomy are "frankly being a little bit paternalistic."

Hercher, L. (2021, July 12). A New Era of Designer Babies May Be Based on Overhyped Science. *Scientific American.* Retrieved from www.scientificamerican.com/article /a-new-era-of-designer-babies-may-be-based-on-overhyped-science/.

Who should pay for the cost of Orchid's program, which requires IVF? Should insurance companies cover the cost of IVF for parents who wish to choose an IVF embryo based upon specific characteristics? Should the insurance company be able to define which diseases or disorders can be considered in PGD? Who decides whether living with a disease is any better or worse or more valuable than living without the disease? Again, consider the sanctity versus the quality of life as they apply to the questions raised in Orchid's program.

Embryonic Stem Cells for Research

The use of **embryonic stem cells** for research raises ethical issues and rigorous debates. In her article *Embryonic Stem Cell Research: An Ethical Dilemma*, Lillian Nwigwe reviewed the ethical issues raised and explained the start of the debate: "The origin of stem cells themselves encapsulates the controversy: embryonic stem cells, originate from the inner cell mass of a blastocyst, a 5-day pre-implantation embryo. The principal argument for embryonic stem cell research is the potential benefit of using human embryonic cells to examine or treat diseases as opposed to somatic (adult) stem cells. Thus, advocates believe embryonic stem cell research may aid in developing new, more efficient treatments for severe diseases and ease the pain and suffering of numerous people. However, those that are against embryonic stem cell research believe that the possibility of scientific benefits of research do not outweigh the immoral action of tampering with the natural progression of a fetal development and interfering with the human embryo's right to live. In light of these two opposing views, should embryonic stem cells be used in research? It is not ethically permissible to destroy human embryonic life for medical progress."

embryonic stem cells Cells that are derived from human embryos or human fetal tissues that are self-replicating.

The debate over the use of embryonic stem cells for research emanates from the fact that the definition of "personhood" is unclear. "Personhood is defined as the status of being a person, entitled to 'moral rights and legal protections' that are higher than living things that are not classified as persons. Thus, this issue touches on existential questions such as: When does life begin? and What is the moral status that an embryo possesses?"

Nwigwe, L. (2019). Embryonic Stem Cell Research: An Ethical Dilemma. *Voices in Bioethics, Vol. 5*. Retrieved from www.doi.org/10.7916/vib.v5i.6135.

Science and technology can manipulate life's early stages, and ethical dilemmas surround society's willingness to accept intervention in the conception–birth process. Religious beliefs are often at the core of debates involving the beginning of life, which is also a key facet of the debate surrounding the use of embryonic stem cells. See Table 11-1 for positions held by various religions about the use of embryonic stem cells for research.

Table 11-1 Religious Positions on Embryonic Stem Cell Research

	Is Embryonic Stem Cell Research Morally Acceptable?			
Religion	Yes	Depends	No	Summary
Judaism	X			After 40 days of development, an embryo is considered human. "Research on embryonic stem cells is morally acceptable since the embryo before 40 days is 'as if it were water' and not an entity with a real soul."
Hinduism		X		It is acceptable "if one intends to do research aimed at healing and improving the lives of patients, but research done for financial gain is not acceptable."
Buddhism		X		The destruction of embryos is not morally acceptable, yet Buddhism does not have an official position on the use of embryonic stem cells for research. Buddhism does not allow for causing pain in any living being, but research on embryonic stem cells can be performed because prior to 14 days, the embryo does not feel pain.
Catholicism			X	Catholicism does not support the use of embryonic stem cells from embryos created exclusively for therapy and research but does support the use of adult stem cells for research. This religion believes that "the moment of conception is also the beginning of the entity of the human person. . . . Thus, the Catholic ethical doctrine does not allow the use of embryonic stem cells from embryos created exclusively for this purpose, by means of assisted reproduction procedures or for the purpose of reproductive cloning."
Protestant			X	The foundation of the Protestant position that does not support use of embryonic stem cells for research recognizes "human beings as entities that will have a relationship first with God and then with others and with itself. Therefore, the human fetus is considered a developing human being that, if not born, will not have these relationships."
Islam	X			The Koran instructs that a fetus acquires "psyche and image at the end of its fourth month of pregnancy." Embryonic stem cell research is acceptable because the embryo cannot be considered a complete human being yet.

Source: Charitos, I. et al. (2021, April 30). Stem Cells: A Historical Review About Biological, Religious, and Ethical Issue. Hindawi. *Stem Cells International*, Volume 2021. Retrieved from www.doi.org/10.1155/2021/9978837.

Cloning and Gene Editing

cloning Identically duplicating an organism.

Science also is investigating how to produce "perfect" specimens through reproductive **cloning**. Technology has reached the point where a fertilized egg can be cloned and implanted for human incubation until birth. In addition, gene editing technology has progressed to the point where scientists believe they can remove certain DNA mutations that lead to disease.

While there are no federal regulations related to human reproductive cloning, several states have enacted laws that prohibit human reproductive cloning. A handful of states prohibit state funds from being used on reproductive cloning. The United Nations and several other countries have also banned reproductive cloning.

Using technology to create a baby with or without personally desired characteristics, however, is not limited to cloning. Other methods, including gene editing, are rapidly becoming viable options, raising several ethical questions for the medical community and society as a whole. Is society willing to allow this to happen? What could be the repercussions of these practices?

One scientist learned firsthand about the repercussions of pushing the ethical boundaries of genetic editing:

Chinese biophysicist He Jiankui, who created the world's first gene-edited babies in 2018, received a three year prison sentence and a $430,000 fine for the unlawful practice of medicine. Two of his colleagues who assisted him received shorter sentences. The Chinese health ministry has banned the researchers from ever working with reproductive technology again. The Chinese science ministry has banned them from applying for research funding. He was fired from his position as an associate professor.

He had used a gene-editing tool called CRISPR-Cas9 [CRISPR is an acronym for Clustered Regularly Interspaced Short Palindromic Repeats], which allows for the removal—or editing—of problematic DNA. Specifically, his objective was to edit DNA in human embryos to make them less susceptible to HIV. This research was condemned globally for many reasons including that the babies were not high risk for contracting HIV.

Scientists have raised concerns that the genetic modifications made by He could be passed down through the generations and present a permanent change to the human race. In addition, the scientists reported that He had not edited the DNA to reflect the exact mutation tied to HIV resistance, and the effects of his edits are unknown.

The Chinese Academy of Science indicated that, "[u]nder current circumstances, gene editing in human embryos still involves various unresolved technical issues, might lead to unforeseen risks, and violates the consensus of the international scientific community."

BBC. (2019, December 30). China Jails 'Gene-Edited Babies' Scientist for Three Years. BBC. Retrieved from www.bbc.com/news/world-asia-china-50944461.

Abortion and the Right to Be Left Alone

Privacy, from a legal perspective, conveys the right to be left alone to make certain personal choices, including whether to abort a pregnancy. In the Tarasoff case described in Chapter 9, the patient forfeited the right to be left alone because he demonstrated an intent to harm a third party. In *Griswold v. Connecticut*, 381.U.S. 479 (1965), *Katz v. United States*, 389 U.S. 347 (1967), and *Roe v. Wade*, 410 U.S. 113 (1973), the U.S. Supreme Court cited several constitutional amendments that establish the right to privacy.

The human right to privacy is grounded in the basic moral tenet that each individual has an incalculable worth. Reflected in the Fourth Amendment of the U.S. Constitution, this right is a core issue of the abortion conflict. On the issue of abortion, one side of the debate holds that an individual's incalculable worth extends to the fetus; the other side holds that the woman's worth—and what she chooses to do with her body—is a high priority.

The well-known abortion decision of the U.S. Supreme Court, *Roe v. Wade*, protects a woman's right to privacy in a first-trimester abortion. This right to privacy allows the woman to communicate with her health care provider concerning an abortion. This decision has been challenged by those believing that having an abortion is tantamount to killing a child. The decision still stands as law, while subsequent case law further defines the interplay of the Constitutional right to privacy and abortions.

Medicolegal Rights of the Fetus

Society's perception of what a fetus is remains full of controversy. Today, fetal rights issues are raised in courts, legislatures, and public debates across the country. Once again, new technology has given us new medical treatments and cures. And, with the new technology comes new ethical questions.

An Alabama mother of six was pregnant when she filled a prescription that eventually caused her to face felony charges. Before the pregnancy, an orthopedist prescribed hydrocodone, an opiate pain killer, for back pain due to her spinal disc degeneration. She had not taken the prescription during the early stages of the pregnancy. As the pregnancy progressed, however, her back pain worsened. Six weeks before she was due to deliver, she refilled her prescription. She later gave birth to a healthy baby boy.

She told her doctor about medications she had taken during pregnancy—including the hydrocodone. Her doctor was required by Alabama law to report this information. When her son tested positive for hydrocodone, and an investigation was launched. The state child services agency cleared her, but the local police and district attorney continued with the case. When her new son was eight weeks old and with all of her children present, seven armed officers raided her house.

As happened in this situation, a woman after carrying a healthy pregnancy and giving birth to a healthy child, can be arrested for being honest with her own doctor. "For many women, this will be the takeaway: don't trust the doctor. When laws incentivize women to be dishonest with their medical providers, or forgo medical care entirely while pregnant, it's not clear how those laws can be said to ensure the safety of a fetus. If anything, they seem to be discouraging the practices that lead to good pregnancy outcomes."

Donegan, M. (2021, July 27). Alabama Is Prosecuting a Mom for Taking Prescribed Medication While Pregnant. *The Guardian*. Retrieved from www.theguardian.com /commentisfree/2021/jul/27/alabama-prosecuting-woman-medication-pregnant.

The Unborn Victims of Violence Act of 2004 made it a crime to harm a fetus while assaulting a pregnant woman during the commission of a federal crime. Adding to this, a majority of states have fetus protection laws and case laws in many others hold that a stillborn child's estate may seek recovery through a **wrongful death** and **survival action** for injuries sustained while in the womb.

While the law protects fetuses from harm during pregnancy, it is clear that frozen embryos do not have the same protections. Who decides when a frozen embryo transitions to a fetus? Should that be a decision of personal ethics or should law or medicine dictate the transition point?

wrongful death Death caused by negligence.

survival action A lawsuit related to a death and brought by the decedent's survivors.

Plaintiffs, who seek to sue for the loss of a frozen embryo, typically file breach of contract and property damage claims, and they avoid wrongful death claims. The nature of the lawsuits brought by these plaintiffs reflect an understanding of the unanimous rejection of wrongful death claims in prior lawsuits. "To date, every court that has considered the wrongful death of an in vitro fertilization (IVF) embryo has rejected that claim on the ground that the term 'person' or 'human being' does not apply to frozen embryos under the meaning of state law (see, e.g., *Gentry v. Gilmore*, 613 So.2d 1241, 1244 [Ala. 1993]); *Jeter v. Mayo Clinic Ariz.*, 121 P.3d 1256, 1261–62 [Ariz. Ct. App. 2005]; *McClain v. Univ. of Mich. Bd. of Regents*, 665 N.W.2d 484, 486 [Mich. Ct. App. 2003]; *Miccolis v. Amica Mut. Ins. Co.*, 587 A.2d 67, 71 [R.I. 1991])."

Daar, J. (2020, September). Legal Liability Landscape and the Person/Property Divide. F&S Reports. Retrieved from www.doi.org/10.1016/j.xfre.2020.08.004.

With one in every 200 pregnancies ending in stillbirth in the United States—about 26,000 each year—there are numerous legal, ethical, and public policy questions surrounding the issue of how to classify those that are stillborn. This extends to questions about record keeping, with lawmakers continuing long-running debates as to whether stillborn children should be documented with birth certificates.

> Last summer, three weeks before her due date, Sari Edber delivered a stillborn son, Jacob. "He was 5 pounds and 19 inches, absolutely beautiful, with my olive complexion, my husband's curly hair, long fingers and toes, chubby cheeks and a perfect button nose," she said . . . "The day before I was released from the hospital, the doctor came in with the paperwork for a fetal death certificate, and said, 'I'm sorry, but this is the only document you'll receive.' In my heart, it didn't make sense . . . we deserved more than a death certificate". . . So Ms. Edber joined with others who had experienced stillbirth to push California legislators to pass a bill allowing parents to receive a certificate of birth resulting in stillbirth . . . 19 states, including New Jersey, have enacted laws allowing parents who have had stillbirths to get such certificates. Similar legislation is under consideration in several more, among them New York . . . But politically, the birth-certificate laws, often referred to as "Missing Angels" bills, occupy uncertain territory, skirting the abortion debate while implicitly raising the question of fetal personhood.
>
> Lewin, T. (2007, May 22). A Move for Birth Certificates for Stillborn Babies. *The New York Times*. Retrieved from www.nytimes.com/2007/05/22/us/22stillbirth.html.

Now that it has been determined that a fetus has rights, can a mother be charged for abuse to the fetus that results in a brain-damaged baby? If fetal neglect becomes a cause of action, would it mean that a pregnant woman is guilty of a crime if she does not eat properly, smokes, or drinks alcohol? Could this be extended to a cause of action against the state for not providing proper food and environment for pregnant mothers who are indigent?

Historically, laws have not been used to punish women for conduct during their pregnancy that might endanger the fetus. In recent years, that trend has seen an increasing number of exceptions. Some exceptions raise questions as to whether such prosecutions actually discourage pregnant women from seeking help for issues related to drugs, alcohol, or mental health.

There has been considerable scientific interest in using the fetus for transplants without much discussion about the rights of the fetus. Think about this issue using the following hypothetical situations:

Suppose an older patient is suffering from the degenerative progression of Parkinson's disease. There is hope that the ravages of the disease may be stopped or reversed by transplanting tissue from the human fetus. Experimentation done with monkeys has shown that symptoms similar to Parkinson's can be controlled by transplanting tissue into the brain of an afflicted adult animal.

1. A neurosurgeon at a large teaching facility wishes to transplant tissues from an aborted fetus into the brain of a former state governor.

2. The former governor's wife wishes to become pregnant by having embryos the couple previously had frozen implanted in her uterus. Then she plans to abort the fetus to allow for the best tissue match.

3. The technique has never been performed in a human before.

Let us now change the facts. We find that the viable fetus is stillborn following a third-trimester miscarriage.

1. A cardiac surgeon wishes to transplant the heart of the stillborn child into an infant born prematurely who will not survive with her own deformed heart for more than 2 days.

2. The preemie has additional deformities of internal organs but no apparent physical deformities.

3. The stillborn child has both internal and physical deformities.

4. Because of the stillborn's physical anomalies, the pathologist wishes to preserve the child's body in formaldehyde to use as a teaching specimen.

Medicolegal Rights of a Newborn

In the spring of 1982, an infant, identified only as Baby Doe, was born in Bloomington, Indiana. The diagnosis at birth was Down syndrome and an obstruction of the digestive tract that precluded normal feeding but was apparently surgically correctable. The parents refused to give consent to surgery, and the hospital took the matter to the court. The superior court concluded that when, as in this case, the parents were "confronted with two competent medical opinions, one suggesting that corrective surgery may be appropriate and the other suggesting that corrective surgery and extraordinary measures would only be futile acts, it was the parents' responsibility to choose the appropriate action without interference by the government." The child soon died.

The case was heavily covered by the press and appeared on television. The media portrayed the child as one who had been denied routine surgical treatment and allowed to starve to death for no reason other than a mild, unrelated handicap. On April 30, 1982, President Reagan sent a memorandum to officials in the government instructing them to take steps to prevent repetition of such an abuse. On May 18, 1982, a notice was sent to most of the nation's hospitals by the Department of Health and Human Services (HHS), explaining that the "discriminatory failure of a federally assisted health-care provider to feed a handicapped infant, or to provide medical treatment essential to correct a life-threatening condition," could be found to violate a federal rehabilitation act. The development of final so-called Baby Doe law took several more years and demonstrated the difficulty of legislating medical issues and the complexity of regulating ethical issues.

Enacted in April 15, 1985, the Baby Doe law is an amendment to the Child Abuse Prevention and Treatment Act of 1974. Public policy behind these regulations prevents withholding of medical care from an infant with one or more noncongenital anomalies by defining the withholding of medical care as neglect. According to the rules, if there is treatment for the condition, it must be provided. There are three exceptions to the policy:

1. When the infant is chronically and irreversibly comatose.
2. When treatment would merely prolong dying.
3. When the treatment would be futile either because the child would not survive or the treatment would be inhumane.

This federal legislation requires the states to establish programs and/or procedures within their child protective service system. It requires response to needs for treatment by infants with disabilities and life-threatening conditions.

While laws can alter the rights of a newborn, so too can new and improved technology, which, in turn, raises new ethical issues. Expensive technology now allows for harvesting, freezing, and storing a baby's umbilical cord in case the child ever gets sick and needs it. Should everyone have the opportunity to store cord blood or is it just for the rich?

"After collection, your baby's cord blood is shipped to either a public or a private blood bank, depending on which you choose.

Public cord blood donations cost the donor nothing and are made available to anyone (including scientists) through a national registry. With public banking, however, you can't always ask for your own baby's cord blood back if a family member needs it." Currently in the U.S., there are approximately 16 public cord blood banks and 147 hospitals that can accept public donations.

"Private [cord blood] banking, on the other hand, costs money but is held for your baby or another family member (most likely a sibling) when or if they may need it. Banks typically charge an initial collection fee of $1,000 to $2,000 per birth, followed by about $150 to $200 per year (storage costs can vary from bank to bank). Insurance doesn't cover private banking, but some cord blood banks offer financial help for families with immediate relatives who have a known blood disorder and would benefit from a stem cell transplant."

Najjar, D. (2020, December 18). Should You Bank Your Baby's Cord Blood? *The New York Times.* Retrieved from www.nytimes.com/2020 /12/18/parenting/pregnancy/cord-blood-banking.html.

Children may be conceived by parents for their assistance in the treatment of a serious illness of another family member. The following is an excerpt from an article in the *Chicago Tribune*:

> Genetic testing of embryos outside the womb has led to the births of five babies selected to produce umbilical cord blood or bone marrow to save the lives of seriously ill siblings, Chicago doctors reported . . .
>
> The controversial procedure, which employs cutting edge genetic tests during in vitro fertilization, expands the possibilities of the creation of so-called "savior babies" to provide stem cells for older children who lack compatible donors for bone marrow transplants . . .
>
> Chicago scientists were able to create babies for five of nine couples whose other children already suffered from bone marrow failure . . .
>
> Umbilical cord blood from one of the babies already has saved a sibling, another transplant is pending, and three of the affected children were in remission and may need the transplants later.
>
> Gorner, P. (2004, May 5). 5 Babies Born to Save Ill Siblings, Doctors Say. *Chicago Tribune*. Retrieved from www.chicagotribune.com/news/ct-xpm -2004-05-05-0405050257-story.html.

Is it ethical to have a child solely for the purpose of obtaining cord blood, bone marrow, or other genetic material to aid another? Is it ethical to do so, if the motivation is financial gain?

There are no correct answers to these complex and difficult ethical questions associated with life's early stages. As a health care professional, it is in your best interest to understand the ethical issues' various positions.

☑ SUMMARY

- There are more than 6,000 known human genetic disorders. Common genetic disorders include cystic fibrosis, sickle cell anemia, hemophilia, and Tay-Sachs disease.
- Testing for genetic information is relatively simple and just requires a DNA sample from solid tissues, blood, saliva, or other nucleated cells.
- While there are no federal regulations related to human reproductive cloning, several states have enacted laws that prohibit human

reproductive cloning. A handful of states prohibit state funds from being used on reproductive cloning. The United Nations and several other countries have also banned reproductive cloning.

- The dilemma of sanctity versus quality of life, as it applies to life's early stages, seeks to examine whether living with a disease or disorder is any better or worse or more valuable than living without the disease.

- The debate over the use of embryonic stem cells for research emanates from the fact that the definition of "personhood" is unclear. Ethical issues regarding genetic research come from legal, religious, and personal beliefs, as well as disparity of options based upon socioeconomic status.

- Ethical questions associated with artificial insemination and assisted reproductive technology are many and include ownership and disposal of frozen embryos, use of an anonymous donor's sperm, eggs, or uterus, should age be considered when performing IVF, among many others.

- The decision of *Roman v. Roman* upheld the terms of the written IVF consent agreement that included a provision to discard the embryos should the parties divorce.

- In *Griswold v. Connecticut*, 381.U.S. 479 (1965), *Katz v. United States*, 389 U.S. 347 (1967), and *Roe v. Wade*, 410 U.S. 113 (1973), the U.S. Supreme Court cited several Constitutional amendments that establish the right to privacy.

- Laws have established protections for the fetus, including the Unborn Victims of Violence Act of 2004. Frozen embryos do not share the same protections as fetuses.

- The Baby Doe Law or Baby Doe Amendment is an amendment to the Child Abuse Prevention and Treatment Act of 1974, and it requires federally funded hospitals and providers must provide care to any impaired infant or be liable for neglect.

SUGGESTED ACTIVITIES

1. Several major religions in the United States have made clear their positions on artificial insemination. Conduct research on three different religions' position on artificial insemination and compare and contrast the basis for their positions.

2. Research a judicial decision about abortion that was issued after the *Roe v. Wade* decision. How does it change or modify the ruling in *Roe v. Wade*?

STUDY QUESTIONS

1. Describe the benefits and detriments of genetic testing.

2. If you or your partner were pregnant and had a family history of a genetic disease, would you have amniocentesis to determine if the fetus had signs of abnormal development? What factors would you consider when determining whether to abort the fetus?

3. Define *sanctity of life* and give an example of an ethical decision based on this philosophy.

4. Define *quality of life* and give an example of an ethical decision based on this philosophy.

5. What are the three exceptions to the Baby Doe Law?

6. What restrictions with regard to the well-being of the fetus, if any, would you place on pregnant mothers? Should a pregnant mother's nutrition be monitored by the government to ensure the fetus is healthy?

7. Some children born with certain congenital conditions experience substantial suffering and pain. If extraordinary means are used to keep these children alive, they may live for a few weeks but not without continual medical intervention. If allowed to die at birth without intervention, they will live a few hours at most. Try to develop philosophies for both sides of this issue.

8. What type of sample is used for genetic testing and from where can the sample be obtained?

CASES FOR DISCUSSION

1. The plaintiff gave birth to a daughter with Tay-Sachs disease. Children born with this incurable degenerative nerve disease do not live long. The plaintiffs claimed that the defendant health care provider was negligent in that he failed to take a proper genealogical history or to properly evaluate their genetic histories. The plaintiffs were Eastern European Jews, a fact that should have put the defendant on notice that there was a high risk the child would suffer from the disease. They also stated that if they had known of the risk involved, they would have taken tests and, if the results were positive, aborted the pregnancy.

2. After 7 years of marriage, a couple learned that in order to have children, they would need to have artificial insemination or adopt because the husband was sterile. They chose artificial insemination and gave birth to a baby boy. The couple separated 4 years after the

child was born, and there were remaining embryos still in storage. The husband wanted them destroyed, and the wife wanted them preserved. What arguments exist for each side?

3. During a first marriage, a woman bore a child after consensual artificial insemination. Her husband was listed as the father on the birth certificate. The couple later separated and then divorced. Both the separation agreement and the divorce decree declared the child to be the offspring of the couple. The wife was granted support and the husband visitation rights. The woman remarried, and her second husband petitioned to adopt the child. The first husband refused his consent. The second husband then suggested that the first husband's consent was not required because he was not the parent of the child. Should the first husband's consent be necessary? What factors would change your position?

4. C.C. had a child who was conceived with sperm donated by C.M. C.C. wanted to have a child and wanted C.M. to be the father but did not want to have intercourse with him before their marriage. He therefore agreed to provide the sperm. After several attempts, C.C. did conceive a child. The relationship between the two parties broke off before they were married, and C.M. wanted visitation rights to the baby. C.C. does not wish to allow visitation rights. What are the arguments for and against allowing visitation rights in this scenario?

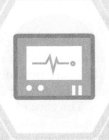

Chapter 12

Death and Dying

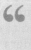 Those who have the strength and the love to sit with a dying patient in the silence that goes beyond words will know that this moment is neither frightening nor painful, but a peaceful cessation of the functioning of the body.

Elisabeth Kübler-Ross, On Death and Dying (1969)

Objectives

After reading this chapter, you should be able to:

1. Identify common influences on an individual's perspectives on death and dying.
2. Summarize the Uniform Determination of Death Act (UDAA).
3. Differentiate among advance directives, living wills, durable power of attorney, and health care proxies.
4. Summarize the basics of the Patient Self-Determination Act (PSDA) of 1990.
5. Define palliative care.
6. Identify the states with death with dignity acts.
7. Explain the need for a do-not-resuscitate (DNR) order from the patient's perspective.
8. Summarize legal and ethical dilemmas related to the decision to keep or remove life support.
9. Summarize legal and ethical arguments for and against euthanasia.

Building Your Legal Vocabulary

Advance directive
Assisted suicide
Cardiopulmonary arrest
Clear and convincing
Durable power of attorney
Euthanasia
Health care proxy
Hospice

Life-sustaining
Living will
Palliative care
Purist
Sanctity
Substitute judgment
Terminally ill

Attitudes Toward Death and Dying

Most health care providers and professionals will, at some point in their careers, care for patients who are dying or who die. The care provided to these terminally ill patients may be customary, such as prescribing medications, taking vitals, or discussing treatment options. The care provided may also be more directly related to death and dying, such as carrying out do-not-resuscitate (DNR) orders or removing life support systems. Ethical issues in health care related to death and dying question both the sanctity and the quality of life.

How we each process death and dying depends on how those influences come together to define our own philosophies about the **sanctity** and quality of life. The issues raised in this chapter are difficult. Your positions on these issues today will be challenged by your experience tomorrow. A variety of influences shape our thoughts and feelings about death and dying, including family, loved ones, religion or spirituality, the media, society, ideas about personal freedom, and life experiences.

Heath care providers, whose first obligation to a patient is to heal, cure, and to do no harm, routinely face questions about death and dying. When a cure is not possible, the health care provider's obligation is to care for and comfort the dying patient. Dr. C. Everett Koop explains his resolution of the conflict:

sanctity The quality of being sacred.

There is this unique tumor of childhood called neuroblastoma in which I have been interested for more than thirty years. Because of this I have developed a broad clinical experience with the behavior of this tumor as it affects the lives of my patients . . . In a given situation I might have as a patient a five-year-old child whose tumor was diagnosed a year ago and who, in spite of all known treatment, has progressed to a place where although her primary tumor has been removed she now has recurrence . . . I know her days of life are limited and that the longer she lives the more likely she is to have considerable pain. She might also become both blind and deaf.

If this five-year-old youngster is quite anemic, her ability to understand what is happening to her might be clouded . . . I can let her exist with a deficient hemoglobin level knowing that it may shorten her life but also knowing that it will be beneficial in the sense that she will not be alert enough to understand all that is happening around her. On the other hand I could be a medical **purist** and give her blood transfusions until her hemoglobin level was up to acceptable standards . . . [S]he would be more conscious of the things happening around her, she would feel her pain more deeply, and she might live longer . . . [A]nd then there are the anticancer drugs which I know without any shadow

purist One who believes in and follows all traditional rules.

of a doubt will not cure this child . . . Would it be better to let this little girl slip into death quietly . . . or should we prolong her life . . . I opt to withhold supportive measures.

Koop, C. E. (1976). *The Right to Live: The Right to Die*, pp. 98–99.
Wheaton, IL: Tyndale House Publishers.

Determination of Death

Ethical, legal, and medical issues arise that require a thorough analysis of the question, "When is a person dead?" The Uniform Determination of Death Act (UDDA) was a response to that question. See Figure 12-1 for some of the reasons why a determination of death can be important. The UDDA is a model act, and it is intended to be a template for state legislations that want to adopt it. The UDDA defines the medical determination of biological death, and it has been adopted by all states with very few modifications.

The UDDA provides the following definition of death: "[a]n individual who has sustained either (1) irreversible cessation of circulatory and respiratory functions or (2) irreversible cessation of all functions of the entire brain, including the brain stem, is dead."

Recent cases that question the Uniform Determination of Death Act, however, have gained attention and fueled debates. In February 2020, Nayim Carter nearly drowned in a pool, when he was 2 years old. When the paramedics arrived, he had no pulse and was not breathing.

Situations Where the Determination of Death Is Crucial
Executing wills and distributing estates A deceased person's will or intestate distribution cannot be made without a determination of death.
Life insurance Life insurance policies require a determination of death before they pay out on the policy.
Tort lawsuits Civil lawsuits that seek to recover damages for someone's death requires a determination of death.
Organ donation A determination of death is required to allow for the harvesting and use of a deceased person's organs.
Criminal matters involving death A determination of death is required to prosecute homicides.

Figure 12-1 Why a Determination of Death Is Important

Nayim was then hospitalized, not responsive and required a ventilator. Nayim's parents refused to authorize brain death tests for a month. They were convinced he needed more time to recover and that God would heal him. When the tests were performed, the results indicated he did not have enough brain activity to sustain life. Nayim's case raised issues about how we currently define brain death, and his case is not an outlier. Nayim passed away in December 2020 while fighting pneumonia. The official cause of death was complications of resuscitated drowning.

Nayim's parent's personal beliefs as to whether their son could recover and whether he was brain dead held more importance for them than the application of the UDDA. In such a case, should the government defer to the parent's beliefs or apply the UDDA? Should science be considered at all given that the parent's beliefs were founded in religion? In response to Nayim's case, Bioethicist Dr. Robert Truog argues that the UDDA needs to be revised to consider this issue and others while also considering the objective evidence raised by science.

> "There have been a number of legal challenges and they continue," said Dr. Robert Truog, the director of bioethics at Harvard Medical and also a professor of medical ethics, anesthesiology and pediatrics. "There is discussion about whether the Uniform Determination of Death Act needs to be revised to address some of these concerns. One (question) is whether patients actually can be considered to be dead based upon the loss of brain function," Truog said. "When other functions may continue. I should be clear that patients who are brain dead have a devastating degree of brain injury, and there's never been anyone who has been diagnosed as brain dead, who has ever had any recovery of consciousness, despite reports that have appeared in the media."
>
> Jones, D. (2021, June 22). Experts Weighs in After Toddler's Death Raises Questions over What It Means to Be 'Brain Dead'. WFTV. Retrieved from www.wftv.com/news/9investigates/experts-weighs-after-toddlers-death-raises-questions-over-what-it-means-be-brain-dead/T4J7WZXEDJCBNEIZNVWSDHCJNI/.

advance directive
A document signed and witnessed according to state statute authorizing one person to make decisions for another, including the authorization or refusal of medical treatment.

Advance Directives

An **advance directive** asserts an individual's right to accept or refuse treatment and gives direction to relatives, friends, and medical professionals. James H. Sammons, former executive vice president of the American Medical Association (AMA), said "From the day [physicians] enter medical school they are taught to cherish and preserve life . . . While physicians should never directly cause death, they must always act in the best interest of the patients, and that sometimes includes allowing them to die." Advance directives can resolve many of the controversies that arise in situations where ethics, law, and medicine collide.

Consider the following: Terri Schiavo, a 41-year-old brain-damaged woman, was the subject of a national right-to-die legal battle. Ms. Schiavo collapsed in her home due to heart failure that led to severe oxygen-deprivation brain damage. Ms. Schiavo's parents, the Schindlers, fought to keep her feeding tube in while Ms. Schiavo's legal guardian, her husband, fought to respect her verbal wish not to be put on life support. The legal dispute between Ms. Schiavo's husband and her parents was exceptionally bitter. The legal battle included legislation passed by Congress that placed the dispute in the federal court system, as well as several appeals to the U.S. Supreme Court, who declined to hear the case.

The Schindlers "can know they have done everything possible under the law in letting government know that they wanted to fight for the life of their daughter," Gibbs said.

In his Supreme Court filing, Gibbs and other lawyers for the parents wrote that removing the tube represented "an unconstitutional deprivation of Terri Schiavo's constitutional right to life."

The Supreme Court's rejection came hours after the 11th U.S. Circuit Court of Appeals in Atlanta, Georgia, rejected the parents' petition 9-2. That court denied three similar requests from the parents last week.

In a concurring opinion of the Atlanta court's latest ruling, Judge Stanley Birch said Congress "chose to overstep constitutional boundaries" by passing a law to force the Schiavo case into federal courts . . .

[T]hree days after Schiavo's feeding tube was removed, Congress passed a bill transferring jurisdiction of the case from Florida state court to a U.S. District Court, for a federal judge to review. President Bush signed it into law the next day. But federal courts refused to overturn the state courts' decision . . .

Florida's 2nd District Court of Appeal heard a week of testimony from five doctors who examined her, including two picked by Michael Schiavo, two by her parents and one picked by the court.

Three doctors, including one appointed by the court, testified that Terri Schiavo was in a persistent vegetative state with no hope of recovery. The two doctors selected by the Schindlers testified they thought she could recover.

The appellate court concurred with a lower court decision that Schiavo had no hope of recovery and that her feeding tube could be removed.

Sosa, N., Franken, B., Phillips, R., Candiotti, S. (2005, March 31).
Terri Schiavo Has Died. CNN. Retrieved from www.cnn.com
/2005/LAW/03/31/schiavo/index.html?iref=newssearch.

Once doctors removed the feeding tube that had kept her alive for more than a decade, it was fewer than two weeks before Ms. Schiavo passed.

In the Terri Schiavo case, the court reaffirmed the **substitute judgment** requirement and found that it was based on **clear and convincing** evidence. In doing so, it allowed the removal of the feeding tube based on permitting her husband to become the decision maker and deciding that he was taking into account her value system and personal belief, as well as her earlier statements about medical treatments. The question was not whether the state had the right to prevent the removal of the tube but that it could not do so without clear and convincing evidence that she would make that same decision if so able. Advance directives are a result of the need for evidence. There are three major forms of advance directives: living will, durable power of attorney, and health care proxy.

Patient Self-Determination Act (PSDA)

The Patient Self-Determination Act, enacted in 1990, requires health care facilities to provide written information to each adult admitted regarding patient rights under state law to make decisions involving the acceptance or refusal of medical or surgical treatment. It also requires documentation of the patient's receipt of this information in the medical record as well as whether a patient has executed an advance directive. Institutions cannot condition care on the provision that the patient execute an advance directive or agree to accept treatment. Health care professionals should know and be able to explain to patients the advance directives options available.

The PSDA governs all hospitals, nursing homes, rehabilitation facilities, home health agencies, and health maintenance organizations and **hospices** that receive Medicare/Medicaid payments. Each entity is required to maintain written policies and procedures regarding advance directives and provide information to patients at the time of admission or enrollment.

Under the PSDA, the regulated facilities must:

- provide written information to patients on admission informing them of their rights under state law to executive advance directives;
- provide written information about how to carry out these rights;
- document whether an advance directive exists for each patient; and,
- educate their staff and community on advance directives.

Living Wills

Most states recognize **living wills**, although state statutes vary in content for the requirement of a valid "living will." Living wills are accepted by the courts, health care providers, the President's Commission for the

---

substitute judgment One person's decision used to make a decision for another.

clear and convincing Legal standard of proof that requires proof that the allegation or contention is far more likely than not to be true.

hospice A medical facility or a home where a terminally ill patient receives palliative care.

living will A will made by a person in which he or she requests to be allowed to die naturally rather than being kept alive by artificial means in the event there is no probable recovery from mental or physical disability.

Study of Ethical Problems in Medicine and Biomedical and Behavioral Research, and lawyers. According to AARP, fewer than 40 percent of American adults have a living will. Living will templates that are valid in your state can be found online.

> There are many reasons to make a living will: to give guidance to your doctors and health care surrogates, provide clarity and closure to your loved ones, prevent conflict or disagreements among family members, and limit the emotional burden on your closest people at the time of your death. Most important is that you remain the captain of your own ship, with the authority to dictate how you want to live and die. Considering that the majority of dying people are unconscious, in distress, or otherwise not able to speak, the living will serves as your voice when you may not have one.
>
> Despite all these reasons, not many Americans have a living will. Well under 40 percent of U.S. adults have created a living will (or similar document). That means that 60 percent are rolling the dice on who will be making decisions for us at the end of our lives. Twenty-five percent report never having thought of end-of-life planning at all. Some simply do not know what the living will is or how it works.
>
> Singleton, A. (2019, August 4). Why All Adults Should Have a Living Will. AARP. Retrieved from www.aarp.org/caregiving/financial -legal/info-2019/what-is-a-living-will.html.

All states have living will statutes. These statutes vary slightly and have differing requirements for the contents and authentication of living wills. A living will is a contract, and it must be executed by a competent person. Its intent is to extend the right to refuse artificial **life-sustaining** procedures into a possible future time of incompetency.

life-sustaining Helping someone to stay alive with medical intervention.

Durable Power of Attorney

The American Medical Association (AMA) suggests the durable power of attorney as a substitute for the living will and suggests further that these be made available in health care providers' offices and hospitals and included as part of the medical record. The AMA compared the living will and the **durable power of attorney** for health care and found that the durable power of attorney covers a broader range of illnesses and situations than the living will. In some states, the durable power of attorney may have a different name, such as medical power of attorney or medical directive.

All 50 states recognize some version of the durable power of attorney, having adopted the Uniform Durable Power of Attorney Act or the

durable power of attorney A document allowing the principal (the person writing the durable power of attorney) to delegate to another person (the agent) the legal authority to act on the principal's behalf.

Uniform Probate Code, or some variation of them. In a durable power of attorney, an individual designates, in writing, another person to act as their decision maker. The document contains the words "this power of attorney shall not be affected by subsequent disability or incapacity of the principal," "[T]his power of attorney shall become effective upon the disability or incapacity of the principal," or similar words indicating the principal's intent that the authority delegated will continue despite disability or incapacity. The authority differs from a regular power of attorney, which terminates upon disability or death.

In most cases, the durable power of attorney is accepted for the clauses of instruction expressly contained within the document. If there is no direction to the agent regarding right-to-die issues, the document is interpreted to mean that the agent has no authority on these issues. Occasionally, the agent may be looked to by a hospital or care provider to assist in a decision, but as a general rule, without instruction for medical treatment, the document cannot be used for that purpose.

Health care durable powers of attorney direct the person appointed to serve as a surrogate in health care decisions under certain circumstances. Again, each state has different requirements, and state bar associations are good resources for identifying these requirements.

Health Care Proxy

health care proxy
Document appointing a specific person to act as a surrogate to make health care decisions for another person under certain circumstances.

All states have enacted legislation empowering patients to use a **health care proxy**. Sometimes known by other terms such as a *directive to health care providers and family* or *surrogates* or some other title, in every case, the legislation provides that the document shall do the following:

1. Identify the principal and the health care agent;
2. Express the intention of the principal that the health care agent has authority to make health care decisions on behalf of the principal;
3. Describe any limitations on the authority of the health care agent;
4. Indicate that the authority of the health care agent to make health care decisions becomes effective upon a determination of incapacity; and
5. Be revoked by notifying the agent or health care provider orally, in writing, or by any other act evidencing specific intent to revoke; by execution of a subsequent health care proxy; or by divorce or legal separation of the principal and spouse when the spouse is the agent.

The Terminally Ill Patient

terminally ill Fatally ill with a condition for which there is no cure.

While advance directives can guide health care for patients unable to make decisions, caring for a **terminally ill** patient presents ethical issues in addition to those raised by advance directives. What is the purpose of providing care to a patient who has no prospect of recovery? In most cases, the objective is to alleviate suffering and ensure the patient is as comfortable as possible. Often in the last months of life, terminally ill patients will receive hospice care that provides **palliative care** and supportive services. Palliative care, which is coordinated medical care intended to provide relief from a seriously ill patient's physical or mental discomfort, is the keystone of medical care for terminally ill patients. Hospice care can take place in hospice-dedicated facilities or in patients' homes.

The National Public Radio program, *This American Life*, featured an episode dedicated to death and taxes. The segment on death focused on hospice care, as seen through the eyes of Nancy Updike, who experienced the natural death of a loved one in hospice. An excerpted transcript of the radio program follows.

palliative care Care intended to keep a patient with a serious or terminal illness as comfortable as possible.

Nancy Updike

. . . I had never seen the kind of expertise these nurses had. They knew death. They seemed to understand it, whereas I, even though I had just watched someone fade away and die right in front of me, all I could think was, what just happened?

. . .

Nancy Updike

. . . But there's a huge difference between dying and the very last part of dying, what Pattie and the other nurses call actively dying, a process that can take hours or even days. But it's different from what comes before. And being familiar with one doesn't mean you'll recognize the other.

. . .

Pattie Burnham

It's a weird thing, because when I came to work at the Kaplan house—and I was a registered nurse and had worked as a nurse for a while—I followed another nurse, Jeanette, for a month. And I was floored by the whole dying process, because it was nothing that I had learned. And I saw Jeanette say to a family—she woke them up and said, he's dying. He's dying right now.

And the man had been there, the patient had been there for a week. And I didn't know what was different. I didn't know what she saw that was different.

And when I asked her to explain it to me and to teach it to me, she said, you'll know. You just need about a month here and you'll know.

Nancy Updike

I talked to a palliative care doctor who told me that the most important thing she got better at with experience was looking for openings that allow you to be helpful, little windows, little moments. With hospice, part of that is trying to

(Continues)

(Continued)

help people take in, bit by bit, the realness of what's happening. Some dying people—no surprise—are not at all OK with the fact that they're dying. And they don't often get a chance to just say so.

. . .

Dying is a constant series of judgment calls and decisions based on options that are very far from what anyone would want. And one thing the nurses are experienced at is trying to make the best of those narrow options.

. . .

But all the stories seemed to be trying to tackle the same huge question. How did we get here?

Pattie Burnham

Grief is one thing. But watching somebody die is a whole other thing.

. . .

Nancy Updike

I asked Pattie if anyone, at the end of that list, says, well, I'm just afraid of dying. I fear death. She said yes. And she listens if they want to talk about it, offers to bring in the chaplain or the social worker.

What else is there? That might be the biggest thing that she and the other nurses know that we don't. They know the limits of what they can do.

Updike, N. (2014, March 25). Death and Taxes. *This American Life.* Retrieved from www.thisamericanlife.org/radio-archives/episode/523/transcript.

Palliative care, including pain management, end of life issues, and emotional support, among others, squarely addresses issues of impending death. In some instances, terminally ill patients are in hospice because they have chosen to forego medical treatment that might extend their lives. In other instances, patients are in hospice because there are no other options. In both cases, most hospice patients find that palliative care allows them to focus on their families, themselves, and other practical issues related to death. What specific ethical issues arise from the care of a terminally ill patient?

The Right to Die

As of 2021, ten U.S. states have enacted death with dignity statutes, including California, Colorado, District of Columbia, Hawaii, Maine, New Jersey, New Mexico, Oregon, Vermont, and Washington, as shown in Figure 12-2. In addition, physician-assisted death was ruled legal by Montana's state

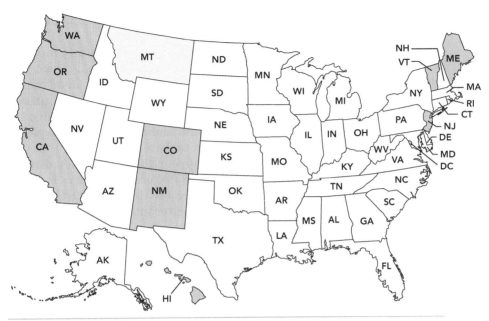

Figure 12-2 States with Death With Dignity Statutes

Supreme Court. The term "death with dignity" is also known as physician-assisted death, right to die, physician-assisted suicide, or aid-in-death acts, among others. Advocates prefer the term death with dignity.

Death with dignity acts allow adults who are residents of the state with the act and who have a terminal illness with fewer than 6 months to live to be prescribed medication to accelerate their death. The acts allow those with terminal illnesses to control how and when their lives will end. Each act has its own specific requirements and protocols.

If refusing treatment may be an appropriate choice, just as choosing treatment may be an appropriate choice, then do health care providers, with the intent of providing a "death with dignity," have the obligation to inform patients of the various ways of dying that are available to them or to assist them with dying? It appears that some health care providers do and that they may have followers ready to assist them in helping patients to die. Michigan health care provider Jack Kevorkian served 8 years of a 10- to 25-year prison sentence for second-degree murder after he administered a lethal injection into a terminal patient. He was released on parole due to good behavior and, perhaps, changes in societal perceptions about a patient's right to die.

Given changes in societal attitudes toward medical intervention in death and dying, the spate of discussion regarding the right to choose medical procedures in the face of death is not surprising.

The right to die debate continues, as do efforts to legalize such action. A contract to murder is an illegal contract and unenforceable under contract law. Each state has at least one statute that makes killing another person a felony. In some states, it is a crime to attempt to commit death by suicide, and in others, it is a crime to aid in a suicide.

Members of the families who have killed another family member with the intent of relieving suffering have been confronted by the criminal justice system. In Florida, a man shot his wife who was in advanced stages of Alzheimer's disease, and he was sentenced to life imprisonment. In Massachusetts, under similar circumstances, a husband suffocated his wife by placing her head in a plastic bag and sealing it with duct tape. He was not sentenced to prison but placed on probation.

The question is this: When does it appear that a patient's disease has progressed to a point where recovery is not possible? There is a possibility that family or others can influence the decision. Further, how will competence be shown? Competence to enter into a contract is a legal issue that may require a psychiatric evaluation.

The diagnosis of Alzheimer's disease can also be challenging for the healthy spouse due to the length of the disease and the cost of treatment. State law requires couples to spend down to a certain level before either one of the parties is eligible for Medicaid. In some states, the family home will be lost to pay the expenses, whereas in others, a lien will be placed on the property to pay off whatever welfare spends during the time of crisis.

The durable power of attorney, living will, and health care proxies are legal instruments that ensure that personal preferences are known when competence is questioned. The moral implications of euthanasia, however, are still questioned by society. The right to choose encompasses a spectrum of decisions related to the following questions: What medical efforts are permissible should a patient experience cardiopulmonary arrest? When is it permissible to remove life support? And, is death by suicide or euthanasia an option?

Do-Not-Resuscitate Orders

cardiopulmonary arrest Cessation of normal functioning of the heart and lungs.

As a result of the treatment of **cardiopulmonary arrest** with cardiopulmonary resuscitation (CPR), patients may be literally brought back to life after the traditional signs of a death have appeared. Whether CPR should be used on every patient is a question that haunts institutional professionals. This decision remains the province of the patient when they have executed an advance directive that includes an order to the health care provider not to resuscitate, a DNR order (in some states, referred to as a directive to health care providers). It is estimated that approximately 80 percent of the 2 million people who die in the United States each year die in institutions. Each institution has professionals trained to respond to a nonresponsive patient with CPR. Is it practicing good medicine to require CPR for every patient, or should it be used like every treatment and prescribed on an individual basis? If CPR is not attempted, is the staff medically abandoning the patient? If an agreement is made between the staff and the patient that this particularly invasive procedure will not be utilized, is the patient psychologically abandoned? These are all ethical and legal questions that must be answered by the practicing professional.

Although awareness of the legal need to have DNR orders in effect, if that is what is desired, has increased, clear guidelines for making those wishes known have not been well established. This can lead to action that is not in accord with the patient's wishes. Sometimes, it takes extraordinary measures to ensure medical care is aligned with one's wishes.

A 70-year-old man was admitted to the hospital. He was unconscious, had a history of serious health problems, and at the time of admittance had a high blood alcohol level. He had no identification on him, and there was no family or friends with him. The hospital staff was surprised when they discovered a tattoo on his chest that read: "Do Not Resuscitate." The health care providers initially did not want to use the tattoo as a directive for medical care since there was no way to confirm that was the intent of the tattoo. The hospital's ethicist saw the tattoo as an "authentic preference," and that the providers' caution in relying on the tattoo "could also be seen as standing on ceremony, and that the law is sometimes not nimble enough to support patient-centered care and respect for patients' best interests." The ethicists' position was corroborated when the hospital located an out-of-hospital DNR that was in agreement with the patient's tattoo.

Willingham, A. J. (2017, December 2). A Man's Tattoo Left Doctors Debating Whether to Save His Life. CNN. Retrieved from www.cnn.com/2017/12/01 /health/dnr-do-no-resuscitate-tattoo-medical-debate-trnd/index.html.

A DNR order only works if the health care provider knows that it exists. Whose responsibility is it to identify whether a patient has a DNR order? What are the ethical issues associated with a provider who refuses to acknowledge a patient's DNR order? What if the provider's refusal is based upon their own personal religious beliefs?

Removal of Life Support

Prolonging life today is often a treatment decision. The provider may make this decision, but it is typically other health care professionals who carry out day-to-day patient care. The withholding of food and water is an indication that the medical community is no longer going to continue nurturing the patient. It is an intentional act. The case involving the removal of the feeding tube from a young woman mentioned earlier in this chapter, Terri Schiavo, became a rallying point for both those supporting the right to die and those supporting the right to life. Over the course of weeks, it led to numerous court actions, legislative action on the state and federal level, direct action by the President of the United States and the Governor of Florida, extensive media coverage, widespread protests, statements from religious leaders, and much more. It underscores the range of opinion and the deep emotional commitments surrounding such issues of life and death. The debate on the removal of feeding tubes shows that there are no easy answers, often just more questions. As the following article shows, even the Catholic Church has had to struggle with the issues involved.

The ethical and moral dilemmas surrounding the end of life can be some of the most difficult and heartrending that most people ever face, and Ms. Schiavo's long coma and the struggle over who should decide what to do about it attracted huge attention and sent off political and social shock waves that still reverberate.

Even the Vatican, whose views on matters of life and death tend to be fairly absolute, had to deliberate for two years over how to answer a request for guidance on cases like Ms. Schiavo's that was posed by American bishops after she died in 2005 . . .

Agence France Presse quotes the question posed by the bishops:

"When nutrition and hydration are being supplied by artificial means to a patient in a 'permanent vegetative state,' may they be discontinued when competent health care providers judge with moral certainty that the patient will never recover consciousness?"

And the answer, from the Congregation for the Doctrine of the Faith, the Vatican office in charge of laying down the law:

"No. A patient in a 'permanent vegetative state' is a person with fundamental human dignity and must, therefore, receive ordinary and proportionate care which includes, in principle, the administration of water and food even by artificial means."

That word "must" makes the answer a pretty stark one: there would seem to be no room left even for a patient's own explicit wishes not to be kept alive in a coma past any hope of recovery, something that many people include in written "living wills" that are meant to spare their loved ones any doubts about such a potentially agonizing decision.

Lyons, P. J. (2007, September 14). Still More Fallout from the Terri Schiavo Case. *The New York Times.* Retrieved from www.thelede.blogs.nytimes.com /2007/09/14/still-more-fallout-from-the-terry-schiavo-case /?scp=2&sq=Terry%20Schiavo%20&st=cse.

It has been legally recognized that individuals have the right to make decisions affecting their own death. Procedures exist to document a dying person's wishes while the person is still considered legally competent.

The ethical conflict in these cases is the tension between the obligation to prevent death and the obligation to prevent suffering.

Euthanasia

Euthanasia, usually refers to an act in which one person kills another, at the request of and for the benefit of the one who dies. Suicide is the taking of one's own life. There is a blurring of the terms **assisted suicide** and *euthanasia*. **Euthanasia**—also known as mercy killing—which is when someone actively assists another to terminate their life at their request. As far back as Hippocrates (460–370 B.C.), "the physician is discouraged from invading the atrium of death" and instructed that, in certain circumstances, "attempts to cure must yield to attempts to comfort." Hippocrates' treatise *The Art* instructs physicians "(1) to do away with the sufferings of the sick, (2) to lessen the violence of their diseases, and (3) to refuse to treat those who are over mastered by their diseases realizing that in such cases medicine is powerless."

There are many arguments made against euthanasia:

1. There could be a mistake in diagnosis.
2. There may be difficulty in determining if euthanasia is voluntary—for example, where there is an undue influence exerted on the patient by a member of the family and/or beneficiary of a will for financial reasons.
3. It could lead to a slippery slope; for example, with the growth of managed care, there may be more financial pressure to hasten death for those who are elderly, uneducated, on welfare, or disabled.
4. Altering the role of health care providers to include the practice of killing patients would bring about a psychological upheaval in the patient–provider relationship, and patients would become less trustful of their provider's role as a healer.

In addition, some examples of euthanasia's slippery slope are from Holland, where there has been a right to die statute since 2002: A gay man in Holland who could not accept his sexuality sought to end his life; a person who was sexually abused and who suffered from severe post-traumatic stress disorder sought to end her life, which prompted a second person who had been sexually abused to seek the same; and a woman who had a pathological fear of germs ended her life via the statute. Who decides what illnesses warrant permission to die in this manner here in the United States? What considerations are factored into the decision?

According to *Black's Law Dictionary*, euthanasia is the act or practice of painlessly putting to death persons suffering from incurable and distressing disease as an act of mercy. It presents legal and ethical problems within the walls of a health care facility as well as without, as shown in the following article:

assisted suicide One person making it possible for another person to commit suicide.

euthanasia An intentional action or lack of action causing the merciful death of someone suffering from a terminal illness or incurable condition.

Eighty-one-year-old Frank Kavanaugh shot his 88-year-old wife in her nursing room bed and then shot himself. Those who knew Kavanaugh maintained that acts were aligned with his long-time advocacy for and on strong convictions that the couple shared regarding personal decision making at the end of life. For Kavanaugh, the shootings were an act of love and loyalty. Some considered Kavanaugh's shootings to be a murder and a suicide. Others considered it to be an assisted suicide and a suicide.

Two days before the shootings, Kavanaugh told his adult son "You know, your mom says she just wants to die." Kavanaugh's son responded, "You know, as an advocate for the right to die and death with dignity, you have to acknowledge that as a legitimate statement." Kavanaugh responded, "You're right."

Peters Smith, B. (2016, June 19). 58 Years of Loving Marriage Ends with Two Gunshots. *Herald-Tribune*. Retrieved from www.heraldtribune.com /news/20160619/58-years-of-loving-marriage-ends-with-two-gunshots.

The issue of euthanasia is a difficult one for society and the courts. The issue of euthanasia also surfaced in the aftermath of Hurricane Katrina in the New Orleans Memorial Medical Center.

The New Orleans community has reacted with fury toward Foti's office and sympathy for head and neck surgeon Anna Pou, MD, and nurses Lori Budo and Cheri Landry, who were arrested in July upon Foti's announcement that his office had uncovered evidence the women intentionally euthanized four patients at Memorial Medical Center in the desperate days following Katrina. Physicians have responded with questions about the evidence Foti has gathered, and laypeople have reacted to what they view as the vilification of health care professionals who didn't have to stay with patients at all and were, many bloggers, editorial letter writers, and radio talk-show callers say, merely trying to ease the suffering of their patients . . .

Foti accuses Pou, an associate professor of otolaryngology at the Louisiana State University School of Medicine, and the two nurses of intentionally administering lethal doses of morphine and the anxiolytic midazolam (Versed) to four patients on Sept. 1, 2005—three days after Katrina hit New Orleans. The four were patients of Lifecare, a long-term acute-care unit located within Memorial Medical Center.

Flooding after the hurricane stranded the hospital, which had no electricity or safe water. Medical and food supplies were nearly gone, and the temperature inside was more than 100°F. Some patients had been evacuated, but most Lifecare patients were physically unable to get out on their own power, and the hospital staff were desperately trying to arrange evacuation.

Within days of the final evacuation of the hospital, rumors began spreading that an unnamed female physician had been seen entering patients' rooms carrying syringes, and that those patients later died. The four patients Foti listed in his complaint against Pou and the nurses included two men and two women, ranging in age from 61 to 90. At least one was paralyzed, two were described as extremely ill, and one was reportedly convalescing.

Foti stated in a press conference that toxicology reports showed lethal amounts of the drugs in the patients' bodies, and that Pou had allegedly told a Lifecare nurse executive that lethal doses were administered to patients too sick to be moved.

"This is a homicide. It is not euthanasia," Foti stated in announcing the case against the women.

Relias Media. (2006, September 1). Arrest of Katrina Doctor, Nurses Stirs Up Strong Support for the Accused. Retrieved from www.reliasmedia.com/articles/122579 -arrest-of-katrina-doctor-nurses-stirs-up-strong-support-for-the-accused.

The Grand Jury refused to indict Dr. Pou and the others for murder and the criminal charges were dropped.

Twenty-nine-year-old Brittany Maynard suffered from terminal brain cancer. She moved to Oregon from California because of its right to die statute. Maynard ended her life on November 1, 2014, but she is partially credited with inspiring the passage of California's right to die statute.

Brittany Maynard, the terminally ill 29-year-old who spent her final days advocating for death-with-dignity laws, took lethal drugs prescribed by her physician on Saturday and died, a spokesman said, "as she intended—peacefully in her bedroom, in the arms of her loved ones."

Maynard, who was diagnosed earlier this year with a stage 4 malignant brain tumor, said last month she planned to die Nov. 1 in her home in Portland, Ore., with help from her doctor. And Saturday, she said farewell, having succeeded at reviving interest—and debate—in a charged subject that had been out of the news for some years . . .

Maynard's journey began on New Year's Day when she was diagnosed with brain cancer. By April, she was told she had six months to live. She looked at treatment options—and side effects. She considered hospice care.

(Continues)

Then she made her decision: doctor-assisted death.

"After months of research, my family and I reached a heartbreaking conclusion," she wrote in an op-ed for CNN. "There is no treatment that would save my life, and the recommended treatments would have destroyed the time I had left."

Bever, L. (2014, November 2). Brittany Maynard, As Promised, Ends Her Life at 29. *The Washington Post*. Retrieved from www.washingtonpost.com/news/morning-mix/wp/2014/11/02/brittany-maynard-as-promised-ends-her-life-at-29/.

Death by Suicide   What happens when rather than getting loved ones involved in euthanasia, terminally ill patients choose death by suicide? Suicide is a traumatic event for the surviving loved ones, who often experience guilt and the feeling that they could have prevented the suicide. There is nothing more that can be done to help the patient after a suicide. The attention of providers and professionals turns to the loved ones to help them deal with their loss. There often is anger, questions about mental health, guilt, and sorrow. In many religions, suicide is prohibited. How does the trauma of the surviving loved ones support arguments in favor of and against euthanasia?

☑ SUMMARY

- Working as a health care professional requires an ability to deal with death and dying on a regular basis. The manner in which a professional handles these matters reflects personal philosophies.

- The Uniform Determination of Death Act, which has been enacted in some form by all 50 states, defines the medical determination of biological death.

- The durable power of attorney, living will, and health care proxy are legal instruments that ensure personal preferences, including health care choices, are known when a patient becomes unable to make the choice themself.

- The Patient Self-Determination Act of 1980 requires health care facilities to provide written information to each adult admission regarding patient rights under state law to make decisions involving the acceptance or refusal of medical or surgical treatment.

- Palliative care seeks to provide relief from pain and signs of a serious illness, regardless of the diagnosis or stage of disease and to improve patients' quality of life.

- As of 2021, nine U.S. states have enacted death with dignity statutes, including California, Colorado, District of Columbia, Hawaii, Maine, New Jersey, New Mexico, Oregon, Vermont, and Washington. In addition, physician-assisted death was ruled legal by Montana's state Supreme Court.

- Whether CPR should be used on every patient is a question that haunts institutional professionals. This decision remains the province of the patient when they have executed an advance directive that includes an order to the physician not to resuscitate, a DNR order.

- It has been legally recognized that individuals have the right to make decisions affecting their own death. Procedures exist to document a dying person's wishes while the person is still considered legally competent.

- Euthanasia usually refers to an act in which one person kills another, at the request of and for the benefit of the one who dies. The moral implications of euthanasia are still questioned by society.

SUGGESTED ACTIVITIES

1. Interview a physician and a religious professional. Document the standards each has about life-support systems and whether they should be used on a terminally ill patient. Note the development of their personal philosophies that has led to their current thinking. Ask what incidents might change their present beliefs.

2. Research the criteria for a pronouncement of death in your state.

3. Use the Internet to find an example of a living will for the state where you live or work.

4. Listen to "Death and Taxes" (Act One – Death), Episode 523 of *This American Life* (April 25, 2014) (excerpted earlier in this chapter) and identify the different types of palliative care described.

5. Look up the durable power of attorney or living will statute in your state. What types of legal protection does your state provide for people using these instruments?

STUDY QUESTIONS

1. Explain your philosophy regarding euthanasia.

2. Why would a patient want a DNR order?

3. What are the factors you consider when identifying your position on the right to die?

CASES FOR DISCUSSION

1. The patient was a man 34 years of age. He left a store and walked toward his car. The defendant, a young man of 18 years, tiptoed behind him and hit him on the head with a baseball bat. He then went into a building, changed his clothes, crossed the street, and entered the store where he worked. When asked why he had hit the man, he said, "For kicks." At the hospital, the patient was placed on an artificial respirator. Two days later, the patient victim's blood pressure, heart-beat, and pulse were not observable; he was unable to breathe when taken off the respirator; and an electroencephalogram did not reveal any cerebral electrical activity. In the opinion of the physician, the patient had reached the stage of irreversible brain death. Two days later, the patient was again taken off the respirator with the same outcome. After consultation with the patient's family, the respirator was removed and his heart stopped. The defendant was found guilty of first-degree murder with the requirement of death satisfied by the proof of brain death. The defendant appealed, stating that "death," as required by the law, never occurred. How should the court rule?

2. For reasons still unclear, the patient ceased breathing for at least two 15-minute periods. She received some ineffectual mouth-to-mouth resuscitation from friends. She was taken by ambulance to the hospital, where she had a temperature of 100°F and was unresponsive to deep pain. She lapsed into a coma. Medical evidence indicated that she suffered severe brain damage, leaving her in a "chronic and persistent vegetative state." The patient was kept alive through the use of respirators and other medical life support systems while her body underwent a continuing deteriorative process. There was no known treatment to improve her condition. Her father requested that life-support systems be withdrawn, but the attending physician refused because the patient did not meet the traditional medical standard for death. Her heart had not stopped nor was she brain dead. If the life-support systems are removed, should the physician be subject to civil or criminal liability?

3. An 83-year-old monk entered the hospital for a routine hernia operation. During the course of the surgery, he suffered cardiopulmonary arrest. When resuscitated, it was found that he was in a chronic vegetative condition. The patient, following his religious convictions, agreed with the Catholic Church's teachings that heroic measures to prolong life were unnecessary. He had discussed those issues in conversations involving other cases and had clearly stated he did not want any extraordinary measures taken to prolong his own life. His guardian asked physicians to remove the respirator that was keeping him alive. They refused. The surgeon asserted that after such a medical procedure was started, it should not be withdrawn. A spokesman

for the hospital stated that the hospital's mission was to do all that it could to maintain life. The guardian then went to court. What should the court decide?

4. At approximately midnight, a patient complained to his wife of a severe headache and lapsed into unconsciousness. Angiograms revealed he had an aneurysm at the apex of the basilar artery. The patient underwent a craniotomy following which a clip was inserted across the aneurysm. The patient never regained consciousness. The patient was put on a respirator. Nutrition was provided through a nasogastric feeding tube. He was later diagnosed as being in a semi-vegetative or vegetative state. Do-not-resuscitate orders were placed in the patient's chart, a gastrostomy tube was inserted, and the nasogastric tube removed. Although the patient's electroencephalogram was abnormal, it did indicate controlled electrical activity generated by millions of cortical nerves, which were normal. Apart from the brain injury, the patient was not terminally ill. The patient's wife, who was also his guardian, requested that the hospital staff remove the gastrostomy tube. They refused, and the matter went to court. Should the court allow removal of the tube?

5. The patient was an 84-year-old bedridden woman with serious and irreversible physical and mental impairment. She was confined to bed and unable to move out of the fetal position. In addition, she suffered from arteriosclerotic heart disease, hypertension, and diabetes, and her left leg was gangrenous to the knee. She had several decubitus necrotic ulcers on her feet, legs, and hips, and an eye problem that required irrigation. She was unable to speak, and her ability to swallow was limited. There was a urinary catheter in place, and she could not control her bowels. Experts determined that she was not brain dead, comatose, or in a vegetative state. Her nephew and guardian wanted to remove the nasogastric feeding tube. Should the court allow it?

Glossary

A

abandon To give up or cease doing.

acceptance An agreement to the terms of an offer.

adjudicate To decide a disputed matter.

advance directives A document signed and witnessed according to state statute authorizing one person to make decisions for another, including the authorization or refusal of medical treatment.

adversary An opponent in a dispute or contest.

affirmative duty An obligation to do or to not do something.

age of majority The age, as determined by state law, at which a person becomes legally able to contract.

agent One who has authority to act on behalf of another.

allocation The act of distributing something.

amniocentesis Test used during pregnancy to diagnose a fetus' genetic disorders and other health issues.

amoral Without consideration of morals.

arbitration A hearing held between two or more parties who disagree on an issue but agree in advance to abide by the decision of an impartial third party.

assault Any intentional act, attempt, or threat to inflict bodily injury on another person with the apparent ability to do so.

assisted suicide One person making it possible for another person to commit suicide.

assumption of risk Voluntary acceptance of a known danger.

autonomy Allowing individuals control over themselves.

B

bargaining unit The labor union, or group of employees with similar interests, authorized to conduct negotiations on behalf of the employees who are members of the union or group.

battery Intentional touching of another person without permission.

beyond a reasonable doubt Evidence so strong and credible that it leaves no more than a remote possibility that there is another explanation for what happened.

bioethics Ethical issues and the implications of the application of biological research.

breach To act contrary to a contractual provision or to fail to perform a contractual provision.

burnout Exhaustion from overwork.

bylaws Regulations adopted by a corporation or association to govern its internal affairs.

C

capitation Payment in a lump sum to providers, HMOs, and health care facilities to deliver health care to a segment of the population.

cardiopulmonary arrest Cessation of normal functioning of the heart and lungs.

censure A formal statement of disapproval.

certification Endorsement by an accredited professional organization that the holder has specific expertise as evidenced by passing an examination.

chemotherapy Drug treatment, most often used in the treatment of cancer, that uses potent chemicals to kill fast-growing cells.

civil The system of law concerned with disputes between individuals or, where the case does not relate to the violation of a criminal statute, between an individual and the state.

clear and convincing Legal standard of proof that requires proof that the allegation or contention is far more likely than not to be true.

cloning Identically duplicating an organism.

collective bargaining Procedural attempt to achieve collective agreements between an employer and accredited representative of a group of employees, to improve the conditions of employment.

common law Law created as a result of judicial decisions.

comparative negligence Negligence measured by percentage, with the determined damages lessened according to the extent of injury or damage committed by the party proven guilty.

concurrent Two or more events happening at the same time.

confidentiality Not disclosing information to those who are not authorized to receive it.

conglomerate A corporation diversifying operations by acquiring varied businesses.

conservator A court-appointed person given authority to manage the financial affairs of an incompetent person.

consideration Something promised that results in making an agreement a lawful, enforceable contract.

conspiracy An agreement among two or more people to undertake an illegal act.

consumer A person who uses products or services.

contingency Something that may occur but is dependent on a different and uncertain future event to happen first.

contract A voluntary agreement, written or unwritten, between two parties that creates an obligation to do or not do something.

contributory negligence Conduct by a plaintiff that is below the standard to which he or she is legally required to conform for his or her own protection.

criminal The system of law concerned with offenses prosecuted by and deemed prohibited by state or federal law, or a person who has been proven guilty of such an offense.

cross-examination Attorney's interrogation of a witness by the other party's attorney.

D

data Pieces of information.

defendant A person or party against whom a civil plaintiff has initiated a lawsuit to settle a dispute; in a criminal matter, a person or party that has been charged with a crime and who is being prosecuted.

defensive medicine The practice of medicine where the main focus is preventing a lawsuit rather than improving the health of the patient.

deposition A sworn verbal statement given out of court in response to questions posed by attorneys involved in the case and transcribed by a court reporter.

deterrence Punishment used to discourage crime.

dilemma Situation where a challenging decision must be made between two or more options.

direct examination Attorney's interrogation of a witness by the party for whom the witness has been called.

directors Those elected and terminated by stockholders to manage a corporation.

disparate impact Disproportionate result that seemingly fair practices or policies have upon a protected group.

disparate treatment A marked difference between the way two things are handled.

dividends Distributed profits of a corporation.

DNA   Molecule within cells that holds genetic information responsible for the development and performance of an organism.

durable power of attorney   A document allowing the principal (the person writing the durable power of attorney) to delegate to another person (the agent) the legal authority to act on the principal's behalf.

duress   Being influenced by threat to do something one would not otherwise do.

E

emancipated minor   A person under the age of majority who is deemed to be completely self-supporting and able to contract.

embryonic stem cells   Cells that are derived from human embryos or human fetal tissues that are self-replicating.

embryos   Fertilized eggs in the early stages of development.

enumerate   To list a number of things.

ethical   Conforming to professionally proper conduct.

ethics   Moral principles that guide a person or a society's choices and conduct.

etiquette   Prescribed code of courteous social behavior.

euthanasia   An intentional action or lack of action causing the merciful death of someone suffering from a terminal illness or incurable condition.

expert witness   A person whose education, profession, or specialized experience qualifies them to testify about their area of expertise as it relates to the lawsuit.

express contract   An explicit agreement between two or more parties.

F

facially neutral   On the surface the matter appears to be impartial.

fee-for-service   Basis of professional billing, either so much per hour or per identified procedure.

felony   A crime that is generally punishable by imprisonment for a sentence longer than a year.

fetus   Unborn, developing offspring from the period beginning 8 weeks (when the major structures have formed) after fertilization of an egg by a sperm until the time of birth.

G

genetic   Resulting from genes or attributable to them.

Good Samaritan   A person who helps another person in distress even though there is no duty to do so.

grossly negligent   Deliberately failing to perform a necessary duty in extraordinary disregard of the consequences to the person neglected.

guardian   A person entrusted to take care of the person, property, and rights of someone too young or otherwise incapable of managing their own affairs.

H

health care proxy   Document appointing a specific person to act as a surrogate to make health care decisions for another person under certain circumstances.

herd immunity   The eradication or slowing of the spread of a disease that occurs when a high enough percentage of the population is immune to the disease and it can no longer spread.

heterologous artificial insemination   An artificial insemination procedure wherein a sperm sample is taken from a donor who is not the partner of the woman seeking to become pregnant.

homologous artificial insemination   An artificial insemination procedure wherein a sperm sample is taken from a donor who is the partner of the woman seeking to become pregnant.

hospice   A medical facility or a home where a terminally ill patient receives palliative care.

I

immoral   Not moral.

implied contract   An agreement not indicated by direct words but evident from the conduct of the parties.

incompetent persons Those who lack the necessary qualifications to perform a duty.

inference A process of reasoning by which a fact is deduced as a logical consequence of other facts.

injunctive relief Remedy preventing or requiring someone to perform or to refrain from performing a particular action.

insurance A contract binding one party to compensate another for specific losses, damages, or injury in exchange for the payment of premiums.

interrogatory Written questions about a case addressed to one party or witness by another party.

interstate commerce The movement of goods and services, or services that rely on the movement of goods, which cross state borders within the United States.

investment Expenditure of resources (money, effort, etc.) intended to secure income or profit.

invitee A person who enters another's property as a result of express or implied invitation.

J

joint venture A group of persons together performing some specific business undertaking that is limited in duration or scope.

judgment A court's decision regarding the rights and obligations of the parties in a lawsuit.

L

larceny Taking the personal property of another with the intent to permanently deprive that person of their property.

legal capacity A person's ability to enter into contracts because no legal disabilities exist.

legal disability Lack of legal capacity for mutual agreement.

legal entity An individual or organization that has legal capacity to contract, incur and pay debts, and sue and be sued.

licensee A person who has express or implied permission to enter another's property.

licensure Completion of basic minimum qualifications required by the state for that profession.

life-sustaining Helping someone to stay alive with medical intervention.

living will A will made by a person in which he or she requests to be allowed to die naturally rather than being kept alive by artificial means in the event there is no probable recovery from mental or physical disability.

M

malice An unjust intention to commit an illegal act to injure someone.

manslaughter The killing of a person without premeditation.

mature minor A person under the age of majority who has the mental capacity to make certain medical decisions without parental consent.

mediation A neutral party meets with parties to a dispute with the intent of persuading them to settle their dispute.

mental incompetence Lack of reasoning faculties needed to enable someone to contract.

minors Persons who are under the age of majority as set forth by state law.

misdemeanor A crime that is generally punishable by a fine or imprisonment of less than a year.

mitigating Make less severe due to considerations of fairness and mercy.

motion The application made to a judge to take a specific action in a case.

murder An act done with intent to kill the victim.

mutual agreement Common agreement and understanding of all parties to a contract.

N

negligence Failure to act with reasonable and prudent care given the circumstances.

negligent act Failure to take reasonable precautions to protect others from the risk of harm.

negligent per se Conduct that is not aligned with the applicable standard of care and without more can be deemed negligence.

negotiated fee schedules The amount an insurance company or other third-party payer will reimburse for a specific medical procedure.

negotiation Exchange and consideration of offers with the objective of reaching an agreement.

nonverbal communication Body language used to communicate something.

notice An announcement of pertinent information to those who have a right or obligation to know.

O

offer A proposal to perform or refrain from a certain action.

officers Persons holding formal positions of trust in an organization, especially those involved in high levels of management.

P

palliative care Care intended to keep a patient with a serious or terminal illness as comfortable as possible.

paternalism Providing for people's needs but giving them no responsibility or control over their destiny.

patient–provider privilege Legal doctrine that protects communications between a patient and a provider from disclosure in court.

peer review Assessment of academic, professional, or scientific work by others who are experts in the same field.

per capita payment Pay equally according to the number of individuals.

perjury A false statement under oath.

philosophy A basic viewpoint of an individual's or a community's value system.

plaintiff A person or party who brings a civil court action against a person or party with whom they have a dispute.

pluralistic Political philosophy wherein people of different beliefs, political parties, and lifestyles coexist and take part equally in the political process.

preimplantation genetic diagnosis Genetic testing used to identify whether a parent's known genetic defect is present in an embryo produced by in vitro fertilization.

premises Physical location, such as an office or building.

preponderance of the evidence The greater weight of the evidence that is more likely than not.

pretrial conference A meeting of the parties and the judge to discuss the readiness for and details of trial process.

principal The employer, or source of authority, of the agent or employee.

privacy Being protected from public scrutiny or having your personal information shared without your permission.

privileged communication A communication (written or verbal) that occurs between two or more people that is protected by law from disclosure in court (see also patient–provider privilege).

probable cause Having more evidence for than against.

product liability A tort making a manufacturer liable for compensation to anyone using its product if damages or injuries occur from defects in that product.

property right A right of ownership to a certain thing.

protected health information Information held by a covered entity (see Table 9-1 for a definition) related to a patient's health status, their health care, or payment for health care.

proximate cause Results as a direct consequence and without which the result would not have happened.

purist One who believes in and follows all traditional rules.

Q

quality assurance Procedures and protocols that maintain a stated level of quality of care received by patients.

qui tam lawsuit A lawsuit alleging fraud and initiated by a whistleblower who receives a share of any recovery as a reward.

R

reasonable care   The amount of care a rational person would use in similar circumstances.

reasonable person   A prudent person whose behavior would be considered appropriate under the circumstances.

reformation   The rehabilitation of a criminal.

registration   Recordation and maintenance of professionals' license-related administrative information.

remedies   Ways to make a nonbreaching party whole after a contracting party has breached.

res ipsa loquitur ("the thing speaks for itself")   Evidence showing that negligence by the defendant may be reasonably inferred from the nature of the injury occurring to the plaintiff.

respondeat superior   Legal theory that holds employer responsible for the behavior of an employee working within the scope of employment.

restraint   Restriction of personal liberty.

retribution   Something given or demanded as a punishment for criminal wrongdoing.

risk management   The practice of considering the risk of actions taken and taking steps to minimize the undesired risks of those actions.

robbery   The forcible stealing of the personal property of another either from their person or in the immediate presence of the victim.

S

sanctioned   Penalized for violating a law or accepted procedure.

sanctity   The quality of being sacred.

scope of practice   The tasks and services that a qualified health care professional is considered competent and allowed to perform pursuant to their license, or, if no license, their education, and experience.

shares   Units of stock giving the possessor part ownership in a corporation.

sociological   Pertaining to human social behavior.

specific performance   The remedy of requiring a party to a contract to perform the contract as specified.

standard of care   The amount of care that a reasonable person in similar circumstances would exercise.

standard of proof   Level of proof required, which is established by considering all evidence and witnesses.

statute of limitations   The law setting a time limit within which one person can sue another.

statutory guidelines   Legislative laws defining legal rights and responsibilities.

stockholders   Those who hold an interest (stock) in a corporation.

strict liability   Responsibility of a seller or manufacturer for a defective product that causes injury.

subpoena   A written order to appear at a specified time and place to give sworn testimony.

subpoena duces tecum   A written order to produce documents or things.

substitute judgment   One person's decision used to make a decision for another.

suit-prone   Likely to sue someone or be sued.

survival action   A lawsuit related to a death and brought by the decedent's survivors.

T

terminally ill   Fatally ill with a condition for which there is no cure.

theft   Taking property without the property owner's consent.

tort   A wrong or injury, other than breach of contract, for which a court will provide a remedy.

trespasser   Someone who enters another's property without express or implied invitation or permission.

U

undue influence   Any improper persuasion to make someone act differently from his or her own will.

utilization review   A process by which hospitals review patient progress to efficiently allocate scarce medical resources.

V

values   Principles of thought and conduct that are considered desirable.

vicariously liable   Legally obligated for the acts of others who are acting as their agent.

W

waives   The act of giving up a claim, privilege, or right.

wanton   An act done with reckless disregard of another's rights or needs.

warranty   A promise that specifically named results will occur.

wrongful death   Death caused by negligence.

Bibliography

Chapter 1

ADANews. (2021, March 24). Inspector General Reports Two Medicaid Fraud-Related Enforcement Actions. *ADANews*. Retrieved from www.ada.org/publications/ada-news/2021/march/inspector-general-reports-two-enforcement-actions-in-march-related-to-medicaid-fraud

Carrns, A. (2021, March 19). *The New York Times*. The Triple Tax Break You May Be Missing: A Health Savings Account. Retrieved from www.nytimes.com/2021/03/19/business/health-savings-accounts-tax-break.html

Centers for Medicaid & Medicare Services. (16 December 2020). Historical. Retrieved from www.cms.gov/Research-Statistics-Data-and-Systems/Statistics-Trends-and-Reports/NationalHealthExpendData/NationalHealthAccountsHistorical

Gorke, J. (2021, March 19). Deploying Healthcare Technology: How Vulnerable Are You? *Forbes*. Retrieved from www.forbes.com/sites/jeffgorke/2021/03/29/deploying-healthcare-technology-how-vulnerable-are-you/?sh=4be7ca4fd050

Holly, R. "We're Rebuilding the Whole Delivery System": Why Amazon Is Betting Big on Home-Based Care. (2021, March 22). Home Health Care News. Retrieved from www.homehealthcarenews.com/2021/03/were-rebuilding-the-whole-delivery-system-why-amazon-is-betting-big-on-home-based-care/

JDSupra. (2021, March 22). Affidavit of Merit May No Longer Be Required for Claims of Vicarious Liability in New Jersey. JDSupra. Retrieved from https://www.jdsupra.com/legalnews/affidavit-of-merit-may-no-longer-be-7077502/

KFF. (2021, February 4). Surprise Medical Bills: New Protections for Consumers Take Effect in 2022. KFF. Retrieved from www.kff.org/private-insurance/fact-sheet/surprise-medical-bills-new-protections-for-consumers-take-effect-in-2022/

Noel, K. (2021, March 24). What Every Doctor Needs to Know About Telemedicine. *AAMC*. Retrieved from www.aamc.org/news-insights/what-every-doctor-needs-know-about-telemedicine

Shepherd v. Costco Wholesale Corp., No. CV-19-0014 (Ariz. Mar. 8, 2021).

Zur, O. (n.d.). The Standard of Care in Psychotherapy and Counseling. *Zur Institute*. Retrieved from https://www.zurinstitute.com/standard-of-care-therapy/

Chapter 2

Backus v. Baptist Medical Center, 510 F. Supp. 1191 (1980).

Brent, N. (2020, August 10). EEOC Files Sexual Harassment Lawsuit on a Nurse's Behalf. *Nurse.Com*. Retrieved from www.nurse.com/blog/2020/08/10/eeoc-files-sexual-harassment-lawsuit-on-a-nurses-behalf/

Bucceri Androus, A. (2021, November 23). What Should a Nurse Do If They Suspect a Patient Is a Victim of Abuse? *RegisteredNursing.org*. Retrieved from www.registerednursing.org/articles/what-should-nurse-do-suspect-patient-victim-abuse/

DEA. (n.d.). Who We Are/About. DEA. Retrieved from https://www.dea.gov/who-we-are/about

Griggs v. Duke Power, 401 U.S. 424 (1971).

Insurance Journal. (2020, September 3). How One Hospital Addresses Sexual Harassment Claims and Culture. *Insurance Journal*. Retrieved from www.insurancejournal.com/news/national/2020/09/03/581423.htm

Jeanine D'Alusio, J. (2020, February 5). Hiring in Healthcare: Interview Questions to Avoid and What to Ask Instead. *Relias*. Retrieved from https://www.relias.com/blog/hiring-in-healthcare-interview-questions-to-avoid-what-to-ask

Medicare Rights Center. (n.d.). The Part D Donut Hole. *Medicare Rights Center*. Retrieved from www.medicareinteractive.org/getanswers/medicare-prescription-drug-coverage-part-d/medicare-part-d-costs/the-part-d-donut-hole

National Council on Aging. (2021, February 23). Get the Facts on Elder Abuse. *National Council on Aging*. Retrieved from www.ncoa.org/article/get-the-facts-on-elder-abuse

Nelson, M. (2021, March 16). Spokane Physician Stripped of License After Reports of Excessive Surgeries. *KREM2*. Retrieved from www.krem.com/article/news/health/spokane-physician-stripped-license-reports-excessive-surgeries/293-14893f1d-7c72-4ddd-b362-61f7672e73bc

Palattella, E. (2021, 15 April). Taylor Miller, Advocate in Erie's Opioid Fight, Dies at 27: "She Fought So Hard." *GoErie*. Retrieved from www.goerie.com/story/news/crime/2021/04/16/taylor-miller-opioid-crisis-heroin-advocate-eries-fight-dies-27-losing-battle/7234867002/

Pattani, A. (2021, January 11). For Health Care Workers, The Pandemic Is Fueling Renewed Interest in Unions. *Kaiser Health News*. Retrieved from www.npr.org/sections/health-shots/2021/01/11/955128562/for-health-care-workers-the-pandemic-is-fueling-renewed-interest-in-unions

Preuss, C., Kalava, A., & King, K. (2021, February 17). Prescription of Controlled Substances: Benefits and Risks. Treasure Island, FL: StatPearls Publishing. Retrieved from www.ncbi.nlm.nih.gov/books/NBK537318/

Substance Abuse and Mental Health Services Administration. (2020, September). Key Substance Use and Mental Health Indicators in the United States: Results from the 2019 National Survey on Drug Use and Health.

Susan H. Jones v. Denis R. McDonough, Case 3:19-cv-00310 M.D. Tenn (2021, March 15).

United Stated Drug Enforcement Administration. (n.d.). Drug Scheduling. *United Stated Drug Enforcement Administration*. Retrieved from https://www.dea.gov/drug-information/drug-scheduling

United States Department of Labor. (n.d.). Bloodborne Pathogens and Needlestick Prevention. *United States Department of Labor*. Retrieved from www.osha.gov/bloodborne-pathogens/evaluating-controlling-exposure

Chapter 3

Constitution and the Bill of Rights. Retrieved from www.archives.gov

Chapter 4

Adams v. State of Indiana, 229 N.E.2d 834 (Ind. 1973).

Associated Press. (2021, April 13). 2 Child Services Workers Fired, Charged in Fatal Abuse Case. *API*. Retrieved from https://apnews.com/article/fairmont-west-virginia-child-abuse-56f66caf6c85a672d22ff64bec1ca55d

Child Welfare Information Gateway. (2017). Making and Screening Reports of Child Abuse and Neglect. Child Welfare Information Gateway. *U.S. Department of Health and Human Services, Children's Bureau*. Retrieved from www.childwelfare.gov/pubPDFs/repproc.pdf

Child Welfare Information Gateway. (2019). Mandatory Reporters of Child Abuse and Neglect. *U.S. Department of Health and Human Services, Children's Bureau*. Retrieved from www.childwelfare.gov/topics/systemwide/laws-policies/statutes/manda/

Children's Bureau (Administration on Children, Youth and Families, Administration for Children and Families), U.S. Department of Health and Human Services. (2019). Child Maltreatment 2019. Retrieved from www.acf.hhs.gov/cb/report/child-maltreatment-2019

DeMay v. Roberts, 9 N.W. 146 (Mich. 1881).

Healy, J., Farr, I., Feiger, & L., Duffy, C. (2019, October 11). One Doctor. 25 Deaths. How Could It Have Happened? *The New York Times*. Retrieved from https://www.nytimes.com/2019/10/11/us/ohio-doctor-overdose.html

Kathleen Waugh v. Genesis Healthcare LLC et al., 2019 ME179 (December 30, 2019).

Klein, C. F. (1995, Summer). Full Faith and Credit Interstate Enforcement of Protection Orders Under the Violence Against Women Act of 1994. *Family Law Quarterly*, 29(2), 253–272.

Medicare Learning Network. (January 2021). Medicare Fraud & Abuse: Prevent, Detect, Report. *U.S. Department of Health and Human Services*. Retrieved from www.cms.gov /Outreach-and-Education/Medicare-Learning -Network-MLN/MLNProducts/Downloads /Fraud-Abuse-MLN4649244.pdf

National Coalition Against Domestic Violence. (2020). Domestic Violence. Retrieved from www .assets.speakcdn.com/assets/2497/domestic _violence-2020080709350855.pdf?1596811079991

National Council on Aging. (n.d.). (2021, February 23). Get the Facts on Elder Abuse. NCOA. Retrieved from www.ncoa.org/article /get-the-facts-on-elder-abuse

Office of the Attorney General, Eastern District of New York. (2015, November 4). Riverhead Physician Assistant Arrested for Conspiracy to Illegally Prescribe Oxycodone. United States Department of Justice. Retrieved from www .justice.gov/usao-edny/pr/riverhead-physician -assistant-arrested-conspiracy-illegally -prescribe-oxycodone

People v. Murray, unpublished decision (Cal App. 2014).

Roe v. Wade, 410 U.S. 113, 93 S. Ct. 705, 35 L.Ed.2d 147 (1973).

Rosman, K. (2021, April 16). The Lost Embryos. *The New York Times*. Retrieved from www .nytimes.com/2021/04/16/style/freezing-eggs -and-embryos.html

The United States Department of Justice. (n.d.). What Is Domestic Violence? Retrieved from www .justice.gov/ovw/domestic-violence. In 2021, the 1994 Violence Against Women Act (VAWA) was reauthorized by Congress. The VAWA provided $1.6 billion to confront the national problem.

U.S. Department of Justice, Office of the Attorney General. (2020, 18 November). Texas Physician Sentenced for Multi-Million Medicare Fraud Scheme. Press release. Retrieved from www .justice.gov/opa/pr/texas-physician-sentenced -multi-million-medicare-fraud-scheme

U.S. Department of Justice, Office of the Attorney General. (2021, 10 May). University of Miami to Pay $22 Million to Settle Claims Involving Medically Unnecessary Laboratory Tests and Fraudulent Billing Practices. Press release. Retrieved from https://www.justice.gov/opa/pr /university-miami-pay-22-million-settle-claims -involving-medically-unnecessary-laboratory

United States Department of Justice. (2021, April 8). Temple Hills Felon Convicted After a Three-Day Federal Trial for Robbery, Brandishing and Discharge of a Firearm, and Being a Felon in Possession of a Firearm. United States Department of Justice, U.S. Attorney's Office, District of Maryland. Retrieved from www.justice .gov/usao-md/pr/temple-hills-felon-convicted-after -three-day-federal-trial-robbery-brandishing-and

Chapter 5

American Medical Association. (2017). Code of Medical Ethics Opinion 1.1.2: Prospective Patients. *AMA*. Retrieved from www.ama-assn .org/delivering-care/ethics/prospective-patients

Belli, Melvin M., Belli for Your Malpractice Defense (1986).

Carter v. Cangello, 164 Cal. Rptr. 361 (1980).

Estate of Reiner, 383 N.Y.S. 2d 504 (1976).

Hand v. Tavera, 864 S.W.2d 678 (Tex.App.-San Antonio, 1993).

Smith v. Sibley, 431 P.2d 719 (Wash. 1967).

St. John v. Pope, 901 S.W.2d 420, 38 Tex.Sup.Ct.J. 723 (Tex., 1995).

Chapter 6

Baumgardner v. Yusuf, 144 Cal.App.4th 1381 (Cal. Ct. App. 2006).

Caburnay v. Norwegian American Hosp., 2011 IL App (1st) 101740 (Ill. App., 2011).

Carroll, A. E. (2015, June 1). To Be Sued less, Doctors Should Consider Talking to Patients More. *The New York Times*. Retrieved from www.nytimes.com/2015/06/02/upshot/to-be -sued-less-doctors-should-talk-to-patients -more.html?_r=1

Console and Associates. (2021, March 25). Bad Bedside Manner or Medical Malpractice? *National Law Review*. Retrieved from www .natlawreview.com/article/bad-bedside-manner -or-medical-malpractice

Goldman v. Kossove, 117 S.E.2d 35 (N.C. 1960).

Katko v. Briney, 183 N.W.2d 657 (Iowa 1971).

Lyons v. Walker Regional Medical Center, 868 So.2d 1071 (Ala. 2003).

McLaughlin v. Mine Safety Appliances Co., 11 N.Y.2d 62, 226 N.Y.S.2d 407, 181 N.E.2d 430 (1962).

McMichael, B., Van Horn R. L., & Viscusi, W. K. (2019 February). "Sorry" Is Never Enough: How State Apology Laws Fail to Reduce Medical Malpractice Liability Risk. *Stanford Law Review*, 71, 341. Retrieved from https://www.stanfordlawreview.org/print/article/sorry-is-never-enough/

McQuitty v. Spangler, 976 A.2d 1020 (Md. App. 2009).

Medscape. (2021). Malpractice: What to Do If You Get Sued: How Plaintiffs Win Their Cases. Medscape.com. Retrieved from https://www.medscape.com/courses/business/100010

Rochester v. Katalan, 320 A.2d 704 (Del. 1974).

Ross-Stubblefield v. Weakland (Ga. App. 2021) std of care.

Ruiz v. Tenet Hialeah Healthsystem, Inc., 260 So.3d 977 (Fla. 2018).

Tammelleo, A. D. (1990, October). Who's to Blame for Faulty Equipment? *RN*, 67.

Thomas v. St. Joseph Hospital, 618 S.W.2d 791 (Tex. Civ. App. 1981).

Torrey, T. (2020, February 7). Defensive Medicine and How It Affects Healthcare Costs. *VeryWellHealth*. Retrieved from https://www.verywellhealth.com/defensive-medicine-2615160

Traynom v. Cinemark USA, Inc., 940 F.Supp.2d 1339 (D. Colo. 2013).

Chapter 7

American Medical Association. (2016, June). Opinions on Privacy, Confidentiality, and Medical Records 3.3.1: Management of Medical Records. *AMA*. Retrieved from www.ama-assn.org/delivering-care/ethics/management-medical-records

Centers for Disease Control and Prevention. (2021, March 26). Goals and Benefits of Data Interoperability. Retrieved from www.cdc.gov/datainteroperability/goals-and-benefit.html

Cordovano, G., McGraw, D., Miri, A. (2020, October 8). How Can Patients Get Medical Records from a Closed Medical Practice? *The Health Care Blog*. Retrieved from https://thehealthcareblog.com/blog/2020/10/08/how-can-patients-get-medical-records-from-a-closed-medical-practice/

Department of Health and Human Services. (n.d.). Individuals' Right under HIPAA to Access Their Health Information. 45 CFR § 164.524. U.S. Retrieved from www.hhs.gov/hipaa/for-professionals/privacy/guidance/access/index.html

Egan, M. (2016, August 9). A Winning Idea: How the Cloud Helps Olympic Athletes Avoid Injury. *GE Reports*. Retrieved from www.gereports.com/a-winning-idea-how-the-cloud-helps-olympic-athletes-avoid-injury/

Gage, S. M. (1981, Spring). Alteration, Falsification and Fabrication of Medical Records in Medical Malpractice Actions. *Medical Trial Quarterly*, 27, 476.

Hippocrates, Hippocratic Oath.

In re Culbertson's Will, 292 N.Y.S.2d 806 (1968).

Johnson v. Wood, 2020-SC-0588_MR (Ky. 2021).

Jones v. Fakehany, 67 Cal. Rptr. 810 (1968).

Mittleman, M. (1980, February). What Are the Chances when Malignancy Leads to a Malpractice Suit? *Legal Aspects of Medical Practice*, 8(2), 42.

Pear, R. (2016, January 16). New Guidelines Nudge Doctors to Give Patients Access to Medical Records. *The New York Times*. Retrieved from www.nytimes.com/2016/01/17/us/new-guidelines-nudge-doctors-on-giving-patients-access-to-medical-records.html

Robeznieks, A. (2021, March 3). Common HIPAA Violations Physicians Should Guard Against. *AMA Website*. Retrieved from www.ama-assn.org/practice-management/hipaa/common-hipaa-violations-physicians-should-guard-against

U.S. Department of Health and Human Services. (n.d.). All Case Examples. *U.S. Department of Health and Human Services*. Retrieved from www.hhs.gov/hipaa/for-professionals/compliance-enforcement/examples/all-cases/index.html#case3

U.S. Food and Drug Administration (FDA). (2020, January 31). 21st Century Cures Act. *U.S. FDA*. Retrieved from www.fda.gov/regulatory -information/selected-amendments-fdc-act/21st -century-cures-act

Woman Leaves Hospital, Finds Out She Died. (2016, June 11). Retrieved from www.nbcwashington .com/news/local/Woman-Leaves-Hospital -Finds-Out-She-Died-382568031.html

Chapter 8

American Medical Association (AMA). (2001, June). *Principles of Medical Ethics*. Chicago, IL: AMA. Retrieved from www.ama-assn.org /about/publications-newsletters/ama-principles -medical-ethics

Chapter 9

Adler, S. (2020, February). Florida Clinic Worker Facing 22 Years in Jail for Wire Fraud and Aggravated Identity Theft. *The HIPAA Journal*. Retrieved from https://www .hipaajournal.com/?s=22+years+in+jail

Adler, S. (2021, January 15). What Are the Penalties for HIPAA Violations? *HIPAA Journal*. Retrieved from www.hipaajournal .com/what-are-the-penalties-for-hipaa -violations-7096/

Bajak, F. (2020, October 1). Hacked Hospital Chain Says All 250 US Facilities Affected. *ABC News*. Retrieved from www.abcnews.go.com /Health/wireStory/hacked-hospital-chain-250 -us-facilities-affected-73374804

Butler, M. (2019, March 12). Hospital Employees Fired for Improperly Viewing Smollett Medical Records. *Journal of AIHMA*. Retrieved from https://journal.ahima.org/hospital-employees -fired-for-improperly-viewing-smollett-medical -records/

Department of Health and Human Services. (2003, April 4). Minimum Necessary Requirement. *U.S. Department of Health and Human Services*. Retrieved from www.hhs .gov/hipaa/for-professionals/privacy/guidance /minimum-necessary-requirement/index.html

Department of Health and Human Services. (2021, June 2). OCR Settles Nineteenth Investigation in HIPAA Right of Access Initiative. *U.S. Department of Health and Human Services*. Retrieved from www.hhs.gov /about/news/2021/06/02/ocr-settles-nineteenth -investigation-hipaa-right-access-initiative .html?language=en

Federal Register. (2000, December 28). 65(250), p. 82465. Retrieved from www.gpo.gov/fdsys/pkg /FR-2000-12-28/pdf/00-32678.pdf

Griswold v. Connecticut, 381 U.S. 479 (1965).

HHS.gov. (ND). Covered Entities and Business Associates. *U.S. Department of Health and Human Services*. Retrieved from www.hhs.gov /hipaa/for-professionals/covered-entities/index .html

HHS.gov. (n.d.). Breach Notification Rule. *U.S. Department of Health & Human Services*. Retrieved from www.hhs.gov/hipaa/for -professionals/breach-notification/index.html

Hippocrates, Hippocratic Oath.

Public Law 104–191.

Roe v. Wade, 410 U.S. 113 (1973).

Tarasoff v. Regents of University of California, 118 Cal. Rptr. 129 (1974).

www.hhs.gov/hipaa/for-professionals/compliance -enforcement/enforcement-process/index.html

Chapter 10

Allen, S., Bombardieri, M., & Rezendes, M. (2008, November 16). A Healthcare System Badly Out of Balance. *Boston Globe*. Retrieved from www.bostonglobe.com/specials/2008/11/16 /healthcare-system-badly-out-balance /j2ushYtZTBiCSxxUtQegbN/story.html

AMA. (n.d.). Medical Tourism: Code of Medical Ethics Opinion 1.2.13. *AMA*. Retrieved from www.ama-assn.org/delivering-care/ethics /medical-tourism

Centers for Disease Control and Prevention. (2021, April 22). The Tuskegee Timeline. *National Center for HIV/AIDS, Viral Hepatitis, STD, and TB Prevention, Centers for Disease Control and Prevention*. Retrieved from https:// www.cdc.gov/tuskegee/timeline.htm

Fressin, F., Wen, A., Shukla, S., Mok, K., & Chaguturu, S. (2021, July 23). How We Achieved More Equitable Vaccine Distribution: Social Vulnerability Analytics Are Necessary,

But Not Sufficient. Health Affairs. Retrieved from www.healthaffairs.org/do/10.1377/hblog20210721.568098/full/

Galewitz, P. (2019, August 12). Medical Tourism Can Save Employers, Patients Money. Kaiser Health News. Retrieved from www.khn.org/news/to-save-money-american-patients-and-surgeons-meet-in-cancun/

Gonzalez, J., Garijo, I., & Sanchez, A. (2020, May 5). Organ Trafficking and Migration: A Bibliometric Analysis of an Untold Story. *International Journal of Environmental Research and Public Health, 17*(9), 3204. Retrieved from www.doi.org/10.3390/ijerph17093204

Health Resources & Services Administration. (2021, April). Timeline of Historical Events and Significant Milestones. *HRSA*. Retrieved from www.organdonor.gov/learn/history

Herper, M. (2020, May 11). Inside the NIH's Controversial Decision to Stop Its Big Remdesivir Study. *StatNews*. Retrieved from www.statnews.com/2020/05/11/inside-the-nihs-controversial-decision-to-stop-its-big-remdesivir-study/

Lytel, J. (2012, October 29). Medical Tourism Doesn't Necessarily Mean Leaving the Country to Get Treatment. *The Washington Post*. Retrieved from https://www.washingtonpost.com/national/health-science/medical-tourism-doesnt-necessarily-mean-leaving-the-country-to-get-treatment/2012/10/29/8d1bf5ce-d679-11e1-b2d5-2419d227d8b0_story.html

Newsome, M. (2021, March 31). We Learned the Wrong Lessons from the Tuskegee "Experiment." *Scientific American*. Retrieved from https://www.scientificamerican.com/article/we-learned-the-wrong-lessons-from-the-tuskegee-experiment/

Piscitello, G. (2021, June 9). These Bonuses for Doctors Create an Immoral Conflict. *CNN*. Retrieved from www.cnn.com/2021/06/09/opinions/financial-incentives-doctors-ethical-concerns-piscitello/index.html

Robbins, R. (2017, September 17). Most Experimental Drugs Are Tested Offshore—Raising Concerns About Data. *Scientific American*. Retrieved from www.scientificamerican.com/article/most-experimental-drugs-are-tested-offshore-raising-concerns-about-data/

Robert, R. et al. (2020, June 17). Ethical Dilemmas Due to the Covid-19 Pandemic. *Annals of Intensive Care, 10*, 84. Retrieved from www.ncbi.nlm.nih.gov/pmc/articles/PMC7298921/

United States Holocaust Memorial. (n.d.). United States Holocaust Memorial Museum Note: Nuremberg Code. Retrieved from www.ushmm.org/information/exhibitions/online-exhibitions/special-focus/doctors-trial/nuremberg-code

Yeginsu, C. (2021, January 19). Why Medical Tourism Is Drawing Patients, Even in a Pandemic. *The New York Times*. Retrieved from www.nytimes.com/2021/01/19/travel/medical-tourism-coronavirus-pandemic.html

Zhang, S. (2017, June 16). The Disputed Death of an 8-Year-Old Whose Organs Were Donated. *The Atlantic*. Retrieved from www.theatlantic.com/health/archive/2017/06/organ-donation-death/530511/

Chapter 11

BBC. (2019, December 30). China Jails "Gene-Edited Babies" Scientist for Three Years. *BBC*. Retrieved from www.bbc.com/news/world-asia-china-50944461

BBC. (2019, September 6). Indian Woman, 73, Gives Birth to Twin Girls. *BBC*. Retrieved from www.bbc.com/news/uk-49575735

Charitos, I. et al. (2021, April 30). Stem Cells: A Historical Review About Biological, Religious, and Ethical Issue. *Stem Cells International*, Volume 2021, Article ID 9978837. Retrieved from www.doi.org/10.1155/2021/9978837

Daar, J. (2020, September). Legal Liability Landscape and the Person/Property Divide. *F&S Reports*. Retrieved from www.doi.org/10.1016/j.xfre.2020.08.004

Donegan, M. (2021, July 27). Alabama Is Prosecuting a Mom for Taking Prescribed Medication While Pregnant. *The Guardian*. Retrieved from www.theguardian.com/commentisfree/2021/jul/27/alabama-prosecuting-woman-medication-pregnant

Gillett-Netting ex rel. Netting v. Barnhart, 371 F.3d 593 (9th Cir. 2004).

Gorner, P. (2004, May 5). 5 Babies Born to Save Ill Siblings, Doctors Say. *Chicago Tribune*. Retrieved from www.chicagotribune.com/news /ct-xpm-2004-05-05-0405050257-story.html

Griswold v. Connecticut, 381.U.S. 479 (1965).

Hercher, L. (2021, July 12). A New Era of Designer Babies May Be Based on Overhyped Science. *Scientific American*. Retrieved from www.scientificamerican.com/article/a-new -era-of-designer-babies-may-be-based-on -overhyped-science/

Katz v. United States, 389 U.S. 347 (1967).

Kolata, G. (2014, February 3). Ethics Questions Arise as Genetic Testing of Embryos Increases. *The New York Times*. Retrieved from www. nytimes.com/2014/02/04/health/ethics-questions -arise-as-genetic-testing-of-embryos-increases .html

Lewin, T. (2007, May 22). A Move for Birth Certificates for Stillborn Babies. *The New York Times*. Retrieved from www.nytimes.com /2007/05/22/us/22stillbirth.html

Najjar, D. (2020, December 18). Should You Bank Your Baby's Cord Blood? *The New York Times*. Retrieved from www.nytimes.com/2020/12/18 /parenting/pregnancy/cord-blood-banking.html

Nwigwe, L. (2019). Embryonic Stem Cell Research: An Ethical Dilemma. Voices in Bioethics, Vol. 5. Retrieved from www.doi.org /10.7916/vib.v5i.6135

Roe v. Wade, 410 U.S. 113 (1973).

Roman v. Roman, 193 S.W.3d 40 (Tex. App., 2006).

Sack, K. (2007, May 30). Her Embryos or His? *Los Angeles Times*. Retrieved from https://www .latimes.com/archives/la-xpm-2007-may-30 -na-embryo30-story.html

Snider, S. (2019, August 27). How Much Does IVF Cost and How Can I Pay for It? *U.S. World News and Report*. Retrieved from https:// money.usnews.com/money/personal-finance /spending/articles/how-much-does-ivf-cost -and-how-can-i-pay-for-it

Chapter 12

Bever, L. (2014, November 2). Brittany Maynard, as Promised, Ends Her Life at 29. *The Washington Post*. Retrieved from www.washingtonpost.com/news/morning-mix /wp/2014/11/02/brittany-maynard-as-promised -ends-her-life-at-29/

Jones, D. (2021, June 22). Experts Weighs in After Toddler's Death Raises Questions over What It Means to Be "Brain Dead." *WFTV*. Retrieved from www.wftv.com/news/9investigates /experts-weighs-after-toddlers-death-raises -questions-over-what-it-means-be -brain-dead /T4J7WZXEDJCBNEIZNVWSDHCJNI/

Koop, C. E. (1976). *The Right to Live: The Right to Die* (pp. 98–99). Wheaton, IL: Tyndale House Publishers.

Lyons, P. J. (2007, September 14). Still More Fallout from the Terri Schiavo Case. *The New York Times*. Retrieved from https://thelede .blogs.nytimes.com/2007/09/14/still-more -fallout-from-the-terry-schiavo-case/

Peters Smith, B. (2016, June 19). 58 Years of Loving Marriage Ends with Two Gunshots. *Herald-Tribune*. Retrieved from www.heraldtribune.com/news/20160619/58 -years-of-loving-marriage-ends-with-two -gunshots

Relias Media. (2006, September 1). Arrest of Katrina Doctor, Nurses Stirs Up Strong Support for the Accused. Retrieved from www.reliasmedia.com/articles/122579-arrest -of-katrina-doctor-nurses-stirs-up-strong -support-for-the-accused

Singleton, A. (2019, August 4). Why All Adults Should Have a Living Will. *AARP*. Retrieved from www.aarp.org/caregiving/financial-legal /info-2019/what-is-a-living-will.html

Sosa, N., Franken, B., Phillips, R., & Candiotti, S. (2005, March 31). Terri Schiavo Has Died. *CNN*. Retrieved from www.cnn.com /2005/LAW/03/31/schiavo/index.html? iref=newssearch

Updike, N. (2014, March 25). Death and Taxes. *This American Life*. Retrieved from www .thisamericanlife.org/radio-archives /episode/523/transcript

Willingham, A. J. (2017, December 2). A Man's Tattoo Left Doctors Debating Whether to Save His Life. *CNN*. Retrieved from www .cnn.com/2017/12/01/health/dnr-do-no -resuscitate-tattoo-medical-debate-trnd /index.html

Index

A

AAMA. *See* American Association of Medical Assistants

abandon and abandonment, 126

abortion, 272
  constitutional right of privacy, 123
  minor's, 122
  Roe v. Wade, 106, 272

abuse
  child. *See* child abuse
  domestic violence, 83, 91–94
  economic, 92
  elder. *See* elder abuse
  emotional, 92
  financial, 90
  fraud versus, 96
  physical, 90–92
  psychological, 92
  reporting of, 30–31
  sexual, 92

ACA. *See* Affordable Care Act

acceptance, 116

accountable care organizations (ACOs), 19

ACOs. *See* accountable care organizations

ADA. *See* Americans with Disabilities Act

Adams v. State of Indiana, 104

adjudicate, 70

Adler, S., 223

administrative law, 70

advance directive, 124, 284–288

adversary, 145

affirmative duty, 162

Affordable Care Act (ACA), 14, 108

agency, 120–121

agent, 7, 120

age of majority, 122

Allen, S., 241

allocation of resources, 236–241
  funding, 250–251
  transplants, 247–251

AMA. *See* American Medical Association

Amazon, 13

American Association of Medical Assistants (AAMA), 137

American Federation of Labor, 58

American Medical Association (AMA)
  Code of Medical Ethics, 94
  confidentiality, 213
  durable power of attorney, 287
  medical records management, 177
  medical tourism and, 255–256
  Principles of Medical Ethics, 195–196, 206

American Medical Technologists (AMT), 137

American Nurses' Association (ANA), 58

Americans with Disabilities Act (ADA), 44–46

amniocentesis, 266

amoral, 197

ANA. *See* American Nurses' Association

Anti-Kickback Statute, 95, 100, 108

apps, 20

arbitration, 72

artificial insemination, 262–265

assault, 71

assault and battery, 106

assisted reproductive technology, 262–265

assisted suicide, 295

assumption of risk, 154, 156

attempted murder, 81

attitudes, death and dying, 282–284

attorneys, release of information to, 184

autograft, 247

autonomy, 251–252

Q

R